I0038269

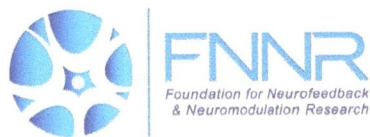

FNNR
Foundation for Neurofeedback
& Neuromodulation Research

Also by Richard Soutar

Longo, R. E., & Soutar, R. (2019). *Mentoring for neurofeedback certification: A guide for mentors and mentees*. Greenville, SC: FNNR.

Soutar, R. (2017). Perspective and method for a QEEG based two-channel bi-hemispheric compensatory model of neurofeedback training. In T. F. Collura & J. A. Frederick (Eds.), *Handbook of clinical QEEG and neurotherapy* (pp. 387-403). New York, NY: Routledge.

Soutar, R., Hopson, J., & Longo, R. (2017). Correlating QEEG and oxidative stress. *New Mind Journal*, Spring, 1-15.

Soutar, R. (2017). Asymmetry as a reliable measure of adult anxiety and depression. New *Mind Journal*, Fall 1-4.

Soutar, R. (2014). An introductory perspective on the emerging application of QEEG in neurofeedback. In D. S. Cantor & J. R. Evans (Eds.), *Clinical neurotherapy: Application of techniques for treatment* (pp. 19-50). New York, NY: Elsevier.

Soutar, R., & Longo, R. (2011). *Doing neurofeedback: An introduction*. ISNR Research Foundation.

Soutar, R. G. (2006). *The automatic self: Transformation & transcendence through brainwave training*. Lincoln, NE: iUniverse.

Crane, A., & Soutar, R. (2000). *Mindfitness training: Neurofeedback and the process.* New York, NY: iUniverse.

Also by Robert Longo

Longo, R. E., & Bingham, B. (forthcoming 2021). *Introducing neurofeedback into your practice.*

Longo, R. E. (2020). My journey into neurofeedback. In J. R. Evans, M. B. Dellinger & H. L. Russell (Eds.), *Neurofeedback: The first fifty years.* Cambridge, MA: Academic Press/Elsevier, Inc.

Longo, R. E., & Soutar, R. (2019). *Becoming certified in neurofeedback.* Greenville, SC: FNNR.

Longo, R. E. (2018). *A consumer's guide to understanding QEEG brain mapping and neurofeedback training.* Bloomington, IN: iUniverse.

Longo, R. E., & Russo, M. (2017). Working with forensic populations: Incorporating peripheral biofeedback and brainwave biofeedback into your organization or practice. In T. F. Collura & J. A. Frederick. (Eds.), *Handbook of clinical QEEG and neurotherapy.* London: Routledge.

Longo, R. E. (2015). The use of neurofeedback to treat traumatic brain injury in sexually abusive youth. In D. S. Prescott & R. J. Wilson. (Eds.), *Very different voices: Perspectives and case studies in treating sexual aggression.* Holyoke, MA: NEARI Press.

Longo, R. E., Prescott, D. S., Bergman, J., & Creeden, K. (Eds.). (2013). *Current perspectives & applications in neurobiology: Working with young persons who are victims and perpetrators of sexual abuse.* Holyoke, MA: NEARI Press.

Longo, R. E., & Prescott, D. S. (2013). Current perspectives and applications in neurobiology: An overview. In R. E. Longo, D. S. Prescott, J. Bergman & K. Creeden (Eds.), *Current perspectives & applications in neurobiology: Working with young persons who are victims and perpetrators of sexual abuse.* Holyoke, MA: NEARI Press.

Longo, R. E. (2013). Traumatic brain injury (TBI): A brief introductory overview. In R. E. Longo, D. S. Prescott, J. Bergman & K. Creeden (Eds.), *Current perspectives & applications in neurobiology: Working with young persons who are victims and perpetrators of sexual abuse.* Holyoke, MA: NEARI Press.

Longo, R. E., & Prescott, D. S. (2013). Ethical responsibilities in neuroscience and neurobiology. In R. E. Longo, D. S. Prescott, J. Bergman & K. Creeden (Eds.), *Current perspectives & applications in neurobiology: Working with young persons who are victims and perpetrators of sexual abuse.* Holyoke, MA: NEARI Press.

Soutar, R., & Longo, R. E. (2011). *Doing neurofeedback: An introduction.* San Rafael, CA: ISNR Research Foundation.

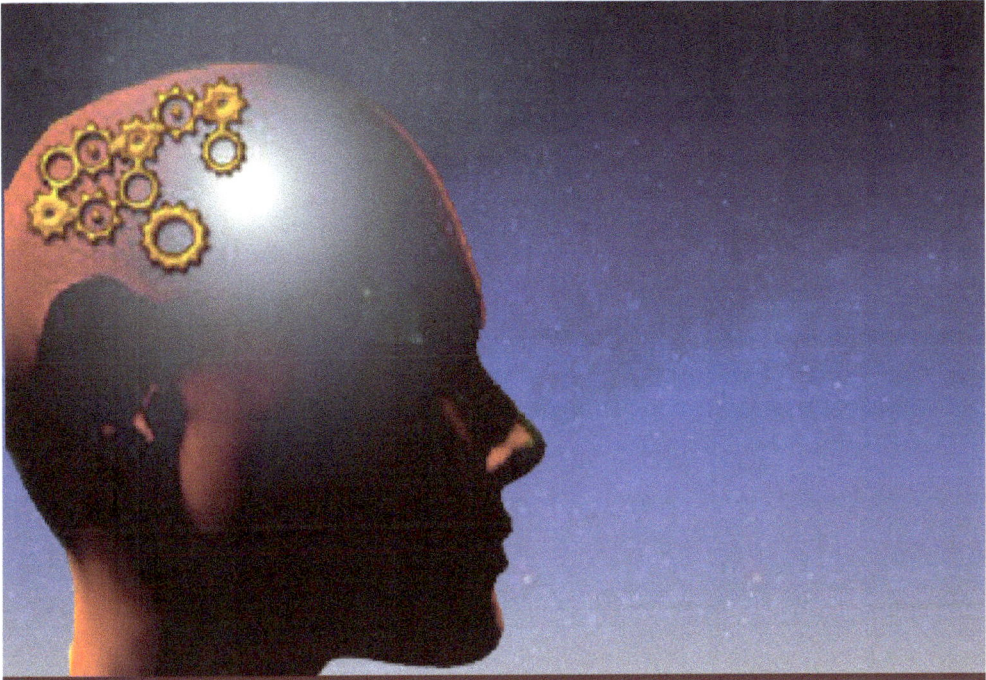

Doing Neurodfeedback:

An Introduction

Richard Soutar, PhD

Robert Longo, MRC

2nd edition

FNNR Publications

Longo, R. E., & Soutar, R. (2020). *Becoming certified in neurofeedback: A guide to the neurofeedback mentoring process for mentors and mentees.* Foundation for Neurofeedback and Neuromodulation Research.

Sokhadze, E., & Casanova, M. F. (Eds.). (2019). *Autism spectrum disorder: Neuromodulation, neurofeedback, and sensory integration approaches to research and treatment.* Foundation for Neurofeedback and Neuromodulation Research.

Martins-Mourao, A., & Kerson, C. (Eds.). (2017). *Alpha-Theta neurofeedback in the 21st century: A handbook for clinicians and researchers* (2nd ed.). Foundation for Neurofeedback and Neuromodulation Research.

Soutar, R., & Longo, R. E. (2011). *Doing neurofeedback: An introduction.* The ISNR Research Foundation.

Hammond, D. C., & Gunkelman, J. (2011). *The art of artifacting.* The ISNR Research Foundation.

Carmichael, J. (2011). *Multi-component treatment for post-traumatic stress disorder, including strategies from clinical psycho-physiology and applied neuroscience.* The ISNR Research Foundation.

Donaldson, S. (2012). *The other side of the desk.* The ISNR Research Foundation.

Thompson, M., Thompson, J., & Wenqing, W. (2009). *ADD centre Brodmann areas booklet.* The ISNR Research Foundation.

Doing Neurofeedback:
An Introduction

Richard Soutar, PhD

Robert Longo, MRC

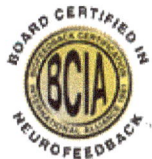

Publisher:

The FNNR

The Foundation for Neurofeedback & Neuromodulation Research 2131 Woodruff Rd, Ste 2100 #121 Greenville, SC 29607 http://www.theFNNR.org

Correspondence: admin@theFNNR.org

Publisher:

The FNNR

The Foundation for Neurofeedback & Neuromodulation Research 2131 Woodruff Rd, Ste 2100 #121 Greenville, SC 29607 http://www.theFNNR.org. Correspondence: Admin@theFNNR.org

Layout Design: Megan Stevens. Correspondence: Publishing@theFNNR.org

Cover concept updated by: Megan Stevens

Doing Neurofeedback: An Introduction.

Second edition, 2021 ISBN: 978-0-9978194-7-2 (print)

Happiness is the highest form of health.

-Buddha

This book is dedicated to all of the clients and patients whom over the years have helped us to better understand the benefits and impact on their lives through participating in neurofeedback services.

We would also like to thank our colleagues, and mentees who have provided us with invaluable ways to help teach others about our field.

And we would like to thank our families who have stood by us and supported our work which has taken time on evenings and weekends in order to better help those we serve and teach.

To all of these people we are humbled and most grateful.

CONTENTS

Health is the greatest gift, contentment the greatest wealth, faithfulness the best relationship.

-Buddha

CHAPTER 1: HISTORY AND PERSPECTIVES IN NEUROFEEDBACK AND QEEG

Quantitative electroencephalography (QEEG or QEEG) brain mapping; and neurofeedback (NFB) training (also referred to as EEG biofeedback, neurobiofeedback, and neurotherapy), are fields still in the early stages of development. QEEG and NFB are practiced by a variety of professionals and innovators from diverse fields who have come together to contribute their expertise to the growth of both areas. Nonetheless, QEEG and NFB enjoy a distinct and unique history.

To truly understand these fields is to comprehend the many competing theories regarding what NFB does to the brain, the disorders it helps, and the best way to employ it. At this time, NFB is still considered experimental in many respects, and practitioners should never make claims of curing a particular disorder. Additionally, the length of treatment varies among patients. NFB usually takes 20-60 sessions on average. Some patients attain results with fewer than 20 sessions, while others may require in excess of 60 sessions for treatment to be effective. When patients reach their treatment goals, an additional 5-10 sessions are often conducted to help set in (consolidate) the NFB training.

At the time of this writing, several methods or styles of neurofeedback have gained popularity. In addition to traditional neurofeedback and Z-Score neurofeedback, full-cap training, infra-slow neurofeedback and sLORETA neurofeedback have become popular. Each of these styles and methods have demonstrated positive benefits and efficacy in treating various symptoms, however, there is no research to suggest that any of the newer methods is more effective or less effective that traditional, 1, 2 and 4 channel training.

QEEG has become more standardized, but there are still several techniques, models, and methods used to gather QEEG data. As professionals, we cannot use QEEG as a diagnostic tool; however, QEEG can help support established or suspected diagnoses. Therefore, it has a differential diagnosis value. Periodic QEEG, or retesting patients once NFB has begun, helps to reassure neurofeedback clinicians that NFB is having the desired effect. Most recently, QEEG has been held up as a valid reliable measure of testing in the New York District Court.

Court Upholds Use of QEEG by Non-Physicians in Expert Witness Testimony

In what amounts to a landmark decision, particularly for quantitative EEG (QEEG) and neurofeedback practitioners, a New York District Court judge has ruled that expert witness testimony based on QEEG evaluations meets what is called the Daubert standard. Daubert is a legal precedent set in 1993 by the

Supreme Court regarding the admissibility of expert witnesses' testimony during federal legal proceedings. It essentially states that trial judges, as "gatekeepers" of scientific evidence, must determine if expert witness testimony is "relevant" and "reliable."

Daniel Kuhn, MD of New York made the case for QEEG and Neuroguide-based interpretations in an affidavit presented to the Court, assisted by Bob Thatcher, PhD The judge's decision in this case also noted that expert witness testimony using QEEG was not the sole domain of neurologists, indicating that other professionals are qualified to testify as QEEG experts. (see: Applied Neuroscience, n.d).

This chapter provides a brief overview of the history and development of QEEG and NFB. A more detailed history of the field can be found in *Mindfitness Training: Neurofeedback and the Process* by Crane and Soutar (2000) and *A Symphony in the Brain*: *The Evolution of the New Brain Wave Biofeedback* by Robbins (2008). A list of similar titles and recommended readings is located at the end of this book. The experts discussed in this chapter have each had a profound impact on the field (Evans, Delinger, & Russel, 2020).

NEUROFEEDBACK EXPERTS

Richard Caton (1842-1926)

Richard Caton was the first to discover changes in the brain's electrical activity in animals after mental activity occurred (Criswell, 1995; Demos, 2005).

Hans Berger (1873-1941)

In 1924, Hans Berger (born in Neuses, Germany) measured EEG on the human scalp. He was the first to record raw EEG tracings (changes in electrical potential measured between two electrodes placed on the surface of the head) on paper. Berger established the (10 Hz) Berger rhythm, and characterized the resultant wave patterns, including alpha and beta waves. His findings were published in 1929.

Wilder Penfield (1891-1976)

Wilder Penfield, a Canadian neurosurgeon, was the first person to do brain mapping in 1928. Penfield worked with patients who suffered from epilepsy. Before operating on patients, he measured the motor cortex and discovered various sites of movement. Penfield stimulated the different parts of their brains with electrodes to locate the cells that set off their attacks while the patients were awake. He learned exactly where each part of the body that was being touched or moved was represented in the brain. Penfield's map became known as the sensory-motor homunculus ("little man"), and his sensory map was depicted in cartoons of the somatosensory and motor areas.

Herbert H. Jasper (1906-1999)

Herbert Jasper developed a standard set of electrode placements on the scalp, so that results obtained in different clinics and laboratories could be compared. This standard set became known as the 10-20 International System.

According to Patent Storm (n.d.):

> In 1949, Jasper's work was adopted for trial at the General Assembly of the International Federation meeting held in Paris. Dr. Jasper's scheme defines a set of electrode placements on the scalp whose relative position will be determined by the dimensions of each individual's head so that electrodes placed on heads of different dimensions will be in comparable locations on the scalp. This system is based on a set of latitudinal and longitudinal arcs upon the surface of an approximately spherical cranium, and positions of electrodes are determined by measurements from standard landmarks (i.e., nasion, inion, and preauricular points) on the skull. Arc length measurements from nasion to inion and from the preauricular point of one ear over vertex to the opposite ear are taken as well as a measurement around the circumference. Electrodes are then placed at locations 10, 20, 20, 20, 20, and 10% along each of these arcs.

Jose Delgado (1915–2011)

Jose Delgado, a professor of physiology at Yale University, developed the brain chip, a device that could manipulate the brain by transmitting and receiving signals to and from neurons. Delgado implanted chips in the brains of animals and subsequently humans. He demonstrated that he could control certain behaviors through brain stimulation. His work was tested in patients who suffered from paralysis, epilepsy, blindness, Parkinson's disease, and other disorders.

Neal Miller (1909–2002) and Leo DiCara (1937–1976)

From Nealmiller.org:

> Neal Miller, Leo DiCara, and their colleagues carried out a series of dramatic animal experiments in the 1960s, demonstrating the operant conditioning of a variety of internal autonomically regulated physiologic processes, including blood pressure, cardiac function, and intestinal activity. Prior to their research, physiologists generally assumed that organisms have control over bodily functions governed by the central nervous system (or "voluntary nervous system"). The internal physiological processes controlled by the autonomic (or

"involuntary") nervous system were regarded as operating beyond conscious awareness or control.

Miller and DiCara used animals paralyzed by curare so that the animals could not produce the desired visceral changes through voluntary activity mediated by the central nervous system. In this paralyzed state their animal subjects were still able to change their visceral functions.

Many of Neal Miller's experiments on curarized animals have not been successfully replicated, yet his animal studies spurred further investigations extending the same operant model of visceral learning to human subjects. More importantly, Miller's research inspired the hope that biofeedback can enable a human being to take a more active role in recovering and maintaining health. Further, it encouraged the dream that human beings can aspire to previously unimagined levels of personal control over bodily states, reaching unprecedented states of wellness and self-control.

Joe Kamiya: A Psychological Model

Joe Kamiya, a psychologist teaching at the University of Chicago, began experiments on brainwave frequencies in the 1960s utilizing a student population and basic medical grade EEG recording equipment. Kamiya attached a sensing electrode to the left occiput of a subject's head where alpha brainwaves are evident. Kamiya presented a tone to the subject, who was then asked to guess whether he or she was "in alpha." Kamiya was able to determine if the subject's guess was accurate through studying EEG readings. Kamiya went on to establish that people could control brainwaves that were previously thought to be involuntary states. Kamiya's findings resulted in the beginning of brainwave biofeedback.

Kamiya's original work reportedly was about anxiety, which is still an interesting topic to the psychology community. Thus, Kamiya's work is characterized as a psychological approach. Kamiya's hypothesis was that increased alpha wave production could lead to decreases in state and trait anxiety. Kamiya's findings strongly supported his hypothesis. In considerable detail, he explored the best methods for training individuals in alpha wave production and its consequences. Unfortunately, not enough people in the field read and learn from his research; instead, they keep reinventing the wheel (Dadashi et al., 2015; Also see: ...Hardt, 1991).

The field of NFB exploded after *Psychology Today* published an article in on Kamiya's work (Kamiya, 1968). The first meeting of biofeedback professionals occurred as part of the 1968 International Brain and Behavior Conference in Colorado. The following year the first specific meeting of biofeedback researchers was held in Santa Monica, California, with 142 people attending. At this meeting the attendees decided to name their group the Biofeedback Research Society—later changed to Biofeedback Society of America and then to the Association for Applied Psychophysiology and Biofeedback. In the 1970s and 1980s, biofeedback research languished. However, several professionals continued to push forward. Over the past decade, NFB and QEEG have flourished once again.

Maurice "Barry" Sterman

Barry Sterman, a professor emeritus in the departments of neurobiology and psychiatry at UCLA, is well known for his experiments on brainwave states in cats in the mid- to late-sixties. Sterman accidentally discovered a specific EEG rhythm state while conducting operant conditioning experiments with cats. While waiting for a food reward, the cats produced the same brainwave pattern in the sensorimotor strip as when they were alert and motionless. Sterman named this spindling 13–19 Hz low-beta frequency EEG pattern "sensorimotor rhythm" (SMR).

In 1967, through serendipitous circumstances, Sterman found that his lab cats, which were trained in the previous unrelated SMR experiment to produce this frequency, increased their resistance to seizure when he exposed them to toxic chemicals that induced epileptic seizures. The results of Sterman's research were subsequently replicated with monkeys and humans.

The combined research of Sterman and others provided the basis for SMR/beta biofeedback training commonly used for ADHD, ADD, and attentional issues. Additionally, SMR/beta training was used for several years on patients with seizures when conventional medication therapies did not work. Subsequently, it was noted that children who were hyperactive experienced improvement in their seizure status, and also had improved behavior. In 1982, Sterman received a research grant from the National Institutes of Health (NIH) to further his research. In this study, the cats were exposed to hydrazine fuel—some cats had seizures, others did not. The cats that had experienced SMR training were more resistant to seizures. Sterman's work led to the discovery that scientists could alter brainwave physiology.

Sterman decided to employ this same procedure on individuals with seizure disorders and learned that it reduced their incidence of seizures. Interestingly, he found that he could reverse the effects of this training and increase seizure frequency as well.

Joel Lubar

Joel Lubar, at the University of Tennessee, pioneered the use of neurofeedback on children with hyperactivity in the 1970s. His major focus involved the use of EEG biofeedback for ADD/ADHD, depression, seizure disorders, Tourette Syndrome and related tic disorders, and certain specific learning disabilities. Joel and Judith Lubar developed a NFB protocol for treating ADHD by decreasing theta and increasing beta (classic landmarks for ADHD).

Lubar's (1995) landmark study provided comparative pre- and post- treatment measurements of several parameters in over 100 individuals with ADHD who improved and in those who did not. The changes noted in the group receiving neurofeedback were nearly equivalent to changes reported for the medication group. Other completed studies have similar findings.

Lubar continued to lead the field in the use of NFB for attentional issues, and later pioneered LORETA neurofeedback, where a signal from the actual brain EEG source is estimated and trained from a 19-electrode montage. Training of this presumably more accurate signal is believed to produce faster and more effective results. Research has yet to be conducted to demonstrate improved efficacy (Coben et al., 2018).

Margaret Ayers (1946 – 2008)

Margaret Ayers's graduate training was in clinical neuropsychology. She used biofeedback therapy for different kinds of medical problems: drug addiction, alcoholism, head injury, stroke, cerebral palsy, and coma. Ayers noted that ADD is often the result of stroke, birth trauma, head injury, or anoxia (a sustained lack of oxygen to the brain). Until her death in March 2008, it was believed that Dr. Ayers performed more NFB sessions than any other individual in the field. She was responsible for the development of digital real-time neurofeedback equipment that sampled EEG at a rate that provided unparalleled definition of the raw EEG and filtered waveforms.

Barry Sterman and Joel Lubar: The Neuropsychological Arousal Model

At the same time that Sterman and Lubar were conducting their work, Margaret Ayers was a lab assistant working for Sterman. She was so impressed with their findings that she struck out on her own to develop equipment and protocols to train the general population. Sterman and Ayers focused on theta reduction rather than beta enhancement. Their approach to EEG training was characterized by Andrew Abarbanel as an arousal model (Andrew Abarbanel PhD, MD,1995)

Since Sterman and Lubar are neuropsychologists in the traditional research mold, this approach is referred as the neuropsychological arousal model. This model proposes that brainwave frequency changes globally in a fairly stereotypical pattern as a consequence of functions related to daily activities. As cognitive processing increases, alpha and theta brainwaves decrease, and beta, or desynchronized brainwaves, increase. As sensorimotor input to the brain decreases, SMR increases and attentiveness decreases. As vigilance decreases, theta waves increase.

Overall, this model appears to be fairly accurate but today we know that the role of theta is far more complex than originally understood. Rather than just being a frequency that was a nuisance arising from poor perfusion contributing to attention deficits, theta is a key player in memory processing as well as cortical activities involved cognitive processing (Meehan & Bressler, 2012). Other exceptions, too numerous to mention here, have been noted as well. It is a good idea to avoid being too rigid with regard to this perspective.

Niels Birbaumer

Niels Birbaumer, a German neuropsychologist whose experience dates back to the beginning of the field in the 1960s, is recognized for his pioneering work in slow cortical potential (SCP) EEG training, which included blind placebo-controlled studies applying the SCP neurofeedback training to epilepsy. His more recent work at the National Institutes of Health (NIH), focused on brain computer interfaces (BCIs), evaluating many approaches to providing control over a computer, and thus a variety of prosthetic devices (Birbaumer, 2006).

A BCI involves acquiring brainwave signals that when amplified and input into a computer can be translated into messages or commands that reflect a person's intentions. It is a system that allows a person to communicate with or control the external world without involving the brain's normal output pathways.

Hershel Toomim (1916–2011)

Dr. Hershel Toomim, a physicist, clinician, and researcher, was a pioneer in the field of psychophysiology and biofeedback and held 22 patents for his inventions. He created the first biofeedback system to use telemetry, enabling patients to walk while disconnected from the central data collecting system. He developed one of the first publicly available neurofeedback units, known as the Alpha Pacer. Dr. Toomim also developed hemoencephalography (HEG)—specifically, biofeedback using an infrared sensor to detect blood flow, or oxygenation, to specifically chosen brain regions.

Elmer Green (1917–2017)

From the Menninger Clinic:

> Elmer Green, PhD, researched and applied biofeedback techniques he developed in his ongoing study of "subtle energies," a field in which he remains preeminent. Dr. Green, the father of autogenic biofeedback training, was the first person ever to receive a National Institutes of Health (NIH) research grant, which was given for his autonomic research program (involuntary internal stimuli) at Menninger in the

mid- 1960s. The techniques he and his wife, Alyce Green, developed were used to train individuals how to achieve more control over their bodies in order to increase their physical and mental well-being.

Green used biofeedback instruments to study Eastern yogis. He discovered that certain yogis could control their internal states merely through meditation and thought. His methods and techniques were adapted by Eugene Peniston and became what is now known as Alpha-Theta training. Richard Soutar (2015) has expanded this approach into a method of neurofeedback known as deep states training.

Eugene Peniston

In the 1980s, Eugene Peniston at the VA Medical Center at Fort Lyon, Colorado, studied the effects of combining Alpha-Theta training with their existing program for alcoholics and published some of the most influential research about neurofeedback (reviewed in Norris, 2017). Five years after participating in the program, 70% of the participants remained abstinent. Peniston researched alcoholism and theta activity, noting that theta—often both theta and alpha—were lower in the back of the brain. He and Paul Kulkosky continued to do groundbreaking research together at the Menninger Clinic on both alcoholism and post-traumatic stress disorder (PTSD). Peniston also consulted and guided Bill Scott on several pieces of research to replicate Peniston's findings.

Paul Kulkosky (1949 - 2019)

Peniston (1998) describes Kulkosky:

> The Peniston/Kulkosky EEG Alpha-Theta neurofeedback protocol is being used by many practitioners to treat alcohol and other psychoactive substance disorders. Some alcohol treatment programs using the Peniston/Kulkosky EEG Alpha-Theta neurofeedback protocol as a primary treatment modality for alcohol addiction have demonstrated that intensive neurofeedback-based treatment has exerted a positive influence on a number of factors which contribute to alcohol intake including stress levels, depressive personality traits, beta endorphin output, resting levels of alpha and theta brainwaves, and prolonged abstinence. Data supporting the efficacy of the Peniston/Kulkosky method are of particular interest for the treatment of substance abuse because successful outcome is being discovered with patients who are difficult to treat in traditional alcohol treatment programs including patients with post-traumatic stress disorder and chronic alcoholic problems.

Bill Scott

From Brain Paint:

> Bill Scott is the principal investigator and first author of an addiction research project that yielded a 79% success rate with Native American alcoholics. This study was with Dr. Eugene Peniston. An interview with Bill by the Psychiatric Times was published as a feature article. Bill Scott has also presented research at the American Association for the Advancement of Science with Dr. David Kaiser. Bill trained the researchers Dr. John Gruzelier and Dr. Tobias Egner (members of Department of Cognitive Neuroscience and Behaviour, Imperial College Medical School) in the use of Alpha-Theta protocols. The results of this research project so improved music abilities among Royal Conservatory of Music students that the Conservatoire has made these protocols a mandatory part of the school's curriculum.

Elmer Green, Eugene Peniston, Nancy White, and Bill Scott: The Alpha-Theta Model

Elmer Green worked only briefly in the field, but left an indelible mark. With a background in biophysics, he experimented extensively with theta wave training—something that horrifies many practitioners today, because much of the emerging paradigm of biofeedback resulted from laboratory analysis of eastern yogis' abilities to control autonomic functions. He related the profound experiences that individuals had with works such as the yogic Aphorisms of Patanjali.

While Eugene Peniston was a managing psychologist at the Menninger Clinic, he enrolled in one of Green's workshops and was so impressed with the technology that he tried it with alcoholics. Paul Kulkosky, his associate, remarked that they noticed many alcoholics had a notable deficit of alpha. They thought that alpha training would help alcoholics while in recovery. When they consistently trained the alcoholics in alpha wave production over a period of several weeks, they found that it accelerated the alcoholics' recovery dramatically. Later they tried the same technique on PTSD patients with similar results. Their published studies were crucial contributions to establishing the early validity of neurofeedback as a psychological tool of considerable adjunctive value at the clinical level (Penniston, 1998).

Nancy White is a past president for the International Society of Neurofeedback and Research; now the International Society for Neuroregulation and Research (ISNR). She originally studied neurofeedback with Adam Crane and began implementing and teaching it extensively. Her workshops inspired many clinicians to adapt the technique. As she worked with people over the years at the clinical level, she refined the technique and eventually developed a theoretical perspective that she detailed in her textbook on the topic.

Bill Scott has achieved more for peer-reviewed research on Alpha-Theta training than just about anyone in the field of neurofeedback. The aforementioned UCLA study is one of the largest randomized controlled trials in the field of EEG Biofeedback, and was conducted during his appointment as a UCLA Staff Research Associate V. In 2005 the results of the study were published in The American Journal of Drug and Alcohol Abuse. He completed a peer-reviewed controlled study of Alpha-Theta training in cooperation with the UCLA Department of Psychology. In it, Bill Scott and David Kaiser have combined both fast- and slow-wave training into a very effective, unique, and comprehensive approach. Unfortunately, few practitioners actually read Scott's research or take workshops to learn his techniques. Despite the amount of high-quality research, many practitioners have misconceptions about Alpha-Theta training; consequently, the approach is underutilized (Scott, Kaiser, Othermer, & Sideroff, 2005).

Alpha-Theta is more attractive to practitioners who are clinically oriented and prefer to interact psycho-dynamically with their clients. It can be used for deep states training and tapping into client issues at a Jungian level. On the other hand, qualified practitioners such as Nancy White will get results with Alpha-Theta-training alone. While success like hers is possible, a fair amount of coaching can assist the client greatly. Alphatheta training has also been used effectively by many successful peak performance specialists such as Rae Tattenbaum.

Within the last few years, practitioners of neurofeedback have taken a second look at deep brain states (Martins-Mourao & Kerson, 2017). Alpha-Theta training has been used in the treatment of alcoholism and other addictions, PTSD, the dysphoric disorders of women musicians, and psychopathic offenders. During this therapy, when the alpha wave amplitude is crossed over by the rising amplitude of theta waves, the state is called the Alpha-Theta crossover state and is associated with the resolution of traumatic memories. This low-frequency training differs greatly from the high-frequency beta and SMR training that has been practiced for over 30 years and is more reminiscent of the original alpha training of Elmer Green and Joe Kamiya.

Beta and SMR training can be considered a more direct physiological approach, strengthening sensorimotor inhibition in the cortex and inhibiting alpha patterns, which slows metabolism (Sterman & Egner, 2006). On the other hand, Alpha-Theta training derives from the psychotherapeutic model and involves accessing of painful or repressed memories through the Alpha-Theta state.

The physiological mechanisms behind these therapies are currently unclear, but the theory is that repressed memories and unresolved traumas exert a stress on the brain that interferes with normal operation. EEGs of alcoholics reveal an inability to produce the alpha waves generally associated with feelings of relaxation and comfort. Theta and alpha waves increase after alcohol consumption. Since drowsiness and relaxation are common effects of alcohol, alcoholics may be self-medicating their abnormally higher level of beta activity and low level of low frequency activity. Many studies demonstrate a high efficacy of Alpha-Theta therapy in treating alcoholism (Martins-Mourao & Kerson, 2017).

Jay Gunkelman

Jay Gunkelman is one of the most experienced clinical and research EEG/QEEG specialists in the world. He started in 1972 with the first state hospital-based biofeedback laboratory and has specialized in EEG for decades. He has authored many scientific papers and a mounting list of books. His depth of understanding of the mind/brain's function is unique. Jay is a popular lecturer world-wide and has occupied leadership positions in the field's professional societies. He is well known for his phenotypes model.

Simply stated, EEG phenotypes are clusters of commonly occurring EEG patterns found in the general population that are believed to be the result of underlying genetics. These phenotypes are purported to play an intermediate role between genetics and behavior (Gunkelman, 2006). In fact, Gunkelman believed that a relatively small number of phenotypes can describe a majority of EEG records in the population.

Gunkelman, now retired, ran a successful QEEG business. He tirelessly carried his equipment all over the world acquiring QEEGs and interpreting them for the neurofeedback community. His insights concerning the relationship between QEEG maps and neural functioning have helped professionals diagnose disorders and determine appropriate medications. Perhaps his most important contribution is his emerging method for determining the best protocols for neurofeedback intervention based on QEEG brain maps.

Robert W. Thatcher

Robert Thatcher is president and chief executive officer of Applied Neuroscience, Inc., a company that provides clinical report analysis, medical and legal evaluations, expert witnesses for court trials, research services, specialized analyses, specialized software pertaining to EEG, and quantitative analysis of the EEG. As president and CEO, Thatcher has both numerous and diverse responsibilities. His work is best noted for his research on head trauma (TBI), QEEG neurometrics, and Z-Scores.

Applied Neuroscience, Inc., has developed a 19-channel instantaneous Z-Score biofeedback program for purposes of neuroimage therapy or neuroimage biofeedback. Patients monitor their own brains in 3-D and in real-time to modify the electrical energies of their brains. Applied Neuroscience, Inc., also has developed a 2- and 4-channel dynamic link library, or DLL, based on the statistics of NeuroGuide for approved industry developers to use in their products. This DLL has provided real-time normative database comparisons for absolute power, power ratios, relative power, coherence, phase delays, and amplitude differences.

BrainMaster® was the first industry developer to incorporate the DLL into a complete biofeedback system. In addition, they developed special techniques for advanced targeting methods and live feedback, and they have published various technical reports and case studies using the new methods.

Thatcher spent a significant amount of time looking at TBI. He noted that at birth, infants' brainwaves are approximately 40% delta, but in adults these waves account for about 5%. Thus, elevated delta is often indicative of TBI. Kirtley Thornton and Dennis Carmody (2008) reported that QEEG identifies TBI approximately 90% of the time.

Thatcher did a great deal of research with head trauma and developed a database that has proven very accurate in diagnosing levels of severity. He also studied EEG and MRI together. This research provided new insights regarding the relationship between grey matter and white matter tissue damage and the resulting consequences in terms of EEG production in the brain. Much of his research focused on coherence. He produced important articles on this topic, which attracted considerable attention in the field of neurofeedback. Presently, Thatcher maintains one of the most widely used EEG databases in the field.

E. Roy John (1924 – 2009)

Dr. E. Roy John was among the world's most recognized researchers in the fields of electrophysiology and biopsychology. He served as a research and development consultant with the Psychological Institute of Atlanta (PSI) and as a clinical consultant with QEEG and EP services offered through PSI. Dr. John and his wife, Leslie Prichep, performed all the initial research on the normative distribution of the human EEG and demonstrated that this distribution was consistent across culture, race, and gender. As a result, he developed the first neurometric database system and published research showing how EEG patterns correlate with various neuropsychological disorders. E. Roy John, in cooperation with the LEXICOR Corporation, supplied the first usable database for the neurofeedback community, NX Link, which provided a standard pattern of normative EEG.

Robert Thatcher and Jay Gunkelman: A QEEG Medical Perspective

Thatcher and Gunkelman probably have done more to promote quantitative EEG analysis (QEEG), or neurometrics, than anyone else in the field. Thatcher worked with E. Roy John developing EEG databases. He presented at the first

ISNR meetings and conversed with neurofeedback providers and researchers. Gunkelman's original training was in the medical side of EEG. He immediately recognized the value of using databases for neurofeedback training. Gunkelman actively taught individuals in the neurofeedback community about the value, importance, and advantages of using and understanding QEEG.

QEEG involves collecting EEG signals from multiple sites (typically from the standard 10-20 International System) on the scalp. These signals are then compared to a normative database to search for deviations from the mean values. These deviations are then usually reported in data tables and in the form of topographic maps. This process gives clinicians a fairly comprehensive picture of what is going on globally and locally in the brain in terms of EEG activity. This information can then be used to decide on an appropriate protocol for training.

Many clinicians like this approach because it provides a clear empirical basis for assessment and protocol decision making. It is also very well grounded in a wider research effort in the neuropsychology community. However, QEEG can be difficult to learn, and it has a longer learning curve than other approaches. It is very technical and often overwhelming to those who are used to more intuitive approaches. In addition, it requires very expensive equipment and databases. Therefore, not every professional is ready to dive into QEEG.

Although many professionals such as Marvin Sams proclaim that it is unethical to provide neurofeedback services without QEEG brain mapping, many others in the field have developed methods for protocol implementation that appear approximately if not equally as effective in results. At present there have not been enough replicated studies to confirm the superiority of one approach over the other. The clear value of QEEG is in assessment and tracking of abnormalities in the EEG.

Siegfried and Susan Othmer

This couple originally became involved in the field of neurofeedback to help their son. They produced some of the early reliable training equipment and developed a large network of affiliated practitioners who utilized their approach. Building primarily on the work of Sterman, they developed a basic and systematic approach to neurofeedback that does not use brain mapping and has proven very effective in dealing with a wide variety of disorders.

Siegfried's background in physics injected some very important challenging ideas into the field regarding research assumptions and theories about the relationship between neural functioning and EEG. At present, these concepts are very much under-appreciated. He is also one of the most outspoken commentators on the political and social implications of the work done in the field of neurofeedback.

Their early recognition of the role that asymmetry plays in proper neural functioning is particularly important. Much of their early technique involved balancing left and right hemispheres with respect to levels of arousal, or symptoms-based training.

Sue developed an innovative bipolar training method that uses multiple sites across the scalp as well as sliding windows of uptraining and downtraining across the frequency spectrum. This new method is more symptom-driven than past methods and results in rapid physiological responses to training. Client reports of changes in sensations, feelings, and symptoms often occur as soon as the session begins and protocols are changed accordingly. Sue developed a very thorough taxonomy of symptoms and protocols that should be used in each case.

Many practitioners like this approach because it is very interactive and provides clear responses to each change. Others have complained that clients don't always know what they are feeling and don't report it effectively. This tendency makes protocol decisions very difficult. Some clinicians have expressed concerns that the protocols are so strong that they may be moving the clients too rapidly. However, it is overall one of the most popular and easy to learn approaches to neurofeedback.

Most recently, the Othmers have focused on low frequency training that involves the use of special electrodes and amplifiers designed for training below 1 Hz. Such training has been termed DC training, sub-delta training, or slow cortical potential training by various researchers and practitioners, and, is hypothesized to affect shifting DC potentials that are the source of EEG activity.

Les Fehmi

Les Fehmi is director of the Princeton Biofeedback Centre and a founding member of the Biofeedback Society of America (now AAPB). For over 30 years, he conducted research and practiced clinically in the area of attention and EEG biofeedback. He developed Open Focus™ training and has specialized in multi-channel, alpha phase-synchrony neurofeedback, which he pioneered. His work is best understood by reading his book on Open Focus methods that he wrote in concert with Jim Robbins (Fehmi & Robbins, 2008).

Adam Crane

Adam Crane is founder of the International MindFitness Foundation, which is dedicated to psychophysiological research and education, with a particular emphasis on developing and making available practical life and performance enhancement strategies and training programs. Since 1971, Crane and the organizations he founded or co-founded have provided leadership in the development of biofeedback hardware and software as well as innovative and effective business models for practitioners.

Les Fehmi and Adam Crane: The Profound Attention Model

Les Fehmi and Adam Crane have both focused on attention as a key to personal development and mental health. Their emphasis on attention is broader in scope than Joel Lubar's. Their approach also involves the metaphysical and the social-psychological. Both have focused on alpha training and synchrony as they relate to attention and influence mental functioning. Synchrony is a special form of brainwave coherence that is discussed later in the book. Fehmi has developed special equipment for training alpha synchrony, but it is not widely distributed at this point. He also has developed some very sophisticated techniques in attentional training.

Currently, Fehmi conducts workshops in these techniques that are experiential in nature and enlightening with regard to how much our perception and consciousness are regulated by our attention. The book *Mindfitness Training: Neurofeedback and the Process* includes Crane's perspective and a sample of his workshop called the Process (Crane & Soutar, 2000). Crane has also worked with others to develop specialized equipment for alpha training and synchrony training, but uses a definition of terms that is slightly different than that of Les Fehmi. In fact, Crane coined the term "profound attention," which he sees as the outcome of both alpha training and the process. He views this form of attentional development as an antidote to many of the modern dilemmas encountered, including mental disorder.

Peter Rosenfeld (1939 - 2021)

Rosenfeld is best known for his depression protocol (1997) correcting frontal alpha asymmetry, a common finding with depression, noting that SMR can alter alpha asymmetry. Elsa Baehr collaborated with Rosenfeld to do research demonstrating the effectiveness of this technique for neurofeedback practitioners, which lead to its widespread clinical use.

Valdeane W. Brown

From Future Health (n.d.b):

> Dr. Valdeane W. Brown is an internationally recognized "trainer of trainers," who teaches and consults widely on personal and organizational transformation and computer systems. With a PhD in clinical psychology and a background in math, physics, computer programming, philosophy, yoga, meditation, and martial arts, Dr. Brown brings a presence and precision to his work, informed by a deep sense of compassion, a profound facility with energy dynamics and commitment to revealing the elegant simplicity inherent in

learning and transformation.

Expanding on the work of others, Brown initially focused on training at C3 and C4. Brown is often misunderstood in the field because he deals in knowledge not understood by most practitioners: nonlinear dynamics and chaos theory. He has developed a technique and a computer program to implement this perspective. His approach involves training both sides of the brain at the same time using multiple frequencies and reinforcement tones. He has provided regular workshops on the topic.

His "Period 3" techniques have three basic stages, where training frequencies are altered at each stage. Some practitioners have doubted the ability of clients to hear and respond to so much feedback activity, but his clients appear to do quite well. Brown maintains that his outcomes are just as good as those who use brain maps, if not better. More recently, Brown has utilized his NeuroCare Pro system to generate a more seamless and automated neurofeedback approach that he has marketed to individuals and practitioners. He feels that his expert system is sophisticated enough that even home users can hook themselves up and effectively train without the guidance of a professional practitioner.

Anna Wise: The High-Performance Mind (1950 – 2010)

Anna did not use EEG biofeedback in the same way that others in the field typically use it. She originally worked with Maxwell Cade, who traveled the world measuring the EEG of reportedly enlightened individuals and other peak performers. Her program was the result of his findings and her insights into his work. Rather than employ operant conditioning directly, she created mental exercises to develop the mind and evaluate progress using specially designed EEG equipment. Her method of "neuromonitoring," as she referred to it, allowed her to work with groups of individuals to access an "awakened mind" state providing profound breakthroughs and insights.

Anna's workshops attracted those interested in deep states training as well as groups working toward insight and spiritual growth. In fact, there is some concern within the community that her approach may not survive. Fortunately, a few individuals are trying to incorporate her approach into their own styles and present similar workshops. Her books, *The High-Performance Mind* and *The Awakening Mind*, are very well-written and provide the best introduction to her work. Both are excellent sources for practitioners.

KEY TRAINERS IN THE FIELD OF NEUROFEEDBACK

Michael (1940 - 2021) and Lynda Thompson

Michael and Lynda Thompson are pioneers in the field of neurofeedback in Canada. They are strong advocates of integrating biofeedback with neurofeedback together in the clinical setting and have led the field in this area, presenting some of the best techniques for utilizing both paradigms. Much of their initial focus was on ADD. They have worked closely with Thought Technology and developed many of their innovative techniques and protocols around Thought Technology equipment. They have published an excellent book on neurofeedback entitled *The Neurofeedback Book*. Over the years they have conducted hundreds of workshops and played a key role in training other practitioners.

Jon Anderson

Jon Anderson has worked with biofeedback and neurofeedback since 1974 and has been one of the key neurofeedback trainers. As a clinician, he has experimented extensively with all of the innovations in the field. He has worked closely with the Stens Corporation and has earned the reputation of being one of the best and most informed instructors available.

Len Ochs

"Len Ochs is a psychologist in private practice, working in biofeedback since 1975 and psychotherapy since 1966. He is considered one of the pioneers in biofeedback—especially in the area of instrumentation development" (Future Health, n.d.b). Len Ochs is most recognized for the development of the Low Energy Neurofeedback System (LENS), which was registered by the FDA in April 2009.

LENS uses a device, under control of a computer program, to produce electromagnetic fields and apply them as brain stimuli. The stimuli are applied by EEG leads that serve as bi-directional conduits for both the stimuli and returning EEG signals. Treatment sessions are very short, typically only a few minutes. Treatments that are too long or use incorrect settings can cause hyper-arousal, headache, irritability, nausea, etc. During treatment sessions, the subject is completely passive; there is no auditory or visual feedback.

LENS treatment is preceded by a diagnostic QEEG brain map to identify zones of the brain where various brainwaves deviate from the norm. Both electrode placement and system settings are determined by the condition being treated and the clinician's interpretation of the brain map.

System settings must be adjusted by the clinician over the course of treatment to accommodate the effects of treatment. The number of treatments needed to improve ADD/ADHD, depression, PTSD, and seizures is claimed to be fewer than for traditional neurofeedback methods.

Richard Soutar

Richard pioneered clinical work with entrainment and QEEG database systems.

He co-developed a hand-held neurofeedback trainer with Dave Siever and collaborated with Brainmaster® developing new concept models for clinical implementation, such as remote/ home training and the Mini-Q. He is best known for his innovative work in deep states training and neuromeditation—the use of neurofeedback to assist in achieving altered states and meditation. Recently, he developed an internet-based Expert Database System for comprehensive clinical use that involves assessment measures along a bio-psycho-social model. It assesses social behavior, cognitive behavior, and physiological symptoms and correlates them with QEEG analysis to rapidly generate a clinically friendly report. This system is a critical step to making QEEG more accessible to clinicians of all types and enhances the visibility of the discipline.

Rob Coben

Robert Coben, PhD received his doctoral degree in 1991 and has been a licensed psychologist in the state of New York since 1994. He is the Director and Chief Neuropsychologist of NeuroRehabilitation and Neuropsychological Services. His experience in rehabilitation neuropsychology includes serving as director for two separate inpatient neurorehabilitation programs, and he is the former director of inpatient and outpatient brain rehabilitation at Staten Island University Hospital. Additionally, Dr. Coben is an affiliate of Winthrop University Hospital, and an affiliated researcher of NYU Medical Center.

Dr. Coben is an associate editor for the Journal of Neurotherapy and Frontiers in Child Health and Human Development, and serves as an editorial reviewer for several prestigious academic journals. His research interests include the study of and treatment applications for Neuropsychology and Neurophysiology in childhood neurodevelopmental disorders, especially autism. Along with Dr. Stevens, Dr. Coben is a co-founder of Integrated Neuroscience Services. Dr. Coben is a member in good standing of the following organizations: American Psychological Association, International Neuropsychological Society, International Society for Neurofeedback and Research, and the American Association of Psychophysiology and Biofeedback

Coben has pioneered a new form of coherence training that may have significant advantages over single channel standard neurofeedback methods used into the present time (Coben et al., 2018b). He is one of the few who has actually compared the two methods and found evidence to support his claims.

Sebern F. Fisher, M.A., BCN

Sebern Fisher came to the field of neurofeedback as a clinical director, a trauma therapist and a skeptic. To her, what was being proposed was high-tech snake oil, but since nearly all of the kids under her care in residential treatment were deemed "untreatable," she thought it was worth a try.

On a rainy March afternoon in 1996, she met her friend, Kathy Zilberman at her home in Great Barrington and trained her brain using a Focus 1000. She was Kathy's first "subject" and they rewarded SMR (12–15 Hz) and inhibited theta (4–7 Hz) for 7 hours over the course of that weekend. The approach Kathy was using is called the arousal/regulation model authored by Susan and Siegfried Othmer with the intended outcome for Sebern of lowering arousal. It was assumed at that point, not accurately, that reinforcing SMR would accomplish this in most brains. Sebern was astonished by what happened. She reported to Kathy, "The brain has a mind of its own. I am quiet in a way I have never felt before—in fact in a way I never knew existed." She saw the landscape and its points of light with stunning clarity and she also experienced a severe migraine (a pre-existing condition), hypomania and pressured speech. Although 12–15 Hz was not calming as had been hoped, it did profoundly quiet what she came to call "ambient fear."

Fisher subsequently pursued training and conversation with every luminary she could find in the field. Many practitioners were just beginning to talk about using neurofeedback to help those brains impacted by early abuse and neglect but these were the people she most wanted to help. She left the field of public mental health because her center could not embrace this new approach. In 1999, she explored the use of FPO2 and other placements at very low frequency rewards to quiet fear, the driver in most severe mental health problems.

Beginning in 2000, she started to write and present on neurofeedback for developmental trauma in both neurofeedback and psychotherapy forums. In 2012, Norton approached her to write a book on her experiences and how she understood them which was published as *Neurofeedback in the Treatment of Developmental Trauma: Calming the Fear-Driven-Brain* (2014).

In her work, Fisher has asked the field of neurofeedback to consider the central role that affect regulation plays in human development and she has asked the field of psychotherapy to open itself to the crucial role of brainwave training in helping people achieve it.

SUMMARY

Most of these practitioners were in the field before brain mapping was available. They and major research facilities developed methods without that important resource. Despite the lower price of brain mapping equipment and databases, many of these practitioners still do not rely on brain maps and are quite successful in their practices. While still recognizing the validity of other approaches, ISNR published a paper recommending the use of QEEG brain mapping for assessment purposes (Hammond et al., 2004). This perspective becomes more understandable by viewing QEEG primarily as an assessment and tracking tool and not the sole basis for protocol determination.

None of the mentioned perspectives is exclusive in the interpretation of neurofeedback. In fact, there is considerable overlap among them. This book weaves these perspectives together, so that the underlying relationships become more obvious.

As they do in most fields, politics surround these perspectives. Also, many technological advancements have been developed for use with these perspectives. However, interesting equipment and programs may or may not work with a specific perspective. Consequently, many practitioners entering the field find themselves purchasing several different pieces of equipment in order to use several perspectives clinically. Others become locked into one expensive piece of equipment and perspective without the ability to change.

Not all perspectives reflect the mainstream research. Learning one type of terminology unique to a cutting-edge perspective can limit dialogue with other practitioners and more mainstream research. In the long run, practitioners are likely to be served best by investigating several different approaches and developing their own "tool boxes."

The Appendices at the end of this book contain a list of leading companies and training programs for those interested.

REVIEW QUESTIONS

1. What series of dramatic animal experiments did Neal Miller and DeCara conduct in the 1960s?

2. Barry Sterman is most known for his work with what experiments?

3. Joe Kamiya is recognized for what contribution to biofeedback?

4. Joel Lubar's major focus of work involves the use of EEG biofeedback for treating what disorder?

5. What did Herbert Jasper develop?

6. What did Hans Berger discover?

7. Which trainer is known for his research and work looking at autism and coherence training?

8. Eugene Peniston is best known for his work using neurofeedback to treat what population?

9. What was Richard Canton the first to discover?

10. Is neurofeedback considered to be experimental?

CHAPTER 2: ANATOMY, ELECTROPHYSIOLOGY, AND THE BRAIN

To understand EEG and its origin, it is best to begin with a study of the basic anatomy and neurophysiology of the brain. Becoming proficient with terms and concepts relating to this topic will make reading the scientific literature easier and contribute significantly to the ability to provide effective neurofeedback protocols.

BRAIN DEVELOPMENT AND STRUCTURES

The human brain goes through a complex process of development starting at birth and continuing through adolescence into adulthood. Even in later adult years, the brain remains plastic and new brain cells are created. The brain develops from bottom to top, right to left, and back to front. It has many structures, regions, and parts, including the cerebral cortex, brain stem, cerebellum, four lobes, two hemispheres, and limbic system. It is vital to know and understand these structures to use EEG and neurofeedback.

The Neocortex and Cortex

Vertically, the brain (also referred to as the triune brain, MacLean, 1977) can be divided into three parts: the brain stem, the limbic system, and the neocortex. The triune brain recognizes that the three major regions of the brain evolved over time, creating separate but interdependent systems: the brain stem and cerebellum (reptilian brain), the emotional brain (limbic system or mammalian brain), and the thinking brain (the cortex).

From a horizontal perspective, the brain can be divided into two parts: the right and left cerebral hemispheres.

P. T. Stein and J. Kendall note that the neocortex is responsible for both cognition and metacognition-the ability to think about thoughts, emotions, and behavior (Stein & Kendal, 2004). The neocortex is responsible for the "executive functioning" of the person. It determines personality, goals, and decisions, and guides the following:

- reasoning
- weighing choices
- concrete and abstract thought
- inductive and deductive reasoning
- cause-and-effect relationships
- delaying actions
- planning

- goal-directed behavior

The neocortex controls cognitive memory that includes facts, figures, faces, names, and dates.

The cortex has six layers. The white matter underneath contains the wiring that connects the cortex for long-distance communication.

Individual Brain Cells Live in "Columns"
Using An Office Analogy:

- The top layers are similar to inter-office memos. Most of the other layers feed into this layer and information processing is integrated at a meta level.
- The middle layers are like the "inbox." Inputs are received from the ascending reticular system and the thalamus for processing.
- The bottom layers serve as the "outbox." In this layer data from the middle layers is directed to modulate activity in the subcortical systems.

Most of the EEG we capture from the scalp is from the top layers. The term used for these EEG producing areas is "dipole layer." The EEG they produce does not register at the scalp until neurons over an area of about at least 6 cm resonate together (Nunez & Srinivasan, 2006).

The neuron (individual brain cell) is the cell body that receives information from other cells connected to its dendrites. The other cells' signals vote on whether this cell should fire a signal. The cell body develops an electrical charge or signal in response to the votes, and then the signal travels down the axon to other cells to vote as well. The waxing and waning of these "voting charges" from layers two and three of the cortex come together to create the EEG.

Neurons live in adjacent cell columns that permeate the cortex layers. Axons spread between adjacent cell columns to create "local" connections (beta-gamma resonances). Axons travel somewhat longer distances to generate regional connections (alpha to beta resonances). Axons travel long distances to generate global connections (delta to theta resonances) (Nunez & Srinivasan, 2006).

Delta, Theta, Alpha, and Beta are the four major brainwaves. To better understand brain waves it may be helpful to think of them the same way one might think about radio stations on the FM frequencies. In a traditional FM radio, each station emits at a specific frequency. For example, 88.5 might be an NPR station in a particular city. FM band widths range from 87.5 to 108 megaHertz (MHz). Hertz are the number of cycles per second. A megaHertz is one million cycles per second.

Then there is power. In an electrical system; electrical power is measured in Volts. Most household items are run on 120 Volts. Major appliances like stoves and clothes dryers run on 220 Volts. Brain waves are measured in microVolts (μV). One volt equals 1,000,000 microVolts.

The distance a radio station can be heard from the transmitting tower is determined by wattage output. Watts refer to "real power". Volt-Amperes refer to "apparent power." Both are the product of voltage (V) multiplied by amperage (A). For example, an electrical device drawing 5 Amps at 120 Volts would be rated at 600 Watts or 600 Volt-Amperes. A light bulb that is 60 Watts is 0.5 Amps.

Hertz are used to measure frequency in brain waves. Delta is typically 1-3 Hz, Theta, 4-7 Hz, Alpha 8-12 Hz and Beta 15 – 30 Hz. The power or "magnitude" of each brain wave and a basic magnitude at each 10-20 site. Each brain wave has a standard power which differs if one's eyes are closed versus eyes opened. For example, the average magnitude at Cz eyes closed is Delta 8 μV, Theta 10 μV, Alpha 14 μV and Beta 7 μV. Thus, Delta, for example, is 1-3 Hz and 8μV.

The charts below are a helpful analogy for looking at frequency and power comparing radio stations and brain waves.

FM Station/ Power

NPR 88.5	Jazz 90.5	Rock 92.3	Talk 94.5
60,000 Watts	10,000 Watts	100,000 Watts	91,000 Watts

Brain Waves /Magnitude (eyes closed)

Delta 1-3Hz	Theta 4-7Hz	Alpha 8-12Hz	Beta 15-20Hz
8 μV	10 μV	14 μV	7 μV

Raw EEG includes all the brain wave frequencies. In neurofeedback and QEEG software raw brain waves are broken down into the individual bandwidths by software known as a fast Fourier transform. The fast Fourier transform is a mathematical method for transforming a function of time (e.g., cycles per second) into a function of frequency; in this case individual brain waves. This is similar to how white light is broken down into rainbow colors by being processed through a prism.

In the cortex, information flows over several major channels or nerve bundles called fasciculae. Information traveling between left and right hemispheres goes through the corpus callosum and anterior commissure. Key pathways for information that traveling from the back to the front are cingulum, uncinate, and arcuate fasciculae. These key pathways are part of two major flow zones that travel from back to front and that meet in the frontal region. These are named the dorsolateral stream or "the where" network and the ventral stream or the "what" network. Convergence zones (such as the posterior temporal region) are major interface zones that bring together information from a large variety of networks.

Recently, it has been discovered that the brain is organized around major "hubs" that help coordinate brain network activity (Hagmann et al., 2008). The majority of these hubs are in the parietal region, the ventromedial frontal region, and the temporal lobes. These hubs are so critical to effective functioning that damage to any one of them results in extensive impairment of whole regions of brain networks. Conversely, damage outside these hub areas remains relatively contained to local areas.

ORIENTATION TO THE BRAIN

The Cerebrum

The cerebrum is the anterior and largest part of the brain. The cerebrum, consisting of two halves or hemispheres, has a primary function of controlling voluntary movements and coordinate mental actions.

The primary difference between the cerebrum and cerebral cortex is that cerebrum is the uppermost largest part of the brain. The cerebral cortex is the outer layer of the gray matter of cerebrum.

The cortex (cerebral cortex) is the largest part of the human brain, making up 80% of the brain's mass, and is a six-layered structure that performs different functions. The cerebral cortex is the gray matter that covers the outermost layer of the brain like the bark of a tree and generates EEG activity. Beneath it is all the white matter that constitutes the wiring between the different areas of the cortex. Subcortical systems include the following:

- limbic system or midbrain (emotion and memory)
- brain stem or hindbrain (survival functions)
- pineal gland (an endocrine gland that produces the hormone melatonin)
- thalamus (sensory and motor functions)
- hypothalamus (regulates sexual drive, thirst, hunger)
- pituitary gland (controls all the other glands)

Neuron cell bodies make up the gray surface of the cerebrum, which is a little thicker than a thumb. White axon fibers, underneath, carry signals between the nerve cells and other parts of the brain and body. "Gray" matter is so colored because of the presence of cell bodies, while "white" matter indicates the presence of myelinated axon fibers.

The cortex is the thinking part of the brain, responsible for people's ability to plan, reason, and consciously "think" about what they do. In other words, the human urges and emotions generated by the limbic system pass through neurological pathways to the cortex, where they are processed. In general, the function of the cortex is higher-level information processing. When it is engaged in this processing, it tends to generate more beta waves.

The cortex has to make sense of and figure out how to respond to and satisfy these urges. This is the most sophisticated part of the brain and can be described from a structural-functional perspective by dividing it into regions or lobes according to their specialization. These lobes are demarcated by indentations called fissures, or sulci. For instance, the back (posterior) section of the cortex is devoted mostly to vision and is called the occipital cortex. The prefrontal cortex (anterior) performs executive functions related to decision making. The temporal lobes (lateral) of the cortex are involved in memory, emotional processing and hearing. The cerebral cortex is highly wrinkled. Essentially, this feature makes the brain more efficient because it can increase the surface area of the brain and the amount of cortical neurons within it (cortical folding). A deep furrow called the interhemispheric fissure divides the cerebrum into two halves, the left and right hemispheres, with each side functioning slightly differently.

The prefrontal cortex, at the front tip of the brain, is the socio-emotional supervisor. It is the part of the brain that helps people stay focused, make plans, control impulses, and make good (or bad) decisions. It also plays a role in mood regulation.

The cingulate, a part of the brain that runs longitudinally underneath and through the middle of the frontal lobes, is the "gear shifter." It allows people to shift attention from thought to thought and between behaviors.

The cerebral cortex is divided into four sections called lobes, the frontal lobes, temporal lobes, parietal lobes, and occipital lobes.

Knowledge of the brain and its functioning continues to expand almost daily. Current research supports much of what has been learned about the brain and its functions through QEEG brain mapping and work with neurofeedback. The following excerpt from *Science Daily* is an example:

Neuroscientists Map Intelligence in the Brain

"Neuroscientists at the California Institute of Technology (Caltech) have conducted the most comprehensive brain mapping to date of the cognitive abilities measured by the Wechsler Adult Intelligence Scale (WAIS), the most widely used intelligence test in the world. The results offer new insight into how the various factors that comprise an "intelligence quotient" (IQ) score depend on particular regions of the brain.

Neuroscientist Ralph Adolphs, professor of psychology and neuroscience, and professor of biology at Caltech, Caltech postdoctoral scholar Jan Gläscher, and their colleagues compiled the maps using detailed magnetic resonance imaging (MRI) and computerized tomography (CT) brain scans of 241 neurological patients recruited from the University of Iowa's extensive brain-lesion registry.

All of the patients had some degree of cognitive impairment from events such as strokes, tumor resection, and traumatic brain injury, as assessed by testing using the WAIS. The WAIS test is composed of four indices of intelligence, each consisting of several subtests, which together produce a full-scale IQ score. The four indices are the verbal comprehension index, which represents the ability to understand and produce speech and use language; the perceptual organization index, which involves visual and spatial processing, such as the ability to perceive complex figures; the working memory index, which represents the ability to hold information temporarily in mind (similar to short-term memory); and the processing speed index.

The authors correlated the four major domains of intelligence (verbal comprehension, perceptual organization, working memory and processing speed, represented by the pictograms) with the lesion maps of over 240 patients. The findings provide the first voxelwise mapping of where in the brain focal damage can compromise intelligence factors.

Somewhat surprisingly, the study revealed a large amount of overlap in the brain regions responsible for verbal comprehension and working memory, which suggests that these two now-separate measures of cognitive ability may actually represent the same type of intelligence, at least as assessed using the WAIS.

The details about the structure of intelligence provided by the study could be useful in future revisions of the WAIS test so that its various subtests are grouped on the basis of neuroanatomical similarity rather than on behavior, as is the case now.

In addition, the brain maps produced by the study could be used as a diagnostic aid. Clinicians could combine the maps with their patients' Wechsler test results to help localize likely areas of brain damage. "It wouldn't be sufficient to be diagnostic, but it would provide information that clinicians could definitely use about what parts of the brain are dysfunctional," Adolphs says (Gläscher et al., 2009; California Institute of Technology, 2009; Svitil, 2009).

THE LOBES OF THE BRAIN

Frontal Lobes

The frontal lobes (see Diagram 1: Lobes of the Brain) are the most anterior part of the cortex. They are located right under the forehead, and are responsible for the following:

- consciousness
- how people know what they are doing within their environment
- executive function
- attention
- motivation
- thinking
- problem solving
- judgments
- planning
- how people initiate activity in response to their environment
- movement and motor execution
- memory
  - short-term memory
  - memory for habits and motor activities
- emotions (current evidence indicates that emotion may be lateralized to both hemispheres)
  - mood control
  - emotional response or inhibition
  - emotional valancing
- language
  - expressive language
  - parts of speech
  - word associations
  - assigns meaning to the words we choose

The frontal lobes have three primary network systems (Chow & Cummings, 1998):

1. The orbital frontal network for processing socio-emotional information

2. The anterior cingulate network for processing attentional information

3. The dorsolateral network for processing memory

They bring together and coordinate information from the limbic system, the posterior processing areas, and temporal lobes. These are important key networks to test and evaluate in clients as they contribute significantly to social and academic performance.

The right frontal lobe controls emotion and expression of language or prosody—the rhythm, stress and intonation of speech reflecting the emotional state of the speaker. Problems occurring in the right frontal lobe can lead to social problems, poor peer relations, and problems with authority. Children with problems in this area may be diagnosed with oppositional defiant disorder or conduct disorder. Elation can also occur when there is damage to or problems with the right frontal lobe. Conversely, depression can occur when there is damage or problems with the left frontal lobe.

Diagram 1. Lobes of the Brain

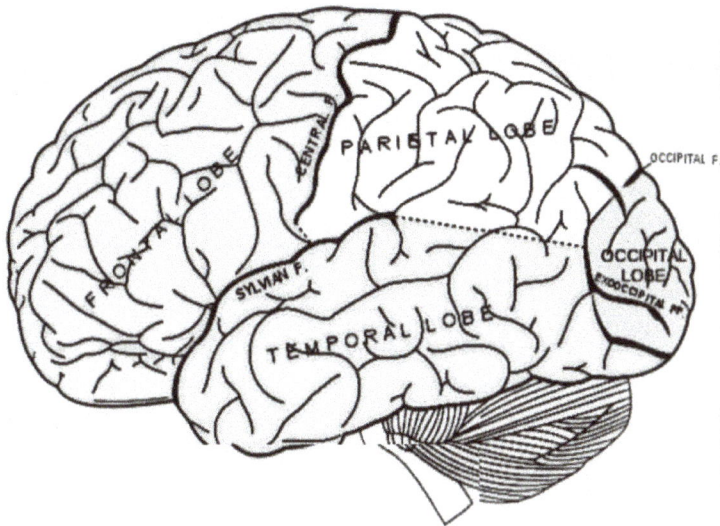

Parietal Lobes

The parietal lobes (see Diagram 1: Lobes of the Brain) are located near the back and top of the head. They are responsible for math and grammar; association between self, the environment, and others; and sensorimotor perception, integration of visual, and somatospatial information.

The parietal lobes are associated with the following:

- movement
- goal-directed voluntary movements
- manipulation of objects
- body awareness
- arousal
- perception of stimuli
- orientation (location)

- location for visual attention
- location for touch perception
- the integration of different senses that allows for understanding a single concept
- recognition
- association
- naming objects

The left parietal lobe governs language, math, and meaning construction, and can reflect language difficulties. The right parietal lobe governs arousal, facial decoding, and receptive prosody. People with Asperger's syndrome often demonstrate a lack of social integration, poor perception of others, and poor perception of self in relationship to others.

The angular gyrus is in the left parietal lobe that lies near the superior edge of the temporal lobe and immediately posterior to the supramarginal gyrus. It is Brodmann area 39 of the human brain (see Diagram 7: Brodmann Areas) and is involved in a number of processes related to language, cognition, reading comprehension, and meaning construction.

Temporal Lobes

The temporal lobes (see Diagram 1: Lobes of the Brain) are located on the sides of the head above the ears, underneath the temples, and behind the eyes. They are connected to the hippocampus, and are involved with the following:

- memory acquisition
- short-term and long-term memory
- emotional valencing
- temper control and aggression
- understanding language
- comprehension
- language function
- perception
- recognition of auditory stimuli and auditory perception
- some visual perceptions
- facial recognition
- categorization of objects and color

The temporal lobes are a major convergence zone. The left temporal lobe governs differentiation in language, receptive language, and auditory processing. When there are problems, especially in the left temporal lobe, people are more prone to temper flare-ups, rapid mood shifts, and memory and learning problems. Dyslexia results from damage to the temporal, parietal, or occipital lobes. Recent research has shown that the temporal lobes also play a role in pain management (Liu et al., 2010).

Occipital Lobes

The occipital lobes (see Diagram 1: Lobes of the Brain) are the smallest of the four true lobes in the human brain. They are located in the rearmost portion of the skull and are associated with visual processing, sequential memory functions, and arousal. In addition, they have connections with the cerebellum that involve the visual vestibular system, which affects balance and the amygdala. The occipital lobes contain most of the anatomical region of the visual cortex.

Diagram 2: Cross Section of the Brain

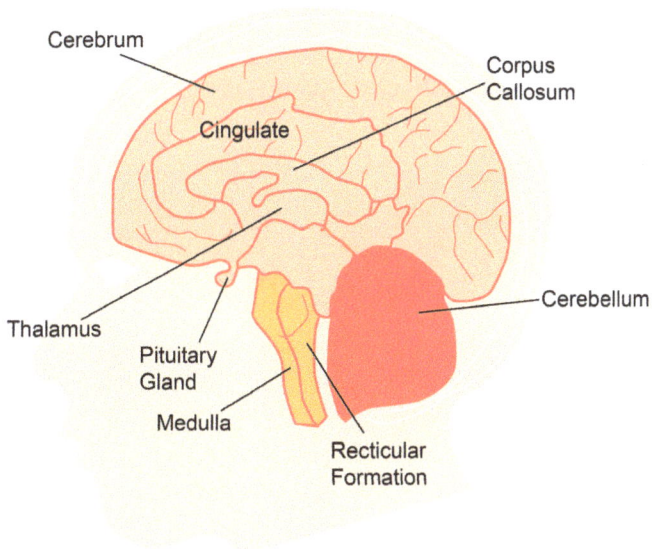

RIGHT AND LEFT HEMISPHERES

The right and left hemispheres are connected by the corpus callosum (a band of approximately 300 million nerve cell fibers, which allows conscious information to be exchanged between hemispheres). It is larger in women than in men and has been identified as critically correlated with emotional intelligence. When children have been severely abused, the corpus callosum is often damaged and smaller than normal as a result. In gifted people, the corpus callosum is often larger than average (Luders et al., 2007). The anterior commissure is another pathway that lies beneath the corpus callosum. It carries unconscious, emotional information between the two hemispheres and is a key pathway for emerging emotional feelings. Each hemisphere of the brain is dominant for certain functions and behaviors. In normal people, the two hemispheres are connected, work together, and share information through the corpus callosum.

The right hemisphere is slightly larger in normal adults, and is responsible for the following:

- emotional quotient (EQ)
- swearing
- early self-concept
- social encoding
- social skills
- face recognition
- emotional processes

    - negative emotions
    - empathy

- nonverbal expression and association
- spatial memory and problem solving
- auditory processing
- musical processing

The left hemisphere is generally responsible for the following:

- IQ
- logic
- verbal association
- verbal expression
- verbal memory
- auditory processing
- word recognition
- math and grammar problem solving

Left-side brain problems often correspond with a tendency toward significant irritability and even violence.

THE BRAIN STEM AND CEREBELLUM

The brain stem connects the limbic system and the thalamus to the spinal cord and helps regulate the basic life functions of the body, such as heart rate, blood pressure, body temperature, respiration, consciousness, and primary states of arousal ranging from sleep to hypervigilance. It also controls the production and release of some neurotransmitters. Neurotransmitter abnormalities are associated with psychiatric disorders such as depression and psychosis (Ziegler, 2002). During deep sleep, the brain stem generates simple delta waves and resonates with cortical generators. The brain stem is the first part of the brain to develop before birth, and brain stem cells are generated directly from the human heart.

The cerebellum (see Diagram 3: The Brain) is located just above the brain stem and controls coordination and motor performance as well as social, emotional, and cognitive functions. The cerebellum accounts for 40% of neurological connections. It coordinates the timing of the entire brain and remembers all the motor sequences for learned behavior. The brain stem is made of the midbrain, pons, and medulla. The midbrain is involved in functions such as vision, hearing, eye movement and body movement.

The anterior part has the cerebral peduncle, which is a huge bundle of axons traveling from the cerebral cortex through the brain stem. These fibers (along with other structures) are important for voluntary motor function.

The pons (see Diagram 3: The Brain) is involved in motor control and sensory analysis. For example, information from the ear first enters the brain in the pons. It is important for regulating levels of consciousness and for sleep. Some structures within the pons are linked to the cerebellum and are involved in movement and posture.

The medulla oblongata is the caudal-most (posterior) part of the brain stem, between the pons and spinal cord. It is responsible for maintaining vital body functions, such as breathing and heart rate.

The cerebellum (Diagram 3: The Brain) is attached to the stem at the back and is involved in maintaining subroutines of the finer aspects of movement, such as dancing, writing, or playing a musical passage. The reticular activation system (RAS) also resides here and has a great deal to do with modulating levels of arousal. Antonio Damasio (1994) argued that consciousness itself emerges in this area of the stem above the area where the trigeminal nerve enters. The reticular formation greatly impacts the power of the EEG at any given time. The RAS and hypothalamus have very dense interconnections controlling many of the basic bodily functions and hormonal functions via the pituitary gland. Irregularities in these functions may be manifest in delta wave abnormalities.

Diagram 3. The Brain

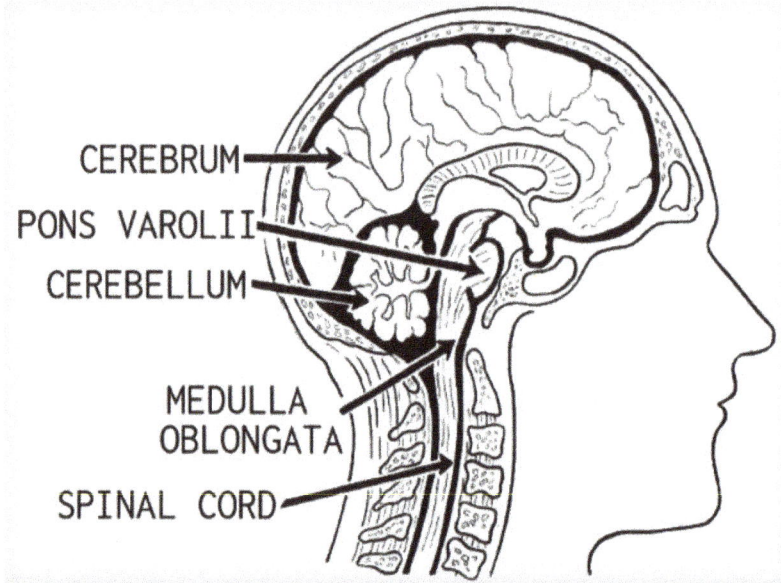

CEREBRUM

PONS VAROLII

CEREBELLUM

MEDULLA
OBLONGATA

SPINAL CORD

Basal Ganglia

The basal ganglia (see Diagram 4: Striatum or Basal Ganglia) are large structures deep within the brain. They control the body's idling speed (anxiety level). The basal ganglia integrate feelings, thoughts, and movement, and help to shift and smooth motor behavior. They allow for smooth integration of emotions, thoughts, and physical movement. When the basal ganglia are overactive, people are more likely to be overwhelmed by stressful situations. They may experience anxiety, panic, increased awareness, conflict avoidance, or heightened fear. Often, they have a tendency to freeze or become immobile in thoughts or actions. These people are at risk for increased muscle tone or tremors that may result in headaches.

Underactive basal ganglia can cause problems with motivation, energy, and get-up-and-go. In addition, increased basal ganglia activity is often associated with anxiety that in turn can intensify pain. Increased left-sided basal ganglia activity is often seen in people who are chronically irritable or angry.

People with basal ganglia problems are often experts at predicting the worst (have negative outlook) and have an abundance of negative thoughts. It is interesting that thoughts affect every cell in the body. In fact, the constant stress from negative predictions lowers immune system effectiveness and increases the risk of becoming ill.

Diagram 4: Striatum or Basal Ganglia

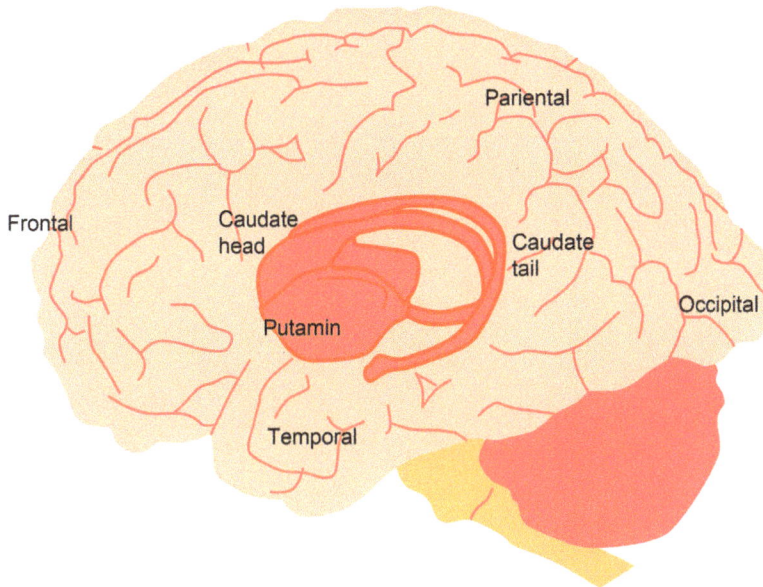

The Limbic System

The cingulate is beneath the outer covering of the cortex, followed by the corpus callosum, and then a collection of smaller structures called the limbic structures. These structures surround the thalamus. The limbic system, which forms a ring around the brain stem, is dedicated to survival and is composed of the thalamus, hypothalamus, amygdala, hippocampus, basal ganglia, cingulate cortex, and septum.

The diencephalons include the thalamus and hypothalamus that mediate arousal, appetite, sex drive, autonomic arousal, muscle tone, and bracing. James Papez, a researcher in the first half of the twentieth century, first identified the limbic system as involved with processing emotional information and memory (Papez, 1937). The primary frequency generated by the limbic system is theta. It appears to emanate especially from a group of structures that make up a circuit at the heart of the system involving the septum and the hippocampus.

The limbic system (see Diagram 5: Limbic System), often referred to as the "emotional brain," is found buried within the cerebrum. From an evolutionary perspective, it is rather old. The limbic system controls autonomic functions with its direct connection to the hypothalamus and is also connected to the cortical and subcortical regions of the brain, through the right orbitofrontal area, which in turn regulates arousal, emotions, and behavior (the socio-emotional part of the brain).

Diagram 5: Limbic System

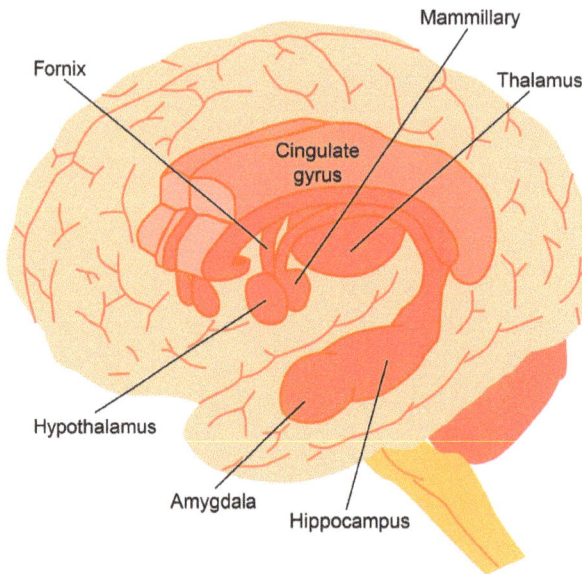

Mammillary

Fornix

Thalamus

Cingulate
gyrus

Hypothalamus

Amygdala

Hippocampus

The limbic system in part regulates and affects perception, experience, and memory. It can be directly affected by psychological trauma. The amygdala is important in memory and has connections to all areas involved with emotions; the hippocampus stores short-term memory. The cingulate gyrus is a neocortical structure with six layers. The thalamus organizes and synchronizes the brain and, like the cingulate, is a key gatekeeper for all incoming sensory information.

The limbic system, especially the hypothalamus, controls the sleep and appetite cycles of the body. The hypothalamus is responsible for translating emotional states into physical feelings, relaxation, or tension. The front half of the hypothalamus sends calming signals to the body through the parasympathetic nervous system. The back half of the hypothalamus sends stimulating or fear signals to the body through the sympathetic nervous system. The back half is responsible for the fight-or-flight response. When the limbic system is "turned on," emotions tend to take over. When it is cooled down, more activation is possible in the cortex. Current research shows a correlation between depression, increased limbic system activity and shutdown in the prefrontal cortex—especially on the left side.

The limbic system and the temporal lobes store highly charged emotions and memories, both positive and negative. Cyclic mood disorders often correlate with focal areas of increased activity in the limbic system specifically and a patchy uptake across the surface of the brain in general. Limbic problems often correlate with cyclical tendencies toward depression and irritability. The importance of understanding the limbic system will be more apparent in the next chapter on EEG.

The Thalamus

The thalamus (Figure 5) is a walnut-sized structure at the center of each hemisphere. It acts as the relay station for incoming sensory stimuli and permits the senses to be used in combination. The structure has sensory and motor functions. All sensory information coming into the body (except olfaction) goes through the thalamus, which is divided up into regions that correspond to different areas of the brain. The sensory information enters this structure where neurons send that information to the overlying cortex. Axons from every sensory system (except olfaction) synapse here as the last relay site before the information reaches the cerebral cortex.

The thalamus has multiple functions. As one thalamic projection may reach one or several regions in the cortex, it is believed to both process and relay sensory information selectively to various parts of the cerebral cortex. The thalamus plays a significant role in regulating arousal, the level of awareness, and activity. It is also responsible for regulating sleep states and wakefulness. Damage to the thalamus can lead to permanent coma, as well as pervasive memory loss.

The thalamus is thought of as the pacemaker of the brain, and its dominant rhythm appears to be alpha. Research suggests that the thalamus may engage and disengage different areas of the cortex through a resonance process involving the use of alpha as a form of braking. Research done by Sterman and Bowersox (1981) also shows that it clearly controls the sensorimotor rhythm (SMR), in a gating system to control information flowing to and from a section of the cortex that controls primary motor functions.

Hypothalamus

The hypothalamus (Figure 5) is a pea-sized structure that lies below the thalamus just above the brain stem and is responsible for certain metabolic processes as well as other activities of the autonomic nervous system (ANS). It synthesizes and secretes neurohormones, often called hypothalamic-releasing hormones. These in turn stimulate or inhibit the secretion of pituitary hormones. It works to maintain homeostasis and is the main center for information exchange between the brain and body, such as the following:

- control of the autonomic nervous system blood pressure
- circadian (24-hour) rhythms and cycles
- emotion

- e.g., anger and aggressive behavior
- thirst
- hunger
- fatigue
- body temperature
- glucose level

The hypothalamus links the nervous system to the endocrine system via the pituitary gland and has extensive links to the brain stem. The amygdala has overriding control in periods of high stress.

Amygdala

The amygdala (Figure 5) is an almond-shaped structure located just beneath the surface of the front, medial part of the temporal lobe. It causes the bulge on the surface called the uncus. It is involved in memory, emotion, and fear. The amygdala is a component of the limbic system that stores memories of fearful experiences (traumatic memories). It monitors incoming stimuli for anything threatening and activates the fight-flight-freeze stress response when danger is detected. The amygdala is responsible for precipitating changes in heart rate, and blood pressure in response to threats. It works via the hypothalamus, brain stem, and the parasympathetic and sympathetic nervous systems. The amygdala stimulates production of brainwave patterns in the basal part of the frontal lobes (prefrontal cortex). The frontal lobe is one of the few structures that can effectively inhibit the amygdala through activation, which appears as increased beta.

Hippocampus

The hippocampus (Figure 5) is a finger-sized cluster of neurons located in the cerebral hemispheres in the basal medial part of the temporal lobe. Like a memory chip in a computer, the hippocampus is the hub of memory and learning. All conscious memory must be processed through the hippocampus. It is also important for converting short-term memory to more permanent long-term memory and for recalling spatial relationships.

The hippocampus is involved with verbal and emotional memory and is vulnerable to traumatic stress. Individuals who become psychologically traumatized (and in some cases physically traumatized, which can lead to psychchological trauma) often suffer from post-traumatic stress disorder (PTSD).

Sherin (2011) notes, "Core neurochemical features of PTSD include abnormal regulation of catecholamine, serotonin, amino acid, peptide, and opioid neurotransmitters, each of which is found in brain circuits that regulate/integrate stress and fear responses." Bremner (2006) states, "Brain areas implicated in the stress response include the amygdala, hippocampus, and prefrontal cortex. Traumatic stress can be associated with lasting changes in these brain areas."

With stress, the hippocampus shuts down the immune system and the Immunoglobulin A (IGA) level goes down, which is related to fear. The hippocampus and particularly the amygdala provide conditioned learning and the ability to learn by association (Kim et al., 2015).

REVIEW QUESTIONS

1. Name three functions of the frontal lobes.
2. Memories are stored in what area(s) of the brain?
3. What is the triune brain?
4. The brain stem is responsible for what function(s)?

Chapter 3: What is EEG?

THE BRAIN AND CLINICAL THEORY

Neurometrics is the quantitative EEG of the brain. The most practical way to consider the brain in relation to clinical theories and applications is to look at it in terms of cortical and subcortical processes (see Chapter 2 for further discussion about brain anatomy and neurophysiology). From an evolutionary perspective, the subcortical structures are older and appear to have a greater overall influence on how the organism conducts its day-to-day business. The cortex, however, is the structure that is most associated with functions considered uniquely human. These two structures appear to work together, to some extent in parallel harmony. When disorders emerge, it is this relationship that is most disturbed.

The goal of this chapter is first to review the basic important anatomical features for those who are less familiar with this topic, and then to explore in deeper detail their structure, function, and the interrelationship of these features as these apply to neurotherapy protocols.

The Somatosensory Cortex/Sensory Motor Rhythm (SMR)

The somatosensory cortex (SMC) is part of two strips of tissue that are dedicated to sensory information and to motor functions. The SMC runs bilaterally across the cortex from ear to ear. Areas of each strip are specifically dedicated to corresponding areas of the body where the information originates and to which it flows back. Information flowing to and from these areas can be controlled through a gating system or "Inhibitory Gate" in the thalamus that opens and closes in response to frequency that is generated by local thalamic oscillators resulting in cortical spindles in the motor system termed Sensory Motor Rhythm or SMR (Sterman, 2006; Sterman & Bowersox, 1981).

The Split Brain

All information coming from the right hemisphere is related to the left side of the body and vice versa. The visual field is divided into two sections, left and right, in each eye. Each left side of each eye goes to the right brain and each right side of each eye goes to the left brain. Although these pathways are not 100% exclusive, they are fairly dedicated. This is important to know when employing entrainment devices to stimulate the left or right hemisphere at specific frequencies.

The Brodmann Areas

The structure of the brain can further be differentiated based on types of cells found in the brain that cluster together in areas or regions. Korbinian Brodmann, a German neurologist, is famous for his system of dividing the cerebral cortex into 47[1] distinct regions based upon their cytoarchitectonic (histological) characteristics (Šimić & Hof, 2015). He created a map that shows these regions, which are relatively stable across species of mammals. These areas are now usually referred to as Brodmann areas (Diagram 6: Brodmann Areas). A Brodmann area is a region of the cortex that is defined based on its organization of cells. Some of these areas were later associated to nervous functions, such as areas 41 and 42 in the temporal lobe (related to hearing); areas 1, 2, and 3 in the post central gyrus of the parietal lobe (the somatosensory region); and areas 17 and 18 in the occipital lobe (the primary visual areas; Korbian Brodmann, n.d.). It is noted that:

> Brodmann areas were originally defined and numbered based on the organization of neurons he observed in the cortex using the Nissl stain. Brodmann published his maps of cortical areas in humans, monkeys, and other species in 1909, along with many other findings and observations regarding the general cell types and laminar organization of the mammalian cortex. (The same Brodmann area number in different species does not necessarily indicate homologous areas.) Although the Brodmann areas have been discussed, debated, refined, and renamed exhaustively for nearly a century, they remain the most widely known and frequently cited cytoarchitectural organization of the human cortex. Many of the areas Brodmann defined based solely on their neuronal organization have since been correlated closely to diverse cortical functions (Brodmann Area, n.d.).

---

[1]   https://en.wikipedia.org/wiki/Cerebral_cortex

Diagram 6: Brodmann Areas

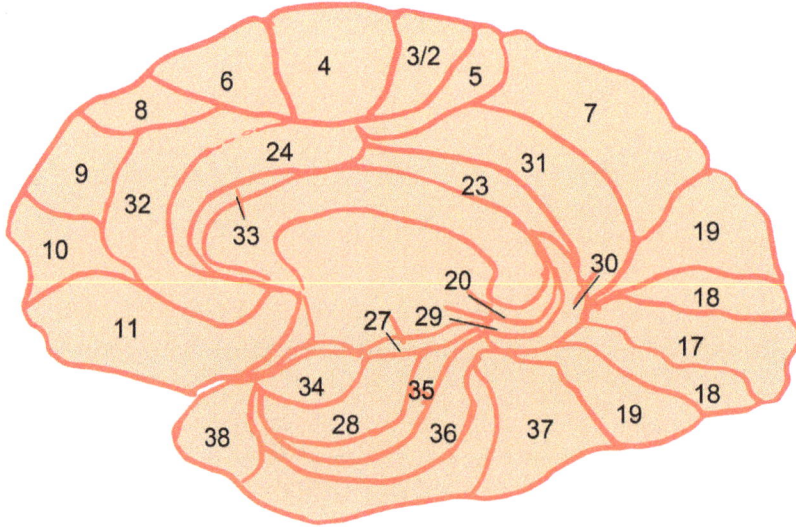

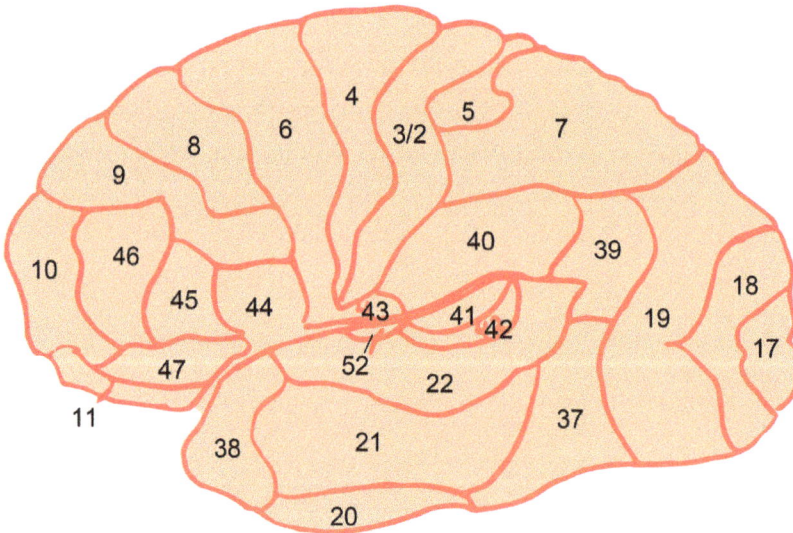

New research based on connectivity and function, in addition to cytoarchitecture, suggests there may be 180 functional regions of the cortex (Glasser et al., 2016)[2].

Two basic divisions of cell type in the brain are neurons and glial cells. Neurons transmit information through electrochemical activity, and glial cells provide maintenance and support for the neurons. Neurons provide the 30 Watts of power the brain generates to carry out its business. Recent research has indicated that the glial cells may play more of a role in information processing than previously thought and are far more than just support cells (Allen & Barres, 2009).

The neuron is profoundly complex, and a basic orientation is necessary in order to understand EEG. The neuron can be divided into four basic components: the dendrites, the soma, the axon, and the synapse.

The soma, or cell body, can be thought of as a simple battery that stores electrical energy by maintaining an electrical charge differential between the inside and outside of its cell wall. It connects to several other neurons through a main fiber that runs out of it called an axon. Diagram 7a: Electrode and Neuron Reception, below, shows an example of a neuron.

Diagram 7a: Electrode and Neuron Reception

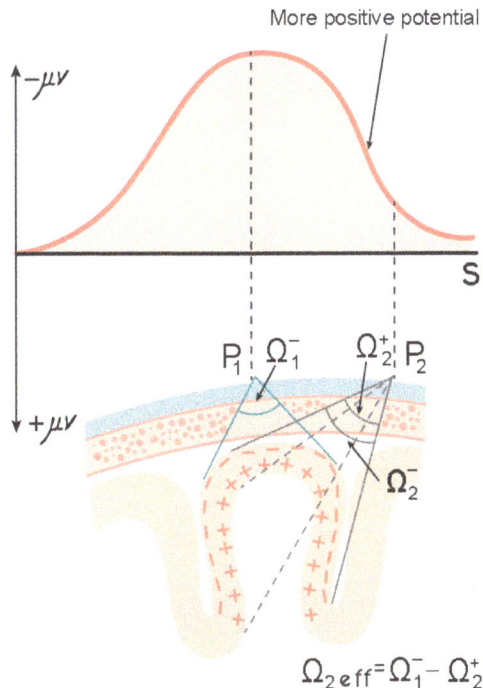

2   http://www.kurzweilai.net/new-brain-map-provides-unprecedented-detail-in-180-areas-of-the-cerebral-cortex. Retrieved November 19, 2018.) (Kurzweil, 2016)

Diagram 7b: Dendrites

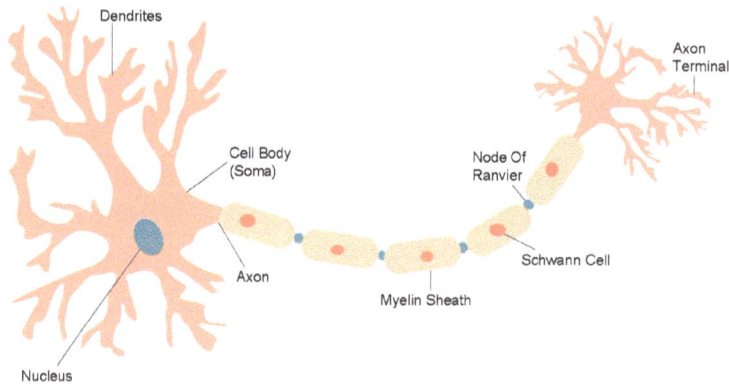

Dendrites are protrusions from the soma that collect electrical signals from several other cell axons. Between the end of each axon and the dendrite of another cell to which it connects is a gap known as the synapse.

The synapse operates like a switch that induces the neuron to fire an electrical impulse. The electrical charge travels down the axon to its own synapse that in turn induces other neurons to fire. This firing is referred to as the action potential. The action potential is an "all or none" event. There is a rest period during which time the neuron recovers, i.e., rebuilds its charge, called the refractory period. Neurons collect impulses from between 5, 000 and 50, 000 other neurons. These impulses either encourage or discourage the neuron from firing. When encouraged, they are depolarized. When discouraged, they are hyperpolarized. The entire cycle from depolarization through recovery takes about two milliseconds.

At the end of each axon is a button-shaped terminal that generates chemicals known as neurotransmitters (see Diagram 8: The Synapse). These are contained in sacks known as vesicles, which migrate to the end of the button when a charge arrives. The neurotransmitters release, flow across the synaptic gap and settle in receptor sites on the receiving dendrite. Receptor sites may increase or decrease over time in response to the average volume of neurotransmitter activity. If excessive neurotransmitter activity occurs over time, the receptors will reduce their population to adjust for the heavy traffic. Heavy alcohol users, for example, may cause excessive amounts of dopamine to cross gaps, eventually causing receptor populations to reduce. If the alcoholic suddenly stops, too little dopamine will be produced with respect to the existing receptor populations. Motor systems will suffer from reduced efficiency. Consequently, the alcoholic's hand may shake like someone with Parkinson's disease. This same process occurs in the hippocampal switching mechanisms that control immune function in response to cortisol levels generated by stress. Prolonged stress degrades the switching mechanism and immune response may be overactive when the stress lifts.

Diagram 8: The Synapse

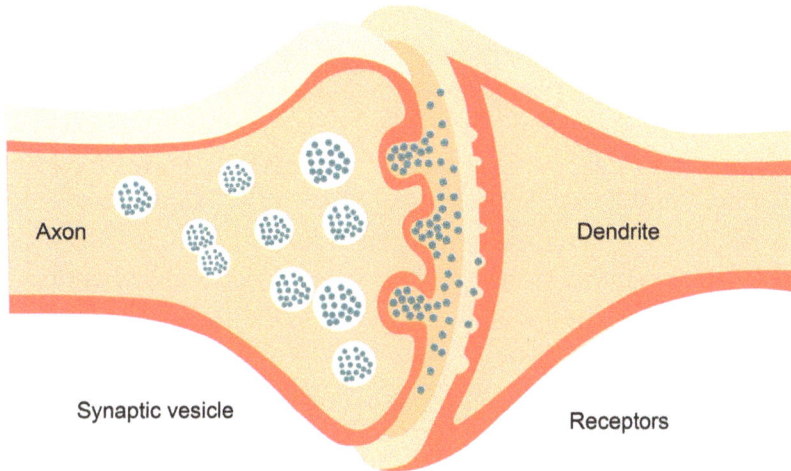

THE NEUROTRANSMITTER SYSTEMS

The Neurotransmitter Systems

Neurotransmitters are the body's chemical messengers and the molecules used by the central nervous system and especially neurons to communicate information. They can excite a neuron generating an action potential, inhibit a neuron from generating an actin potential or modulate large groups of neurons over extended time periods. Neurotransmitters come in the form of small amine molecules, amino acids and neuropeptides and are often classified accordingly. The neurotransmitters that modulate are referred to as monoamines or neuromodulators and there are six major ones you typically hear about the most. They are dopamine, norepinephrine, serotonin, acetylcholine, histamine and GABA. The body may have hundreds of neurotransmitters and accounts vary but only somewhere between sixty and a hundred have been identified, depending on how they are classified. Much of the research in pharmacology focuses on these neuromodulators because they have such far reaching effects on physiological symptoms, mood and behavior and in the past drug companies were willing to fund extensive research on them. As a consequence, many neuroscientists gravitated toward large funded projects and universities followed suit resulting in an overemphasis on research on the effects of these neuromodulators and related topics.

More recently, the efficacy of many psychotropic drugs regulating the neuromodulators has been called into question (Whitaker, 2010) and the big money research has waned with many investigators turning toward other technologies such as Transcranial Magnetic Stimulation, Pulsed Electro Magnetic Fields or pEMF, Laser, Photo Bio Stimulation, Heart Rate Variability and Photic Stimulation.

There is a growing trend in scientific investigations into the area of electronic medicine and biofeedback practitioners, including neurofeedback practitioners have been in the forefront of this exploration for decades. Nevertheless, clinicians doing neurofeedback need to understand the basics regarding how these important neurotransmitters are impacted by oxidative stress, how this influences behavior, and how this is reflected in the QEEG. Neurofeedback alters and conditions states of arousal and consequently conditions neuromodulator activity resulting in structural changes in the brain (Ghaziri, 2013) and this has been confirmed by replicated studies. This in turn impacts the effect of psychotropics on the brain and the resulting side effects that occur. As a clinician you need to be able to explain what is happening to your clients and fellow health practitioners in terms familiar to them and who may be over a decade behind in their reading and understanding of contemporary research (Morris et al., 2011).

Table 1: Major Neurotransmitters

Neurotransmitters	Type	Source, Major Influence Areas, Associated Disorders
Dopamine	biogenic amine inhibitory	substantia nigra: attentional networks, hedonic centers, schizophrenia, ADHD, addictions
Serotonin	biogenic amine inhibitory	Raphe nuclei: mood centers, sleep cycles depression, addictions
Norepinephrine	biogenic amine excitatory	locus coeruleus: general arousal levels, attentional networks
Acetylcholine	cholinergic	acetylcholine nuclei: memory networks, memory problems
GABA	amino acid inhibitory	global: general arousal levels, anxiety disorders
Histamine	biogenic amine	global

Diagram 9: Norepinephrine System

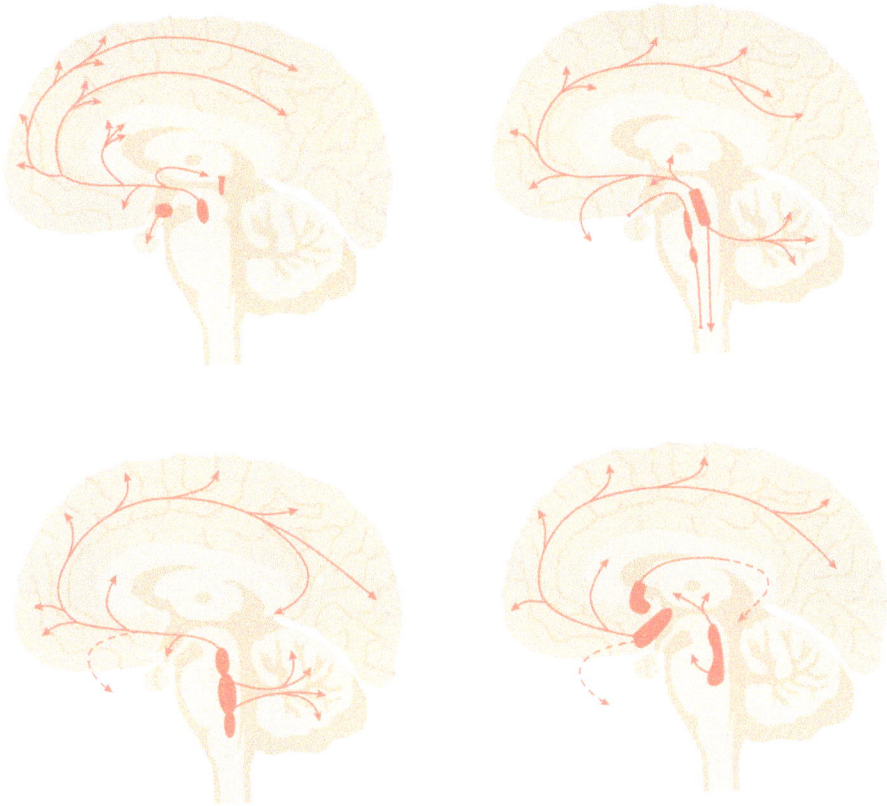

The Neurotransmitter EEG Connection

An approximate correlation between EEG activity and neurotransmitter activity appears to exist but the relationship is quite complex and it is clear that there is no one to one correspondence between a given component band such as beta and a given neuromodulator such as dopamine. In fact, dopamine influences both alpha and beta (Melgari et al., 2014). EEG activity and neurotransmitter activity reflect different fundamental levels of activity in the brain. The correlation is not precise. However, there is clearly a functional relationship that is useful to consider, since so much intervention and research is directed toward the neurotransmitter systems. The use of drugs also alters EEG activity; it is important to be aware of this alteration when reading EEG and taking baselines (see Table 2: Drug Effect on EEG).

Table 2: Drug Effect on EEG

Drug/Type	Impact/Effect on EEG
Barbiturates	Increase 25–35 Hz beta amplitude
Benzodiazepines	Increase beta
Caffeine	Increases beta and decreases slower waves
Marijuana	Effects EEG for three days by increasing global alpha
SSRIs	Decrease alpha and increase beta

From a neurotherapy perspective, the attentional system drives processing in the awake brain. This system is referred to differentially in the neuroscience literature as the External Attention System (Chun, 2011), the Salience Network (Menon, 2013) and the Orienting Network (Peterson and Posner, 2012). Much of psychological literature focuses traditionally on the effects of stimuli on the brain and it is the external attention system that identifies salient stimuli and directs neural activity into processing the percepts related to that stimuli and evaluate its consequences for behavioral responses. Fundamentally it is through this basic attentional process that we find food and detect danger. Behaviorism is fashioned around this fundamental notion that environmental stimuli elicit behaviors that arouse the organism to action or sooth it into rest. In neurofeedback we are harnessing the salience network through operant conditioning in order to influence and condition functional states to permanently alter structure and function of the brain (Ghaziri et al., 2013; Levesque, 2006). Replicated studies have shown the strong relationship between EEG activity and the BOLD signal (Rosa et al., 2010). Altering EEG activity corresponds to altered BOLD signal and therefore brain activation and altered network configurations related to altered states of arousal and processing. The neurotransmitter systems are intimately involved in this process and reflect many aspects of but it in a complex fashion. Future research into the complex relationship between EEG activity and neurotransmitter activity will continue to provide us with guides to action and refinements in protocols.

CORTICAL SYSTEMS: PYRAMIDAL CELLS, CELL COLUMNS, AND LAYERS

The cortex is comprised of groups of cells referred to as cell columns or macrocolumns, which are several millimeters in diameter. These columns are composed of functionally related groups of cells that run vertically through the six layers of the cortex (as discussed in Chapter 2). The exact nature of these columns and the area of their physical extension are still under debate.

From an EEG perspective, it is when these columns are in the process of firing together that the wave fronts become recorded as EEG. Nunez (2006) indicates, however, that EEG cannot be used to specifically measure activity at the macrocolumn level of activity. In fact, synchronous activity of about 60,000, 000 pyramidal cells or 600,000 macrocolumns is required to generate a readable EEG signal at the scalp. This amount of activity is defined as a single "dipole layer" and is typically 6 cm squared in size. This is roughly half the size of Broca's area.

It should be apparent that traditional EEG measures only broad areas of activity. Therefore, it has limited spatial resolution (as compared to the spatial precision of MRI). The summated dipoles (active current flow around a cell) that generate a dipole layer are from a particular type of cell, a pyramidal cell. It is the pyramidal cell that is most responsible for the generation of the pre- and post-synaptic potentials that are detected by the EEG (see Diagram 11: Cell Columns).

Pyramidal cells outnumber all other cell types in the cortex and have a special orientation to the six layers of the cortex. Atypical dendrites (dendrites that emerge from the apex of a pyramidal cell) extend vertically through the layers and basal dendrites extend horizontally.

Diagram 10: Cell Columns

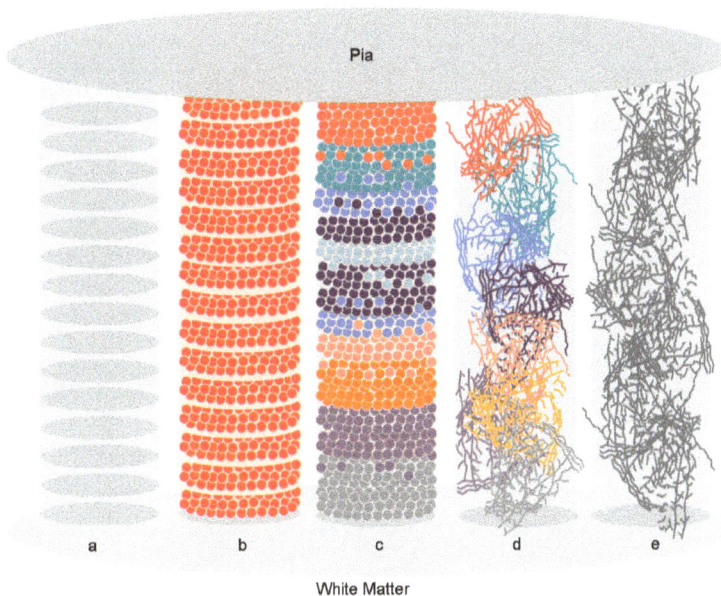

Pia

a   b   c   d   e

White Matter

The axon of the pyramidal cell extends downward out of the grey matter and becomes part of the white matter (see Diagram 11a: Axon and Cell Columns, below). So, the input to these cells comes from the upper layers and their output extends downward through their axons. The larger cells exist in the lower layers and occupy layers 2, 3, 5, and 6. Stellate cells aid communication between pyramidal cells within the cortex and are called interneurons. Stellate cells, which exist mostly in layer 4, are neurons with several dendrites radiating from the cell bodies, giving them a star-shaped appearance. The three most common stellate cells are the inhibitory interneurons found within the molecular layer of the cerebellum, excitatory spiny stellate interneurons, and inhibitory aspiny stellate interneurons.

Inputs to the cortex come from the thalamus and from other areas of the cortex (association fibers) and enter in layer 6 at the base. Thalamic input fibers generally end in layers 4 and 3. This apparently makes them the main input layers. Association fibers tend to input in layers 6, 5, 3, 2, and 1.

Diagram 11a: Axon and Cell Columns

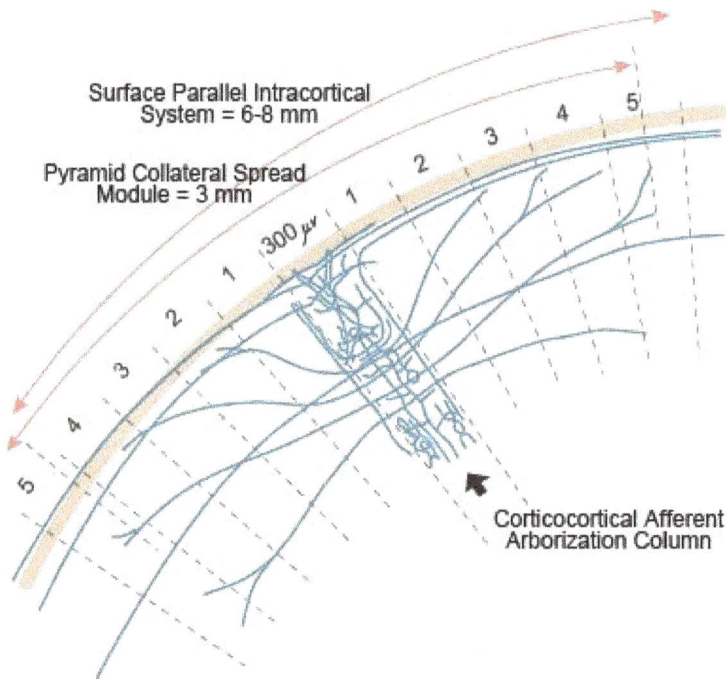

Diagram 11b: Fiber Systems

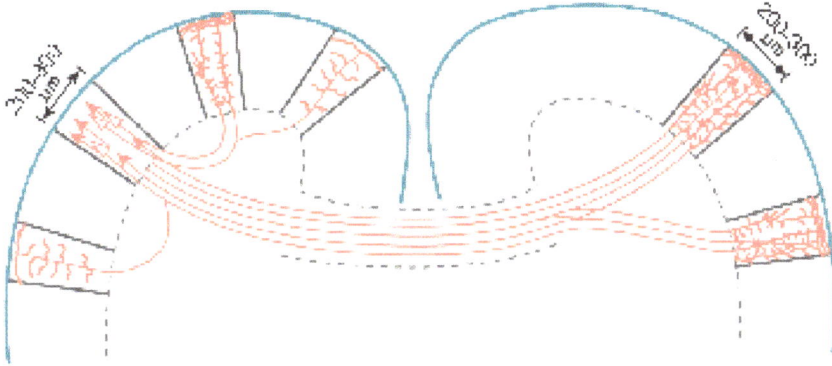

Outputs from cells in layer 6 generally go to the thalamus while those in layer 5 go to subcortical nuclei. Most outputs go to other cortical areas. Layers 2 and 3 generally reinput back to the cortex, so outputs generally go to three areas: cortex, thalamus, and subcortex.

FIBER SYSTEMS

The wiring of the cortex is composed of axons (white matter) that run in bundles along specific pathways. It is important to understand this wiring because it is through these bundles of fibers that areas of the brain are functionally connected for intermodal and cross-modal operations (in QEEG this is referred to as coherence). It is the summation of these operations that generate coordinated behavior and perception. When looking at a brain map, it is easier to understand what areas may be affecting other areas and the consequences of hyper- and hypocoupling between cell ensembles. Phase and coherence analysis in QEEG attempts to assess the level of connectivity in these pathways.

There are two basic association subcortical fiber systems (see Diagram 12: Subcortical Fiber Systems) that are involved with intracortical (situated or occurring within a cortex and especially the cerebral cortex[3]), communication or cortico-cortical (cortex to cortex) exchange. The two types include short association fibers, which connect adjacent areas or gyri of the brain, and the long association fibers, which connect more distant regions. There are three basic long association fiber systems. The cingulum is within the cingulate gyrus and connects frontal and parietal lobes with parts of the temporal lobes. The uncinate fasciculus connects the orbital lobe (the lower surface of the frontal lobes over the eyes) and other parts of the frontal lobe with the anterior temporal lobe. Parts of it also connect with the occipital lobe. The arcuate fasciculus connects parts of the frontal lobe with the temporal lobe as well, especially

---

3   *https://www.merriam-webster.com/medical/intracortical*

Broca's area and Wernicke's area, which relate to expressive and receptive language processing in the left hemisphere.

Another fiber system, the commissures, connects the hemispheres and is known as the corpus callosum and the anterior commissure. These fiber systems are concerned with short-term memory functions, including the transference of learned tasks between hemispheres. As noted in Chapter 2, severe damage can occur to this area of the brain as the result of child abuse.

Diagram 12: Subcortical Fiber Systems

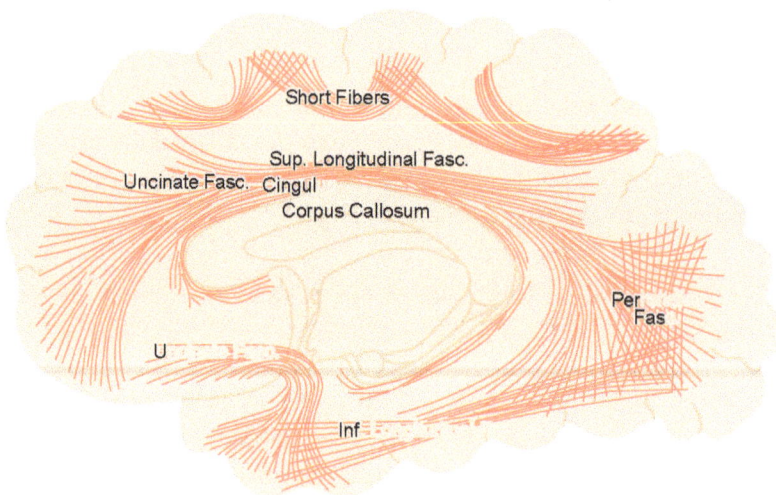

BRODMANN'S AREAS: CONNECTING THE DOTS

As noted above, Brodmann analyzed the brain based on the congregation of cell types in different areas of the brain. These brain areas are frequently used by neurologists to associate function with location. Table 3: Brodmann Areas and Localization of Function shows the Brodmann areas as they relate to function and EEG. The International 10-20 System of electrode placement is shown in Diagram 13: 10-20 System of Electrode Placement. In the 10-20 System the "F" such as in F3 stands for frontal, the "C" for central, "P" is for parietal, "O" is for occipital and "T" is for temporal. The "z" indicates midline locations on the scalp. Today, neuroimaging is resulting in a new mapping system, but it has not yet been entirely integrated into neurology and neuropsychology.

Thalamic Projection Tracts

The projection tracts are fiber systems that bring information into the cortex from the thalamus as well as output information and are known as the corona radiata. One group of projection tracts connects the frontal cortex to the thalamus. A second group of projection tracts connects to motor neurons through the reticular formation. Another group connects parietal, occipital, and temporal fibers to the spinal cord. Two other groups of projection tracts connect to auditory and optical functions in the temporal and occipital lobes, respectively.

Diagram 13: 10-20 System of Electrode Placement

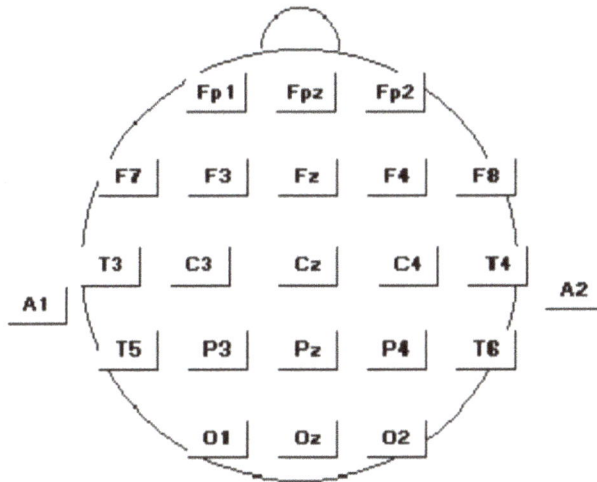

THALAMIC PROJECTION SYSTEM

The thalamus is divided into sections that connect to specific related areas of the brain, through axons extending to and from pyramidal cells in the lower cortical layers. These axons appear to set up resonances between the thalamus and the cortex. Oscillating neurons in the thalamus send signals in specific frequency ranges to the cortex, which in turn sends feedback to the thalamus. A constant dialogue is established where different sections of the brain engage and disengage as the cortex coordinates its various modules into organized behavior.

Early researchers felt that alpha rhythms were primarily generated by the thalamus alone (Anderson & Anderson, 1968), but newer theories contend that while alpha rhythms spontaneously emanate from thalamic neuronal oscillator circuits, their shifting patterns are driven through interaction with the cortex. The alpha range represents a functional idling frequency that turns off or "desynchronizes" as different sections of the brain become active. The on-task activity appears to involve gating mechanisms in the beta range. Lower frequency activity in theta appears to be related to resonances with subcortical activities, particularly in the limbic system.

Table 3: Brodmann Areas and Localization of Function

SITE	BRODMAN AREA	FUNCTION
Fpz	10, 11, 32	Emotional inhibition, oversensitive, impulsive Motivation & attention
Fp1	10, 11, 46	Cognitive emotional valence—lateral orbital frontal Irritability, intrusive, depression Social awareness—approach behaviors
Fp2	10, 11, 46	Emotional inhibition—lateral orbital frontal Impulsivity, tactlessness, mania Social awareness—avoidance behaviors
F7	45, 47, 46	Working memory—visual & auditory Divided & selective attention—filtering Broca's area—semantic short-term buffer (word retrieval)
F8	45, 47, 46	Prosody Working memory—spatial & visual, gestalt Facial emotional processing Sustained attention
F3	8, 9, 46	Short-term memory—verbal episodic retrieval Facial recognition, object processing Planning & problem solving—Wisconsin Card Sort (rigidity)
F4	8, 9, 46	Short-term memory—spatial/object retrieval Vigilance area—selective & sustained attentional area
Fz	8, 6, 9	Personality changes Intention & motivation—poverty of speech, apathy Possible anterior cingulate—internal vs. external attention Basal ganglia output
C3	3, 1, 4	Sensory & motor functions
C4	3, 1, 4	Sensory & motor functions

SITE	BRODMAN AREA	FUNCTION
Cz	6, 4, 3	Sensory & motor functions
T3	42, 22, 21	Language comprehension—verbal understanding Wernicke's area—inner voice Long-term memory—declarative & episodic processing Event sequencing—visualization Amygdala/ hippocampal area
T4	42, 22, 21	Personality—emotional tonality (anger, sadness) Categorization & organization Visualization and auditory cortex
T5	39, 37, 19	Meaning construction—angular gyrus Acalculia Short-term memory
T6	39, 37, 19	Facial recognition—emotional content, amygdaloid connection
P3	7, 40, 19	Digit span problems, information organization problems Self-boundaries excessive thinking
P4	7, 40, 19	Visual processing—spatial sketch pad, vigilance Personality—excessive self-concern, victim mentality Agnosia, apraxia, context boundaries, rumination
Pz	7, 5, 19	Attentional shifting perseverance Self-awareness, orientation association area Agnosia, apraxia
O1, O2	18, 19, 17	Visual processing, procedural memory, dreaming
Oz	18, 17, 19	Visual processing, hallucinations

NewMind Neurofeedback Center

Thalamic Gating

Barry Sterman has pioneered work demonstrating the gating system by which sensory information is directed toward the motor cortex or blocked through thalamic oscillators. As a consequence of these findings, Sterman experimented with individuals with seizure disorders. He dramatically reduced the frequency of seizures through SMR training. Joel Lubar (Lubar & Bahler, 1976) later applied these findings with considerable success to individuals with ADHD. Sterman found that seizure activity continued to decline over a decade after patients quit training. Lubar also found that individuals with ADHD continued to show improvement after training.

NEOCORTICAL DYNAMICS: OSCILLATORS, WAVEFRONTS, AND NETWORKS

Oscillators

Oscillators are groups of neurons that work together to generate rhythmic pulses of electrical activity. According to Buzsáki (2006), they form momentary cohorts of activity, called cell assemblies, networking together for 30—100 ms or more. They are associated physiologically with glucose and oxygen consumption and neurometabolic coupling, which is controlled by local cells called astrocytes (Freeman, Ahlfors, & Menon, 2009). These neurons fall under the category of simple Limit Cycle Oscillators. They shift the frequency and phase of their pulses in response to a stimuli and this results in the setting and resetting phase activities leading to the coherence activity we record in QEEG. The phase lock and shift activity is the result of a phenomena known as Attractor Itinerancy (Miller, 2016). The term itinerancy is used if a system switches rapidly between distinguishable patterns of activity that last significantly longer than the switching time. A good example is the heartbeat. The Attractor is the dominant rhythm that the beats maintain. This type of oscillatory activity is also responsible for communication between gamma and theta frequencies. These oscillatory activities occur throughout the brain. Their interaction results in oscillatory hubs in both the cortex and the thalamus as well as key subcortical structures such as the septal hippocampal oscillators related to memory processing.

The oscillating neuronal activity of the brain is self-organized and emerges through harmonic interface in a fashion we are only beginning to understand. It operates according to dynamical principals that are described as non-linear and bordering on chaos. We can see this kind of self-organized emergent activity throughout nature in weather systems and in human social activity such as emerging markets in economic activity and memes on the internet. For neurofeedback practitioners It is not crucial to understand the details of nonlinear dynamics and EEG oscillators but it is important to understand that it is the basis for electrical activity in the brain and that it operates on a level of complexity that borders on the chaotic. In the future we may see this as the basis for cybernetic interface and we are already harnessing it with many technologies including Neurofeedback.

Theories of how EEG arises and propagates itself are still evolving. The EEG at the surface of the cortex (see Diagram 14: EEG Wavefronts) reflects the summated activity of ensembles of cells in the form of extracellular current flow, the physical substrate supporting oscillatory activity. This summated activity is due apparently to synchronously activated postsynaptic potentials from vertically oriented pyramidal cells. Nunez & Lopes de Silva (1995; 2006) proposes that this summated activity forms standing wavefronts that hover over the surface of the cortex and scalp. According to his calculations, these wavefronts are so large that there is no neutral site to place a reference electrode that would allow for an approximately infinite resistance between the wave sources required for a true reference site. Thus, the ear lobes have been chosen as common reference points for databases as a good compromise (rather than the nose, another good compromise).

The contribution to the EEG recorded at a specific site has been theoretically determined by Nunez (1995) and involves the following definition:

$$f(n), b \ (BQ)$$

where:

f = frequencies,

n = spatial patterns (corresponding frequencies and overtones);

b = multiple frequencies in the same medium interacting;

B = global control parameters (neurotransmitter activity); and

Q = local control parameters (physical electrical activities causing state transitions).

If all of this seems complex and overwhelming, it is to even the best neuroscientists. A simpler heuristic to keep in mind comes from the neurology community and suggests that approximately 40% or more of the total global EEG, or volume-conducted EEG, is being recorded at any given electrode location. So, when you train locally, keep in mind that you are training globally as well unless you are using sLORETA and you have an artifact free session.

Diagram 14: EEG Wavefronts

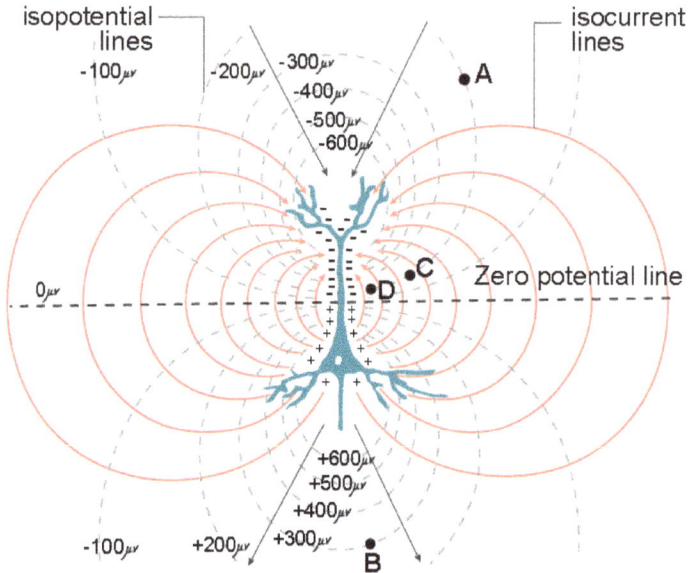

Clearly the area of approximately 3 square centimeters (approximately the size of a quarter) of activity monitored by an electrode draws its characteristics from a complex mixture of local and distant activity. Consequently, local activity is merely a peculiar reflection of the sum of activity occurring in the brain at that moment. To assume that the activity noted is primarily a reflection of the local activity would be erroneous. To assume that distant activity is or is not affected by local recruitment of EEG is an unsound conclusion. To consider local recruitment to be affecting primarily the local area is equally unsound. Nunez & Lopes de Silva (1995; 1996) and Freeman (2003) note that the complexity of the EEG is such that we do not at present have the mathematical models to untangle it.

In terms of EEG training, this has important implications. Texts on neurology clearly state that the impact of any one area of the brain on others is so complex as to be difficult to untangle in any given situation as well. The brain consists of a complex system of networks. Research on these networks in the brain is not always in agreement. However, what is known and agreed upon is the complexity and interactivity of networks within the brain. Neurology texts rely primarily on the physical behavior of the organism to determine what sections of the brain are most impacted by focal lesions. They find it difficult to predict the specific consequences of damage to one area of the brain. This is also in part due to the great variance in the anatomy of individual functional locations.

Thus, one must be careful when doing neurofeedback training designed to target a specific region of interest (ROI). Anatomical variation even causes difficulties in averaging site findings in functional MRI research as well and is part of the daily challenge of neuroimaging teams trying to match an individual's personal anatomy with a standardized MRI atlas library. This MRI procedure is referred to as image segmentation. It is good to keep in mind that in the EEG world Homan et al., (1987) found at least a 10% variance between anatomical location and the 10-20 system. This has profound implications for how we use the Talairach atlas with sLORETA and the level of accuracy we should expect in terms of source localization of current source activity. This must be considered in conjunction with how artifact confounds accuracy and new emerging understanding that BA areas are far more functionally complex in structure and fiber pathway intersections than previously understood (Zilles et al., 2002). They are not as homogenous in structure and function as previously believed. Linking a functional activity to only one Brodmann area is bordering on electronic phrenology. Function is highly distributed in the brain. It should be considered as system (Freeman, 2003).

Correcting the "system" to correct its deviant attributes or symptoms is consistent with the highly effective and research-based paradigm that is emerging in contemporary healthcare known as Functional Medicine. Targeting specific ROIs with complex neurofeedback technologies is interesting theoretically but is highly innovative and experimental and there is very little research to demonstrate it has any advantage over better researched standard "system" based neurofeedback (Coben et al., 2018). These technically complex methods appear to be effective but there is no clearly demonstrated advantage based on any existing research. These methods may not be doing what we think they are doing and in the manner we believe they are doing it. They are also very expensive and have a sharp learning curve creating a perceived barrier to entry into the field by those interested. Those entering the field should consider learning the basics of standard neurofeedback as proposed in the BCIA Blueprint of Knowledge before engaging in the more experimental technologies in the field. There are many advantages to starting out with the simple basis.

The more recent research on brain connectivity fiber pathways involves mathematical simulations based on Hagmann's (2008) mapping of the hubs, nodes, and pathways of the cortex. These simulations are correlated with MRI and anatomical observations of real head injury cases. They indicate that damage to hubs and nodes has more extensive impact than damage to any other areas and the effects on those areas that are secondarily impacted are complex in pattern and difficult to predict according to leading investigators Alstott, Breakspear, Hagmann, Cammoun, & Sporns (2009). Since hubs and nodes only occupy a relatively small area of the cortex, lesions may frequently have only local consequences but on occasion very extensive bilateral consequences. In light of this, it may be dangerous to assume that training EEG in one specific site based on symptom or anatomical identity will affect all individuals with similar problems in the exact same manner.

The problem becomes even greater when DSM diagnoses are relied on to guide intervention, since they are based on constellations of general behavior patterns rather than specific behaviors used as cues by neurologists. The DSM is a symptom-based method of developing a diagnosis, and a phenomenologically based diagnostic classification scheme. When the DSM-V was released, it was immediately challenged due to the lack of science supporting its contents and diagnostic recommendations (Khoury et al., 2014). Furthermore, multiple subtypes in terms of EEG with respect to many of the DSM diagnostic categories have been found. For instance, Chabot (1998) believes he has isolated eleven subtypes of ADHD and other researchers have reported five possible subtypes of schizophrenia. Another example is traumatic brain injury (TBI). TBI symptoms are so varied that they can resemble the symptoms associated with several disorders including but not limited to ADD, ADHD, depression, anxiety, and PTSD. Many prescribers do not ask patients if they have ever had a head injury when prescribing a medicine to treat the symptoms of one of the above disorders.

Quantitative EEG brain mapping can indicate abnormal brain function in a specific location using a dynamic electrophysiological perspective. QEEG cannot yet—and may never—predict specific behavioral deviance with accuracy, although general categories of EEG patterns have been found highly correlated with specific DSM categories of disorder. NewMind Technologies is presently involved with a collaborative project with the University of North Carolina to collect data comparing dimensions of social behavior with dimensions of QEEG analysis. We expect some predictive relationships to emerge. It should be kept in mind that training based solely on QEEG does not guarantee results. Training at a specific site may not permanently alter activity in that site. On the other hand, it may alter activity, but predicting its effects on other more distant sites is not possible. Therefore, a general catalogue of training patterns for different symptoms may prove more effective in guiding training—although QEEG interpretation may be most effective in determining the general problem from an EEG perspective.

Often, professionals will ask, how does EEG compare to other measures?

EEG can identify activity not captured by MRI, such as documenting the consequences of axonal shearing from a TBI that influence processing in a disruptive manner and generate chronic symptoms.

PET and fMRI provide better spatial resolution than EEG and MEG (magnetoencephalography), but poorer temporal resolution. MRI shows responses in terms of seconds while EEG shows responses in terms of milliseconds.

Global, Regional, & Local Activity

Wavefronts can develop as a result of activity involving small local areas as well as multiple areas covering the entire brain. These wavefronts resonate back and forth between various regions of the brain depending on their phase relationships and have come to be referred to as resonant loops. Researchers have divided this activity into three categories: local, regional, and global resonant loops.

The first type of resonant loop is called a local resonant loop and takes place between local cell columns that are known as macrocolumns (see cortical systems above). There is a great deal of resistance between adjacent cell columns. The brain carefully regulates interaction between local cell columns to avoid too much excitation and seizure activity. In fact, the brain has powerful inhibitory mechanisms in place and much of the electrical activity is dedicated to inhibition. There is a constant dialectic between excess excitatory activity and excessive inhibitory activity. It appears that the brain is delicately balanced between seizure and coma (Austin, 1998).

The resonances between local cell columns usually occur at frequencies above 30 Hz and are often called gamma. They are beyond the range of many present day QEEG databases. Much of the activity in this frequency range has been associated with excessive mental chatter and disorders such as schizophrenia. It is also the range of a great deal of scalp EMG. It is often difficult to distinguish between gamma and scalp tension. In fact, many researchers believe it is difficult, if not impossible, to increase the amplitude of this frequency range significantly through training (Muthukumaraswamy, 2013; Whitham et al., 2008)

Resonances around 38–42 Hz are known as Sheer rhythms (Friedemann et al., 1994; Sheer, 1976) and appear to be related to learning. Rhythms of 40 Hz are also thought to be related to activation processes associated with DC current activity in the brain that involves consciousness.

Resonances that develop between cortical cell columns that are several centimeters apart are called regional resonances. The exchange of communication between cortico-cortical sites would also dominate this range as well as cortico-thalamic sites. These resonances result in alpha and low beta activity. It appears that these involve the idling and engagement of cell columns as they process information incoming as a result of attentional activities and conscious articulation.

Global resonances develop as a result of activity between distant sites of the cortex and fall into the theta and delta range. Many of the sites involved in this frequency range are believed to include subcortical functions. Hippocampal-septal activity in the limbic system is known to generate a significant amount of theta activity. Theta activity is associated with coordination of cortical networks, memory, and emotional processing as well (Buzsáki, 2006). Presently, it appears that gamma activity, by exciting cortical cell assemblies, is coordinated through timing mechanisms that are associated with theta and may provide a basis for understanding the "binding" mechanisms in the brain.

Robert Thatcher (personal communication) argues that these global resonances are related to meta-functions such as personality functions that are integrative in nature. In addition, we know that theta involves daydreaming and rumination activities. These may be more primitive forms of processing related to subcortical functions. Subcortical theta inputs dominate the Default Mode Network that process predominantly self-referential activities in the parietal region. This is one of the reasons theta activity is highest in this region. Delta's primary function appears to be related to sleep, yet it is very much a part of waking cortical activity and plays a key role in stimulus identification and processing through the external attention system (Knyazev, 2012). This is the reason delta is dominant in the eyes open frontal EEG record when processed through digital filters. Although it is in the background, research in QEEG suggests that lack of delta may indicate a lack of continuity in white matter fibers, which could be thought of as low connectivity between networks.

The pattern below (Diagram 15: Expanding EEG Waves) is adopted from Nunez's (1995) book on neocortical dynamics and shows the theoretical pattern of expanding EEG waves generated from local sources over fractions of a second.

Diagram 15: Expanding EEG Waves

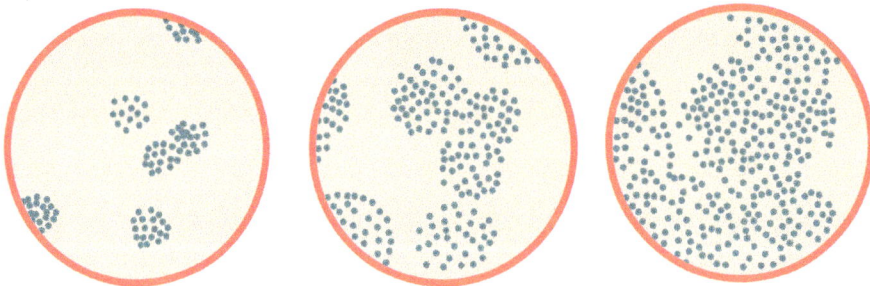

These patterns tend to establish relatively stable patterns that last longer and are called standing waves. The patterns in Diagram 16 (see Diagram 16: Stereotypical Patterns of High and Low Amplitude Locations) are characteristic of those found during an alpha baseline. They indicate stereotypical patterns of high and low amplitude locations seen in a brain map and may reflect the patterns of neural network activation.

Diagram 16: Stereotypical Patterns of High and Low Amplitude Locations

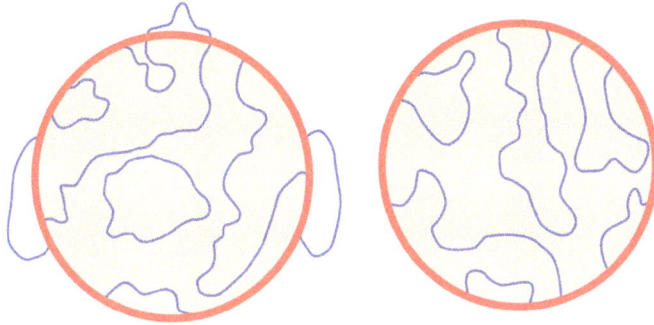

Hypercoupling, Hypocoupling, and Coherence

The resonant loops we have discussed appear to favor different frequencies based on the number of resident synapses and the amount of delay characteristically involved with those neurons. *Hypocoupling* in the brain involves smaller loops and higher frequencies, indicative of anxiety and seizure and correlates roughly with increases in norepinephrine and dopamine and decreases in GABA. *Hypercoupling* is said to occur when brain activation decreases, slow waves increase, serotonin and dopamine levels decrease, and depression and increases. Hypocoupling, therefore, characterizes a high level of cerebral activation and arousal that is often reflected in conscious or awake information processing states. As the brain becomes engaged in hypercoupled activity, activation decreases and slow wave activity increases while the brain moves toward an increased resting state and sleep.

Too much hypocoupling moves us toward excess activity, anxiety, and seizure. Too much hypercoupling moves us toward reduced activity, depression, and coma. Excessive hypocoupling shows up in positive schizophrenia and anxiety with excessive activity in the 23–38 Hz range. Excessive hypercoupling is found in negative schizophrenia and ADHD with excessive activity in the 1–8 Hz range. Increasing the average level of activity in the 9–15 Hz range to reduce activity in the upper and lower frequency ranges is often an important goal of training. Recent research suggest that hyperconnectivity in a brain circuit may predict psychosis (Cao et al., 2018).

Coherence describes the relationship between two localities in the brain. As cell ensembles fire and generate wavefronts, their frequencies often match up as they resonate together. The more they resonate together, the more their timing becomes synchronized. The peaks and valleys of their waveforms begin to match each other and they become phase-locked. When the two waves become perfectly overlapped we say they are synchronous (see Diagram 17: Wavelength and Phase). This is a special case of coherence, and is referred to as state phase coherence in electronics theory. The peaks and valleys of the waves match up in lock step.

When the peaks and valleys of the waves match up in lock step, their phase angle becomes zero. The degree to which they phase lock is often spoken of in terms of an average phase angle. When locations are 180 degrees out of phase, their peaks are occurring at opposite times. In neurometrics, coherence refers to the degree in which two locations have a consistent phase angle. When their phase angle is consistent, they are considered to be in a high level of communication. When coherence is too high, there is a lack of differentiation between functional areas. When coherence is low, there is a lack of communication between functional areas.

Diagram 17: Wavelength and Phase

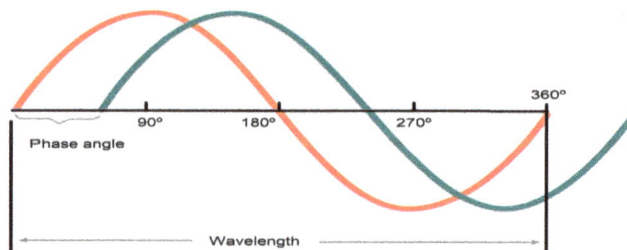

Technically, the whole issue is more complex, and there is considerable disagreement in the definition of EEG coherence. EEG coherence is formally defined as the covariation of phase over time with respect to a mean value based on a database. According to Duane Shuttlesworth (personal communication), the late E. Roy John chose the definition of covariance of power between various sites in the left and right hemispheres. To confuse issues more, Sterman has introduced a similar measure he calls comodulation, which is the covariance of frequency over time with respect to a mean value based on a database.

Nunez & Srinivasan (2006) indicates that coherence measures are highly contaminated by volume conduction over interelectrode distances of up to 10 cm. This would invalidate a large portion of the connections displayed on the average QEEG. Roberto Pascual Marqui (2007), who developed low resolution tomography (LORETA) imaging at the Key Institute, echoes these concerns in his latest research and argues that coherence is a two-dimensional measurement. By this he means that typical measures of coherence disregard the important influence of inputs and feedback from multiple sources. David Kaiser, who co-developed the Sterman Kaiser database, goes further and says that it is one-dimensional (personal communication). He also indicates that two-dimensional coherence is confounded by possible contributions from a third-dimensional source involving thalamic mediation (personal communication). David Kaiser and Paul Nunez argue that coherence should be based on Laplacian transforms to be accurate. Thatcher argues that this practice only distorts phase measures upon which coherence is based. Taking these arguments into account, it may be best to consider coherence as a vague but general measure of connectivity.

Phase is defined as the degree to which the peak and trough cycles of two sites agree, what is often referred to as phase angle in electronics. Coherence is derived from phase since it measures how consistent this relationship is over time. Symmetry, on the other hand, is the covariance of amplitude at two different sites. Training coherence and phase differences between two locations is becoming popular, especially with traumatic brain injury (TBI) and learning disabilities (LD), even though there is little research on the topic. Jonathan Walker, a neurologist from Texas, was originally one of the leading proponents and most experienced clinicians in this area. He and Joe Horvath experimented extensively with coherence training. Horvath published his findings and indicated that coherence training by itself was likely to result in many negative side effects if not done carefully and correctly (Horvath, 2009). He found training delta and then theta coherence issues in sequence usually lead to significant changes that precluded the need to train higher frequencies. He reported that training alpha and beta coherence was especially fraught with peril with respect to side effects and wasn't often required. Several manufacturers now offer equipment with two or more channels or even full 19 channel training programs that have this capability. Mark Smith (personal communication), one of the early key developers of Z-Score training, observes that zscore training of coherence that includes power or magnitude training at the same time reduces the risk of side effects but there is little research on this topic. Rob Coben (2018) has also developed a method of multichannel coherence training that takes into account the contributions of all channels combined and has shown it to be highly effective, especially when combined with amplitude training. He has published research utilizing a control group design indicating it may be more effective than standard single channel training.

It should be noted that we have tens of thousands of pre- and post-brain maps showing major changes from coherence due to training in the amplitude (magnitude) domain. One domain affects the other domain (i.e., power or magnitude has an effect on coherence and coherence has an effect on power). The research question that needs to be answered regards the advantages that might be gained by training coherence. Although coherence and power (or magnitude) are mathematically different and independent dimensions, functionally they are not different. The brain is a dynamic system that derives power and magnitude as a consequence of phase activity (Srinivasan & Nunez, 2006).

Brainmaster® Technologies was the first to developed an innovative approach to training using a DLL (dynamic linked library) to link live EEG training to the Neuroguide database. This technology was referred to as "Z-Score training." This method allows coherence to be trained within specific parameters based on the normative database. This assures that coherence will be trained within very carefully defined limits, so that it cannot easily be trained too high or too low. As coherence training has attracted growing interest, as noted above, many clinicians have noted serious unintended side effects. The Z-Score training method appears to minimize this problem.

The Othmers have proposed that their Infra-low sub delta protocol techniques result in a form of "anti coherence training" that encourages plasticity in networks that are too high in coherence. Siegfried has also indicated that they may move away from the bipolar montages. They presently use a two-channel version of this approach that might be more precise and controlled. Currently, however, the Othmers are doing sub-delta or "infraslow" training (EEGInfo, n.d.).

Comodulation

Barry Sterman and David Kaiser have developed the connectivity measure known as comodulation. It is mathematically derived from the covariance of power of two electrode locations. This measure looks at the correlation of magnitude between locations. Although it is not presently represented in other database systems, it appears to be a very valuable correlate of disorder and capable of predicting specific functional problems. There is not very much research employing this measure at present, but it may prove more robust than coherence in the future.

Connectivity

Connectivity is a hot topic in neurofeedback and QEEG at present. Many arguments surround issues regarding what are the best measures of connectivity and how to obtain and represent them. Freeman (2009) defines connectivity along two dimensions: effective and functional. Functional connectivity indicates the actual existing integration of hubs, nodes, and networks at baseline or rest. Effective connectivity concerns how well modules and networks communicate "under load" or during a task. This difference is reflected in a baseline EEG vs. EEG during training. A QEEG typically shows functional connectivity unless it is done during a task, such as reading. A healthy EEG distribution during a resting QEEG indicates good functional connectivity with respect to the default mode of operation. This important emerging research in the neuroimaging community profoundly validates the use of both QEEG as an assessment measure and neurofeedback as a remedial intervention.

The most recent efforts in the development of many EEG database systems are to develop a three dimensional measure of connectivity, such as Hudspeth's Neurorep System and the Key Institute's LORETA. There may be mathematical, spatial, and temporal limits to this agenda. Thatcher is focusing more on measuring network configurations based on phase locking, which appears to be a more realistic solution. The NewMind database system, on the other hand, focuses instead on EEG as a measure of activation and uses multivariate analysis to determine this dimension. This is more in line with the present approach of the neuroimaging community and is grounded in 100 years of postmortem studies and clinical observations in neurology.

All of the above issues must be ultimately taken into account when considering what is a valid measure of connectivity and the significance of connectivity itself with regard to assessment and training. Clearly this is a long-term project for the QEEG community and will not be resolved in the near future. This should guide us to be cautious when we evaluate any claims made with regard to the representation of connectivity.

Traditional Bandwidths

Traditionally the EEG spectrum is divided into bandwidths with the names alpha, beta, theta, and delta. (Alpha is further broken down into lo-alpha and hi-alpha, and beta is further broken down into lo-beta, beta, and hi-beta). In the past, these have been used as if they were the only possible ones to consider, although others such as gamma were discussed. The waves in these bandwidths have a specific shape or morphology that helped to identify them.

Electroencephalographers traditionally count the number of wave peaks in a second and look at the wave shape to identify the wave type they are viewing. So there are two components to the analysis: frequency and morphology. Most people in neurofeedback tend to rely mostly on frequency. This can be misleading at times, especially with respect to alpha because alpha can be as slow as 3 Hz or as fast as 15 Hz and is primarily identified by morphology. Below are some samples of typical wave types. To learn them all requires considerable study. Courses in EEG technology are offered at local colleges and can be helpful to gain a better understanding of EEG.

The first wave type presented is rhythmic delta (Diagram 18: Non-Rhythmic Delta) and is usually considered to be from 1.5 to 3.5 or 1 to 4 cycles per second. It is a normal type of delta you would expect to find in your EEG and is predominantly present in deep sleep. The second type of delta is non-rhythmic and is abnormal (see Diagram 19: Non-rhythmic Delta). It is often present when individuals move their eyes around or shift around in their seats. It may also be present in areas with white matter lesions. According to Robert Thatcher (personal communication), and based on his research with EEG and MRI, high levels of localized delta on a brain map may indicate white matter damage as well.

Diagram 18: Rhythmic Delta

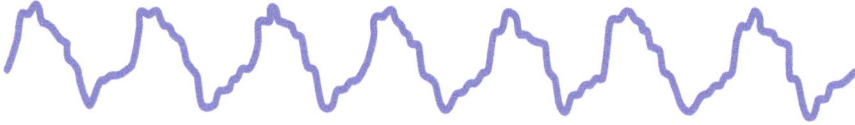

Diagram 19: Non-Rhythic Delta

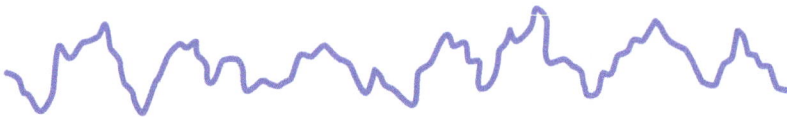

The next sample is rhythmic theta and irregular theta (Diagrams 20 and 21). Rhythmic theta is a normal variant that is present in the waking EEG and is found in a bandwidth between 3.5 and 7.5 or 4 and 7 cycles a second. You will often see it increase as individuals get drowsy or start daydreaming while training. Five cycles per second theta has been found to be associated with memory functions. According to Thatcher (personal communication), high amplitude focal theta may be associated with damage to the cortex. Theta spikes are common when individuals blink. This can be a problem for eyes-open training, especially in front of the motor strip.

Diagram 20:Rhythmic Theta

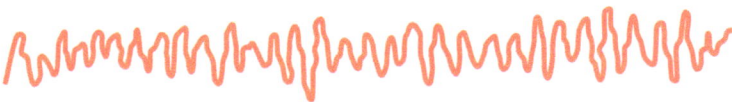

Diagram 21: Non-Rhythmic Theta

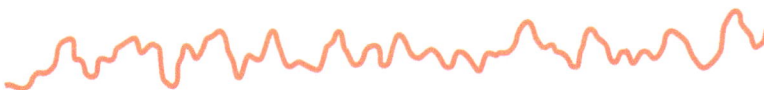

Diagram 22: Normal Alpha Wave shows the smooth-flowing EEG pattern of the alpha wave. It resides generally in a frequency band between 7.5 and 12.5 cycles per second (or 8–12 Hz). Alpha may go as low as 3 cycles per second according to Frank Duffy (1989). Recent research by Hughes and Crunelli (2005) supports this position as well. Many medically trained professionals consider the alpha spectrum to go as high as 14 cycles per second. When 14 Hz alpha occurs over the motor strip, it becomes SMR. This sample waxes and wanes in what looks slightly like spindles. This is common in alpha. Alpha represents the brain in a resting or neutral state, yet it is prepared for action. It is often referred to as the idling frequency.

Diagram 22: Normal Alpha Wave

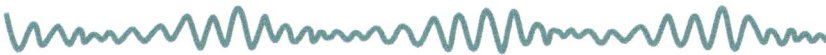

The low-amplitude rapidly fluctuating sample (see Diagram 23: Typical Spindling Beta Wave), shows the beta wave. It is sometimes called desynchronized EEG. It is frequently considered any frequency above alpha and indicates cortical processing. We see beta occur when people problem-solve or think carefully about a topic. When individuals worry constantly, it appears in higher amplitudes. It takes the brain a great deal of energy to produce these higher frequencies, so they tend to always be lower in amplitude than the lower frequencies. Their amplitude is also attenuated more than lower frequencies as they pass through the skull and scalp. According to Marvin Sams (personal communication), real beta occurs in spindles. If it does not, then it is artifact. Continuous sinusoidal beta that is focal may indicate a lack of inhibitory control over an area.

Diagram 23: Typical Spinding Beta Wave

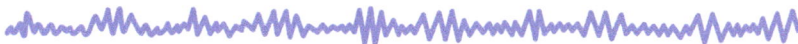

Finally, there is a sample of abnormal waveforms known as sharp waves and spikes (see Diagram 24: Sharpe Waves and Spikes). These waves may often be associated with seizure activity. They are both usually very high in amplitude and fairly random in their occurrence. The spike is very narrow, whereas sharp waves tend to be a little wider.

Diagram 24: Sharp Waves and Spikes

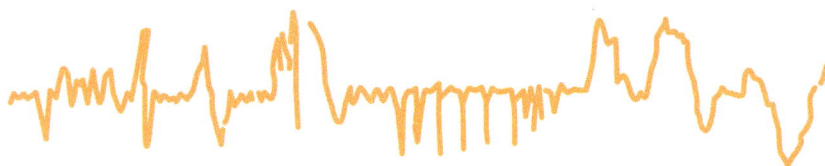

This section has been a brief review of what is frequently referred to as morphology of waveforms. Amplitudes and frequency are considered in the spectral analysis often focused on in neurofeedback, but morphology is often overlooked. Important clues can come from the EEG wave shapes themselves regarding organic problems. At the same time, clinicians must keep in mind scope of practice when considering morphology and take care with regard to expressing any medically related opinions resulting from their engagement with this aspect of EEG assessment. For those interested in more detail on the topic of morphology, Tiff Thompson of Neurofield provides regular and valuable workshops on morphology.

Nonlinear Dynamics and EEG

As noted above, it is clear that the brain maintains a careful balance between seizure and coma. Most of its activity is inhibitory in nature. A contained maelstrom delicately balanced would be a good description. Seizures often appear like thunderstorms or spreading wildfires in the brain. The brain appears to maintain its balance between hypo- and hypercoupling by constantly returning to a balanced state centered around 10 Hz while performing waking activity (also known as Berger rhythm). This center is so robust that healthy individuals never deviate from a mean resting alpha of 10 Hz by more than .5 Hz on average (Neidermeyer & Lopes de Silva, 2006). The standard deviation from the mean of 10 Hz is, therefore, .5 Hz. This is a very tight range. Sterman's research with pilots reveals that too much average time outside this range exhausts individuals. Their task performance level degrades quickly. For instance, individuals suffering from thyroid and liver conditions often have an average alpha frequency of around 7 Hz or 8 Hz. These individuals are usually fairly depressed and can barely perform. It is clear that their neurotransmitter systems are severely depleted, possibly from too long a period in hypocoupled states of anxiety.

Theories of nonlinear dynamics state that complex systems move through iterations or cycles, which are so complex that their patterns are very difficult to determine. They appear to be almost random, yet a high level of order is maintained over long periods of time. These systems usually have at least one center of focus or balance, or attractor state, through which they maintain continuity and reference. Whirlpools in a stream are a good example. Although there are complex current flows, the whirlpool remains fairly stable in configuration and location. By using this model for EEG activity, it is easy to draw a correlation between 10 Hz alpha and the attractor state postulated in nonlinear dynamics theory. It has been proposed that this attractor state reflects the health of the entire system and that dysregulation leads to more average time away from this standing attractor state in the brain. This theory is somewhat supported by Sterman's research and the work of David McCormick (1999), Hughes and Crunelli (2005), Silberstein (Nunez, 1995), and other clinical observations.

Ron Ruden (1997) also proposes that the brain, as a consequence of stress and trauma, actually grows networks that lead to progressively more dysregulation and greater deviance from the existing attractor state. This dysregulation generates greater noise in the system and consequently more dysfunctional behavior. This generates a shift in the attractor state that Ruden calls neohomeostasis. Neohomeostasis, therefore, reflects an actual physical growth of dendrites, which generates an organic abnormality in the brain with respect to its intended pattern of development. New neural networks contributing to such a new configuration may involve closed loops that protect the neohomeostasis and may be reflected in obsessional rumination patterns and delusional thinking. Recent articles by David McCormick (1999) also suggest that dysrhythmias causing shifts in the normal functioning of thalamocortical loops lead to disorder. In addition, the work of Joseph LeDoux (1996) indicates that old networks never die, but that new inhibitory networks need to be grown to alter and manage these "networks of trauma."

Hemispheric Dominance and EEG

Past research shows that there are normative patterns of bilateral amplitude (Bruder et al., 1997; Davidson, 1995; Forbes et al., 2008; Fox, 1991:1994; Gold et al., 2012; Heller & Nitschke, 1998). An amplitude or frequency asymmetry can have significance. Alpha tends to be highest in the right hemisphere while beta tends to dominate in the left. It is unclear what role theta plays in this picture, but having a roughly equivalent theta in both hemispheres appears to be the favored position at present. Lubar (1991) has observed that individuals with high theta do show differences in behavior and disorderly features. Too much theta on the left tends to result in lack of organization, while too much theta on the right results in impulsivity. According to the research of Richard Davidson (2000), the left hemisphere appears to be related to approach behaviors and the right hemisphere to avoidant behaviors. Too little alpha in the right hemisphere correlates with negative behaviors associated with patterns of social withdrawal. Individuals with depression appear to have this pattern. Too much beta on the right is highly correlated with mania as well. In the last decade, research has continued to support this perspective.

There is also a pattern of EEG from front to back. Fast waves in the beta frequencies tend to be higher in amplitude with respect to slow waves in the front of the brain than in the back while slow waves, like alpha and theta, tend to be higher in amplitude with respect to fast waves in the back than the front. Most of the databases indicate an EEG spectral pattern similar to that found at Cz, except the spectrum shifts toward the fast waves going frontally and toward the slow waves going occipitally. Consequently, theta is still highest at Pz. Individuals with ADHD tend to have too much theta in the front. Depression tends to appear as too much alpha frontally.

When individuals have more than one disorder, the brain may have asymmetries left to right and front to back, resulting in the appearance of four quadrants of asymmetry, as shown in the NxLink QEEG map segments displayed in Diagram 25: Asymmetries.

Each globe represents the head as seen if you are looking down from above. The top of each globe is the front of the head and the bottom is the back, so in cognitive disabilities (learning disability, LD), excessive high amplitude delta is higher in the back than in the front. With ADHD, excess theta is higher in the front and tapers into normal range moving toward the back. Depression appears as high amplitude alpha in the center or the front. Anxiety can appear as excess beta in the front or the back (see Diagram 25: Pre/Post Rolandic Asymmetries).

Diagram 25: Pre/Post Rolandic Asymmetries

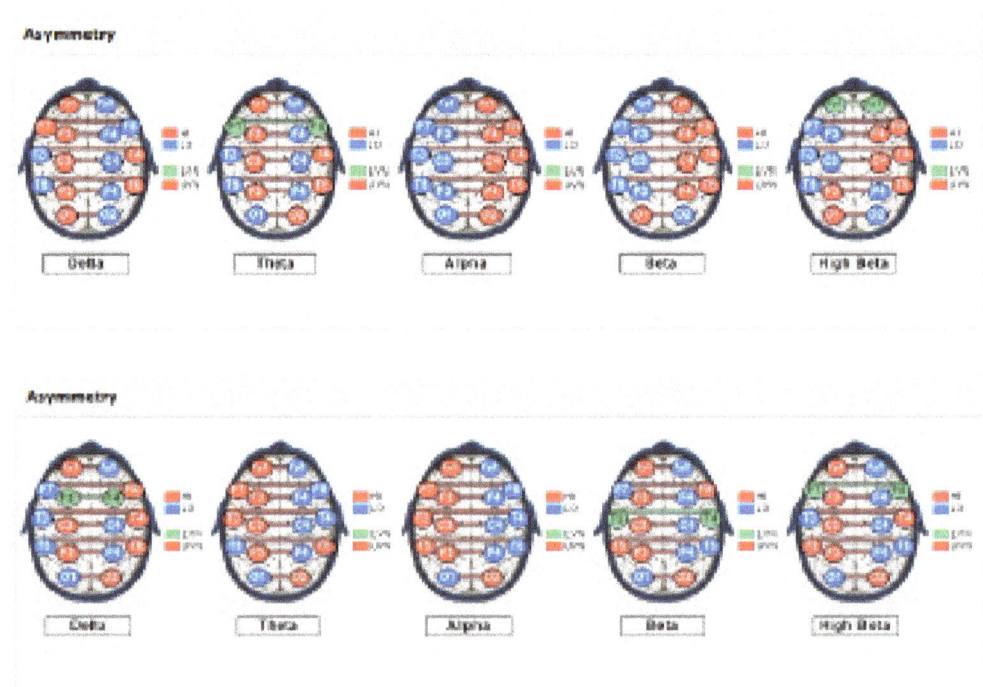

88

Additional Points to Note:

- Two-instrument artifact is a condition where two different devices, such as EDR and EEG, are used in the same location. When the electrodes are too close, the result is electrical contamination that distorts the signals being detected by both devices.

- Optical isolation is used in some equipment to enhance safety and reduce artifact. Typically, the signal is processed through a pre-amplifier, converted into light, and sent through a fiber optic cable that uses a short optical path to transfer the signal to the main amplifier while keeping it electrically isolated. Since the electrical signal is converted to a light beam, transferred, then converted back to an electrical signal, there is no need for electrical connection between the source and destination circuits.

- EEG alpha asymmetry refers to the observation that alpha is typically higher in magnitude in the right hemisphere than in the left. This is usually an enduring condition that indicates an individual with a stable and positive affect, but nevertheless can reverse itself when such an individual experiences a temporary negative mood. Individuals who chronically experience negative moods usually demonstrate alpha higher in the left hemisphere than in the right.

- REM sleep characterized by sudden eye movement and EMG.

Diagram 26: Pre/Post Rolandic Asymmetries

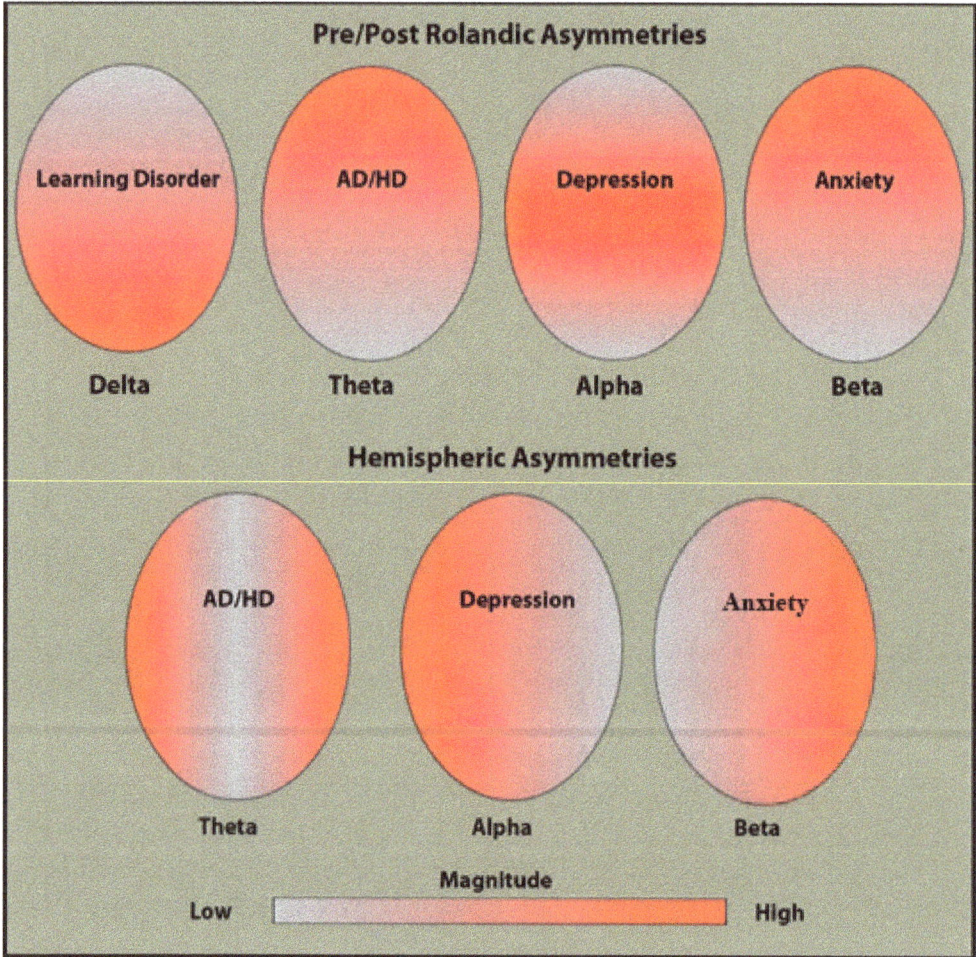

Pre/Post Rolandic Asymmetries

Learning Disorder — Delta
AD/HD — Theta
Depression — Alpha
Anxiety — Beta

Hemispheric Asymmetries

AD/HD — Theta
Depression — Alpha
Anxiety — Beta

Magnitude
Low — High

REVIEW QUESTIONS

1. What is the Berger rhythm?

2. Brodmann is best known for the development of what system?

3. What system is used for electrode placement?

4. What are examples of traditional electrode placement cites using the 10-20 International System?

5. What is an action potential?

6. Can EEG invalidate MRI?

7. Do PET and functional MRI provide better space and resolution than EEG and MEG?

8. What produces EEG alpha asymmetry?

9. What constitutes REM sleep?

10. What is neurometrics?

CHAPTER 4: ELECTROPHYSIOLOGY OF DISORDERS & QEEG ASSESSMENT

Paradigms of QEEG

Since the last addition was published much has changed in the field of neuroimaging and it has broad implications for QEEG. This has resulted in a significant re-evaluation of theories related to QEEG from our perspective.

Up to this time there has been an effort by most in the field of neurofeedback to identify QEEG patterns that correlate with categories of disorder based on the diagnostic manual. The first examples were presented by E. Roy John (John, 1989) showing typical patterns he was finding in anxiety and depression as well as schizophrenia. There was considerable excitement and hope that each disorder would have a unique map pattern. Unfortunately, when he and Robert Thatcher looked at map patterns of schizophrenics they found five sub-types instead of one standard pattern (John, 1990). Alper et al. (1998) uncovered two patterns for OCD. Things went from bad to worse as Chabot (1996) found 11 subtypes of ADHD and possibly more. This has continued to be the case for most disorders in the DSM. The New York Medical University Database developed by John and first marketed as NxLink in 1996 (now Brain Dx) has a discriminant that attempts to identify various disorders based on map pattern but falls short in actual clinical application. Most of the medical and psychiatric staff at various hospitals and clinics where I attempted to deploy it requested I discontinue using it as it was incorrect in most cases and caused confusion in documenting client history. In recent times the reason has become more clear. The diagnostic categories themselves have serious if not fatal flaws (Nemeroff & Weinberger, 2013) and NIH is showing little interest in funding research using these categories. The neuroimaging community has abandoned them almost entirely (Kudlow, 2013). We are chasing ghosts of an era now giving way to more modern technological discoveries.

Early in the field the dominant emerging general model of disorders from a neurofeedback or EEG perspective was probably first proposed by Siegfried Othmer (Evans & Abarbanel, 1999). It was a more systems based model in that it saw the various disorders as a consequence arousal dysregulation that could be corrected by neurofeedback. There was support for this perspective based on correlations between electrophysiology and neurotransmitter activity as reported in the literature and expanded upon in Nunez's book in a chapter by Silberstein (Nunez, 1995). In this model excess dopamine and noradrenaline, with reduced GABA, was associated excess fast wave and reductions in dopamine and norepinephrine resulted in excess slow wave activity. Consequently symptoms emerge when the brain is operating too fast or too slow.

Diagram 27: Brain Too Fast and Brain Too Slow

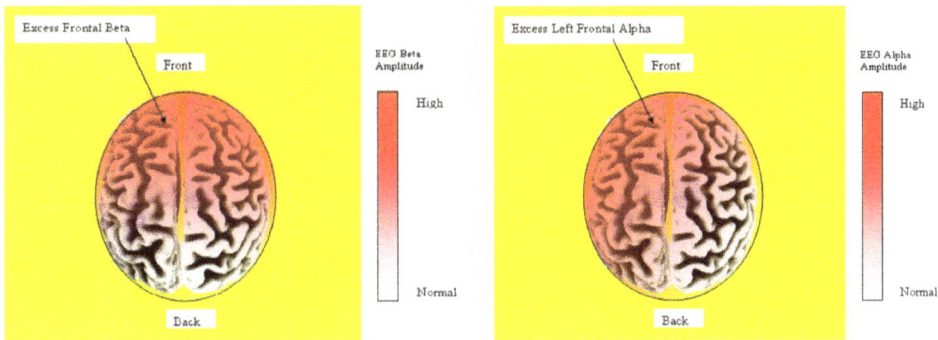

Excess Frontal Beta

Front

EEG Beta Amplitude

High

Normal

Back

Excess Left Frontal Alpha

Front

EEG Alpha Amplitude

High

Normal

Back

Consequently, disorders are placed tentatively along a spectrum in a pattern that appears to be in agreement from clinical observation. Anxiety disorders, mania, and OCD show up as excessive frontal fast-wave activity while depression, ADHD, and Tourette's syndrome are associated with excessive frontal slow-wave activity. The specific features of these disorders will be discussed in a later section but Diagram 28: A Spectrum Model of Mental Dosorders by Brain Function.

Parallel to this perspective is the emerging understanding that inflammation plays a major role in the brainwave patterns we are seeing in QEEG. The blood brain barrier is more vulnerable than previously assumed and subject to infiltration due to a wide variety inflammatory processes including any sub-concussive event (Wu et al., 2013). The neuro-inflammatory process can also be initiated by the impact of Toxic Stress on both the brain and the internal organs (Alkadhi, 2013; Enciu et al., 2013). The resulting loss of normal healthy sleep patterns can multiply and accelerate these factors (Walker, 2017). This accelerates the natural oxidative stress that occurs in the brain resulting in initial excess fast wave activity and excitotoxicity followed by a gradual loss of energy, decreasing beta activity and increasing slow wave activity (Soutar et al., 2017).

Brain Too Fast: The red shaded area on the left shows the front of the brain as being overactive and producing too much beta (See Diagram 27: Brain Too Fast and Brain Too Slow). More recent research shows excessive left frontal beta as being associated with anticipatory anxiety, right frontal beta with panic or reactive anxiety and posterior beta associated with negative rumination (Engles et al., 2007). This activity is also associated with excess glutamate production and a diminished ability of the brain to either clear it or convert it back to glutamine. The result is growing inflammation and neuronal apoptosis (Wang & Michaelis, 2010).

Brain Too Slow: The red shaded area on the right shows the front of the brain as being underactive (especially the left side) and producing too much alpha. (See Diagram 27: Brain Too Fast and Brain Too Slow). We have concluded from our clinical experience that much of the depression we see is end-stage anxiety. Most depressed individuals have experienced elevated levels of anxiety for years and have depleted their neurotransmitter systems by the buildup of glutamate and inflammation (see Chapter 3) to the point where the brain is shutting down to protect itself, hence the high-amplitude, low-frequency alpha. This is congruent with the research on learned helplessness and agrees with the research of Joseph LeDoux on the effects of anxiety on the brain (LeDoux, 2015). More recent research reveals that excessive excitotoxicity resulting from chronic overarousal combined with poor sleep triggers a proinflammatory response in the brain to building glutamate levels. This reduces mitochondrial output and depletes energy resources for generating beta frequencies with the outcome of a growing alpha predominance (Belanger et al., 2011; Lin & Beal, 2006).

Many neurotherapists these days tend to treat symptomology or EEG features rather than DSM categories because the categories do not always correlate with EEG features. Gunkelman and Johnstone (Johnstone et al., 2006) urged practitioners to look beyond the standard DSM categories and look at the electrophysiology of disorders in terms of phenotypes. An even more sophisticate approach may be to treat sources of symptoms or the system as a whole as in Functional Medicine. As previously mentioned, we often find that there are several EEG subtypes for each category of behavioral disorder. Behavioral typologies and EEG do not always agree. For instance, an individual may score very high on the Beck Depression Inventory and have either excessively high-amplitude, low frequency alpha 8–9 Hz or excessively high-amplitude, high-frequency alpha 11–14 Hz (anxiety, exhaustion, moving toward entrenched depression). The most effective protocol may be different for different individuals, even though each individual may have depression. Our earlier model of the spectrum of disorders breaks down as shown in Diagram 28: A Spectrum Model of Mental Disorders by Brain Function.

Another more recent approach to interpreting QEEG, which several hundred clinics have adopted, is to view what is going on in the brain as a continuous process of energy loss due to oxidative stress and its impact on mitochondrial ATP production. The brain requires far more energy to produce beta for higher cognitive processing functions than for alpha, theta or delta. As energy production decreases, higher frequencies are lost and we see slower frequencies progressively dominating. From this perspective we can categorize symptomology based on physiological entropy and the resulting functional losses at different stages of reduced energy output. Those interested in the details of this theoretical approach should see the article Correlating Oxidative Stress and QEEG (Soutar, 2017).

TRAUMA AND ITS IMPACT ON THE BRAIN

Reviewing all the available literature on QEEG is beyond the scope of this book. However, there are some basic principles and scientific findings that we would like to review to make the use and comprehension of QEEG more practical from a clinical perspective.

The brain is often negatively impacted when a person is traumatized. Trauma can result from a variety of experiences, which include, but are not limited to the following:

- actual physical injury to the head or traumatic brain injury (TBI)
- neglect, physical abuse, sexual abuse
- exposure to traumatic events such as the death of a sibling or parent, the killing of a family pet or farm animal, natural disasters, life-threatening experiences, and others

Teicher, M. (2007) notes that abuse during childhood, particularly childhood sexual abuse, is a risk factor for development of impulse control disorders, and can lead to a cycle of violence and perpetration. Early stress can exert enduring effects on brain development that may underlie many of the consequences of sexual abuse. Research also shows the negative effects of childhood sexual abuse on development of the hippocampus, corpus callosum, prefrontal cortex, and visual cortex (Anderson et al., 2008). This abuse further leads to the potential for lifelong physical health problems (Anda & Felitti, 2018).

Diagram 28: A Spectrum Model of Mental Disorders by Brain Function

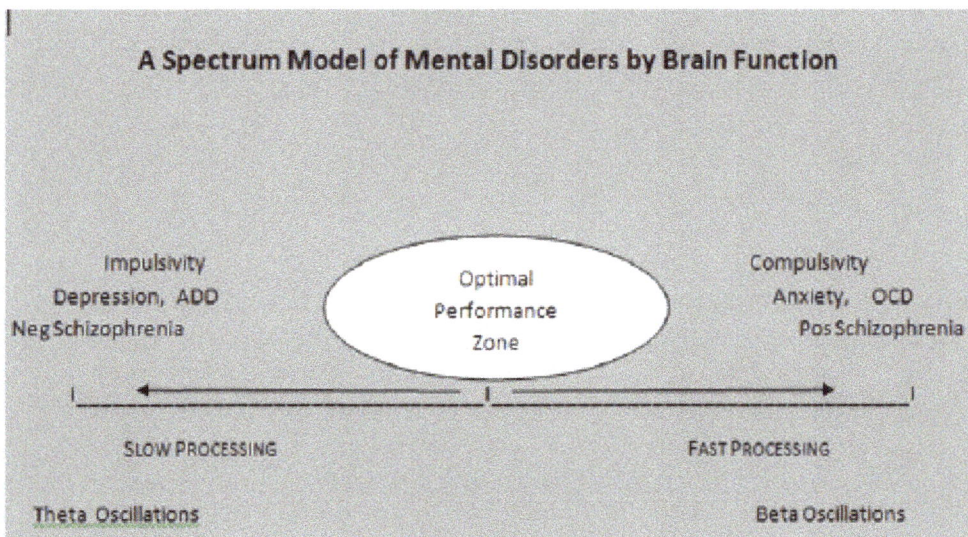

A Spectrum Model of Mental Disorders by Brain Function

Impulsivity
Depression, ADD
Neg Schizophrenia

Optimal
Performance
Zone

Compulsivity
Anxiety, OCD
Pos Schizophrenia

SLOW PROCESSING

FAST PROCESSING

Theta Oscillations

Beta Oscillations

The Training & Research Institute, Inc. (2004) in Albuquerque, New Mexico, notes that childhood physical, emotional, and sexual abuse and neglect can cause antisocial behavior by overexcitation of the limbic system, the primitive midbrain region that regulates memory and emotion, and the prefrontal cortex, which is associated with judgment, consequential thinking, and moral reasoning. They note the following seven points:

1) The left hemisphere is responsible for regulation and oversight of logical responses to a situation and control and mediation of emotional responses generated by the right hemisphere.

   The impact of childhood abuse or neglect results in diminished control of emotional response, resulting in poor or inappropriate reactions to emotional situations, angry outbursts, self-destructive or suicidal impulses, paranoia, psychosis, and a tendency to pursue intense ultimately unstable relationships.

2) The prefrontal cortex is the internal editor of emotional states, consequential thinking, moral reasoning, and reactions to emotional crisis.

   The impact of childhood abuse or neglect results in increased potential for depression and delinquent and criminal behavior.

3) The corpus collosum creates communication between the right and left hemispheres.

   The impact of childhood abuse or neglect results in a significantly smaller corpus collosum, causing nonintegrated, inappropriate responses to everyday situations. (The larger the corpus collosum, the more one is in contact with one's emotions.)

4) The temporal lobes regulate emotions and verbal memory.

   The impact of childhood abuse or neglect results in poor modulation of emotions, and an increased chance for temporal lobe epilepsy.

5) The hippocampus (part of the limbic system) is responsible for the formulation and retrieval of verbal and emotional memories.

   The impact of childhood abuse or neglect results in lower performance on verbal memory tests, possible continued emotional and memory problems, and concerns during the adult years.

6) The amygdala (also part of the limbic system) creates emotional content for

memories, mediating depression, irritability, and hostility/aggression, and governing reaction and responses to fear. The amygdala can be considered as the "watchdog" of the brain.

> *The impact of childhood abuse or neglect results in a significantly smaller amygdala, raising the risk for depression, irritability and hostility/aggression; and is also responsible for incorrect emotional "memories," absence of fear conditioning, and an increased chance of psychopathic tendencies.*

7) The purpose of the cerebellar vermis is to modulate production and release of neurotransmitters. The cerebellar vermis has a significant number of receptor sites for stress-related hormones.

> *The impact of childhood abuse or neglect results in an increase in potential risk for psychiatric symptoms such as depression, psychosis, hyperactivity, and attention deficits, and in rare cases, psychotic symptoms are possible.*

EEG PROFILES OF VARIOUS DISORDERS AND ASSOCIATED PHYSIOLOGY

Below are some basic explanations of EEG and disorders based upon overall brain functioning. A more detailed list of disorders and their association to QEEG appears towards the end of this chapter. Keep in mind that QEEG appears to correlate more with disorders that have strong physiological correlates such as anxiety, depression, OCD, Bipolar Disorder, etc., likely for the reasons cited above.

BRAIN TOO FAST

See Diagram 27: Brain Too Fast and Brain Too Slow.

Anxiety

Usually, excessive fast waves (beta) occur frontally and spread globally as anxiety levels increase. This pattern is usually interpreted as excessive frontal processing activity, especially worry as noted in the research by LeDoux (1996; 2015) and indicates that the cortex typically speeds up mental activity to suppress amygdalic over-arousal, perhaps blocking medial forebrain bundle circuits. Frequently, this pattern may appear as reduced slow-wave amplitudes rather than elevated beta.

Beta dominance in anxiety usually has more beta in the right hemisphere than in the left, indicating an effort by the brain to increase the right frontal area to inhibit limbic activity (Gold et al., 2012; Soutar, 2018).

Research indicates that the right amygdala and right frontal region is most sensitive to negative stimuli and plays a key role in emotional processing (Le Doux, 2015). Theta is also frequently low in amplitude when anxiety is present. Higher amplitudes in right frontal beta are often indicative of growing panic while posterior beta is associated with rumination (Engles et al., 2007). In general, the frontal beta is usually indicative of worry. Posterior beta is indicative of rumination. Globally elevated beta is suggestive of trauma or PTSD, as beta blocks input from the limbic system (input from the limbic system shows up in theta). When we see increases in beta, alpha usually drops out because of the classic EEG desynchronization as fewer networks are in idling mode. Anxiety, ironically, often creates attentional problems and from a symptomology standpoint looks like ADD and ADHD (Solomon et al., 2014). Consequently many anxious children get misdiagnosed as having ADD and the receive methylphenidate medication which can make their anxiety symptoms worse when it wears off.

Daniel Amen is a renowned clinician and author who specializes in SPECT scans for diagnostic purposes. He believes (Amen, 1998) a connection between basal ganglia activity and anxiety exists. Since the dopamine circuit plays a central role in basal ganglia activity, and appears elevated in conditions where the brain is running too fast, there seems to be a connection between an overactive attentional network and high dopamine levels.

The basal ganglia have strong efferent connections with the premotor strip through the ventral anterior thalamus. The basal ganglia also connect up to the cingulate and associational networks through the intralaminar nuclei. These same nuclei receive efferents (axonal fibers) from the motor strip and feed information in a loop back to the basal ganglia. The 10-20 locations of Cz and Pz seem to be important areas of possible influence on the attentional system and the dopamine system. Adjustments to this system may be driving the rest of the cortical system, especially in terms of neuromodulator activity.

Fibromyalgia

Fibromyalgia looks very similar to anxiety except beta amplitudes increase toward the rear and alpha amplitudes increase toward the front (Mueller et al., 2001). This phenomenon is often called "the backwards brain." This pattern also shows up in chronic fatigue and other physiological disorders. LORETA maps show this activity to be in the posterior cingulate. Standardized low-resolution brain electromagnetic tomography (sLORETA) is a QEEG method of analyzing the EEG and determining the exact source within the cortex of any group of frequencies (Pascual-Marqui, 2002).

OCD

A meta-analysis of the literature indicates that the only basic distinction reflected by OCD brains is a bilateral difference in hemispheric speed, although presentations by Leslie Prichep, PhD of NYU include discussions of a common high beta background (Hanson et al., 2003). There appear to be alpha and theta subtypes of OCD, with the alpha subtype being less responsive to existing medications. Many clinicians report excessive fast-wave activity around Fz and interpret it as an overactive cingulate. The cingulate has been implicated as central in the attentional network with regard to discriminating internal from external stimuli. Gunkelman (Johnstone et al., 2003) have identified a phenotype of OCD manifesting as frontal beta spindles. The discriminator theory of consciousness and LeDoux's (2015) short-term memory and consciousness theories come into play here. The cingulate may be getting stuck and locking on networks that are rigidly and repetitively engaging and processing internal stimuli that are threatening due to excess dopamine activity in the basal ganglia (see Chapter 3). The cingulate also connects the frontal and parietal lobes to the parahippocampal gyrus and the temporal lobe. The basal ganglia loop through the intralaminar nuclei may be locking up the whole system in response to overactive inputs from the fear centers in the amygdala.

The question is, where is the best place to intervene in the loop? Fz and Pz seem to be the best candidates from clinical reports. Cz SMR is used successfully by the Othmers (1994, 2008). In addition, research from UCLA by Jeffery Schwartz (2002) indicates the caudate as a key player. He believes he has isolated a worry circuit within the anterior cingulate that fails to appropriately manage internal dialogue related to worry.

The only case where OCD did not appear in the pattern thus far describe showed up as excessive focal alpha in absolute power at Pz. This makes sense, as focal damage to this area often results in perseveration problems. Pz also has direct connections through the lateral dorsal thalamus to the cingulate and the basal ganglia have efferents running through the interlaminar nuclei to Pz connecting motor functions with associative functions. Sherlin and Congedo (2005) have done research indicating that OCD can appear as deviant beta activity anywhere along the cingulate.

Hammond (2003) trained two cases of OCD with a complex series of protocols that resulted in improved symptoms based on MMPI and Y-BOCS.

Surmeli & Ertem (2011) trained 36 subjects with QEEG guided NFB and found 33 improved based on post testing using Yale-Brown obsessive-compulsive scale (Y-BOCS) and the MMPI. Follow up 26 months later showed 19 subjects had maintained their improvements.

BRAIN TOO SLOW

See Diagram 27: Brain Too Fast and Brain Too Slow.

Depression

Depression is the beginning of the slowing of the brain reflecting reduced energy and inflammatory processes. It is a state involving progressive levels of withdrawal behaviors, consequently we refer to it as an inhibited state. By viewing the alpha and beta symmetry you can determine how entrenched the depression has become and whether the client is also shifting back and for the between anxiety and depression states. Depression initially appears as growing alpha asymmetry with high-amplitude alpha frontally and centrally in the eyes open map which then appears more regularly in the eyes closed map. More specifically, alpha dominance in depression is in the left hemisphere. The alpha is often lower in the normal frequency ranges and progressively dips into the 8-9.5 range Hz range but may also drop down as low as 7 Hz when thyroid issues are present. The lower frequency may indicate how old and entrenched the depression is. On some equipment, depending on filter settings, this may look like high theta. Alpha is the doorway between the limbic system and the cortex. When alpha is low, the door is usually closed. It is easy to confuse depression with head injury and ADD and the alpha asymmetry helps make the distinction more clear. Recent research is indicating that TBI often precipitates depression as it deeply impacts the endocrine system.

Depression is highly co-morbid with ADD (20-50%) as is anxiety (47%) as well (McIntosh et al., 2009). Margaret Ayers (personal communication) originally argued that most ADD is really associated with anoxia, stroke, birth trauma, or head injury, which makes sense from an EEG morphological perspective. Beta may still be dominant in the right hemisphere in depression, locking the depression in place with the older anxiety that generated it. The ISI will show both anxiety and depression symptoms high in these cases. To help distinguish between ADD and the contribution of depression to inattention, we use the TOVA or the NewMind Attention CPT and the Beck Depression Inventory or the NewMind ISI. Slowing in the frontal lobes is classic ADHD. Often we see elevated delta and theta in the frontal areas (however, elevated delta in the frontal areas can be indicative of TBI or heavy metal toxicity as well).

Atypical Depression

At this point, it is important to discuss atypical depression or depression with anxiety. From our perspective, all depression begins with anxiety (unless it is a result of physical trauma or chemicals). As we have said, as the anxiety matures, the beta amplitude increases on the right and depletes neurotransmitter systems and generates inflammation as the brain slows. As it slows, alpha amplitude increases and moves to the left, shutting down executive function. This process reduces the desire to interact with others protects the brain from further social interactions that might stimulate further fear and anxiety.

During this transitional phase, the symptoms of depression appear with the pre-existing anxiety. As the depression matures, the alpha increases in amplitude and slows in frequency, reducing processing. Statistical analysis of our database indicates that depression symptoms actually begin to manifest when the right hemisphere is about 80% beta dominant with respect to the left hemisphere (Soutar, 2018). The beta on the right blocks the process from reversing at a certain point and depression becomes profound. Eventually the beta migrates back to the left hemisphere to compensate for the high levels of left hemisphere alpha. This is why increasing beta on the left helps unblock chronic depression, although increasing alpha to the right in the atypical depression is often better.

The original research done on this model was done by Richard Davidson (2000). Peter Rosenfeld worked with Elsa Baehr (1997) on research showing that training to correct asymmetry can reduce symptoms of depression. Baehr went on to work with Tom Collura to develop a simplified version of this protocol involving increasing alpha on the right while inhibiting it on the left using powerful inhibits. Choi et al. (2009) later demonstrated with a control group design that training alpha asymmetry reduced symptoms of depression as well. Research in this area continues to reveal the efficacy of this approach to neurofeedback. This and other basic protocols are outlined in Chapter 6.

SPECTRAL ANALYSIS

Spectral analysis graphs are available on most EEG equipment systems (see Diagram 29: Spectral Analysis). They have become very sophisticated and often provide real-time analysis. Using spectral analysis for reviewing the changes in EEG amplitudes over time and in relation to different tasks can be very useful. Lubar (1991, 1999) notes that individuals with ADD have an increase in slow-wave (2–8 Hz) activity when intentionally processing information such as reading and math. Correlating changes reflected in the spectral analysis graph with activities recorded at the same time can reveal hidden dynamics and confirm diagnoses or indicate progress in training.

In conjunction with TOVA scores, progress can be thoroughly documented as clients progressively learn to use the correct circuitry to process information. In fact, on-task spectral analysis graphs probably can provide far more than baseline measures. Presently, QEEGs may include clients engaging in reading and math exercises in order to identify attentional and processing problems by seeing how these exercises alter the EEG. Unfortunately, this kind of analysis may be time consuming and difficult to employ in a clinical setting.

Diagram 29: QEEG Brain Map (NewMind Technologies)

Brain Map Date: 10/9/2020

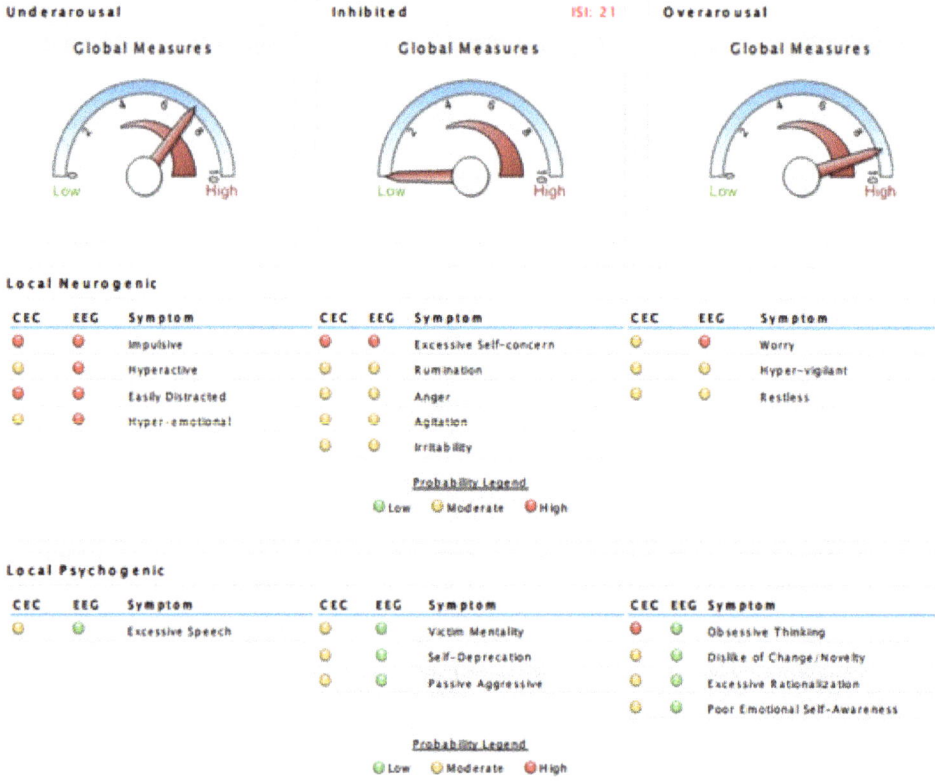

Underarousal   Inhibited   ISI: 21   Overarousal

Global Measures   Global Measures   Global Measures

Low   High   Low   High   Low   High

Local Neurogenic

CEC	EEG	Symptom		CEC	EEG	Symptom		CEC	EEG	Symptom
●	●	Impulsive		●	●	Excessive Self-concern		○	●	Worry
○	●	Hyperactive		○	○	Rumination		○	○	Hyper-vigilant
●	●	Easily Distracted		○	○	Anger		○	○	Restless
○	●	Hyper-emotional		○	○	Agitation				
				○	○	Irritability				

Probability Legend

● Low   ○ Moderate   ● High

Local Psychogenic

CEC	EEG	Symptom		CEC	EEG	Symptom		CEC	EEG	Symptom
○	●	Excessive Speech		○	○	Victim Mentality		●	○	Obsessive Thinking
				○	○	Self-Deprecation		○	○	Dislike of Change/Novelty
				○	○	Passive Aggressive		○	○	Excessive Rationalization
								○	○	Poor Emotional Self-Awareness

Probability Legend

● Low   ○ Moderate   ● High

Doing Neurofeedback: An Introduction

Brain Map Date: 10/9/2020

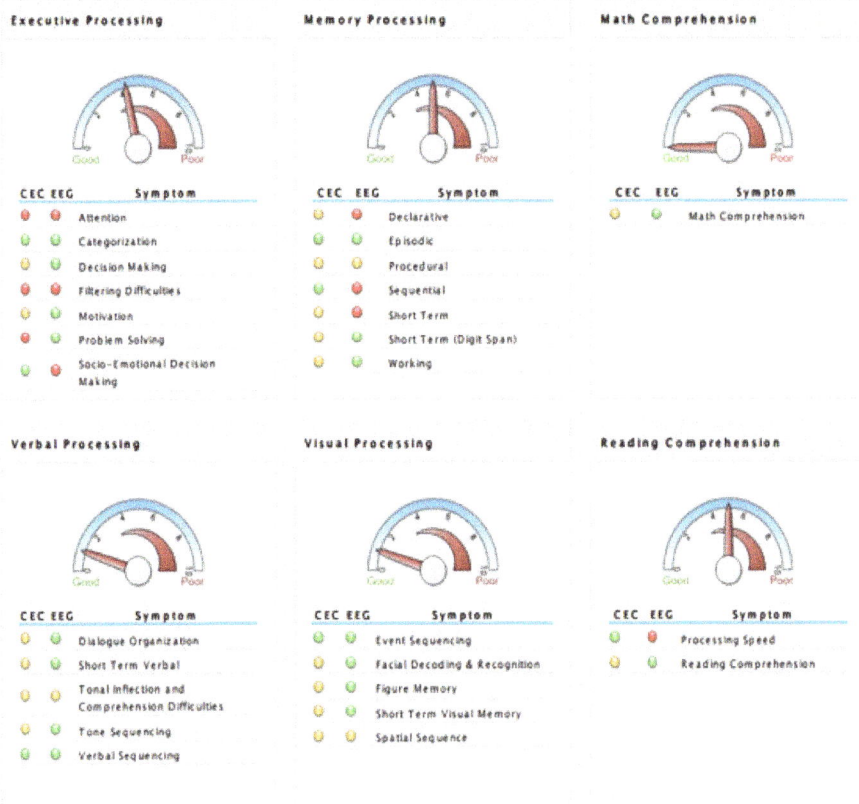

Executive Processing

CEC	EEG	Symptom
●	●	Attention
●	●	Categorization
●	●	Decision Making
●	●	Filtering Difficulties
●	●	Motivation
●	●	Problem Solving
●	●	Socio-Emotional Decision Making

Memory Processing

CEC	EEG	Symptom
●	●	Declarative
●	●	Episodic
●	●	Procedural
●	●	Sequential
●	●	Short Term
●	●	Short Term (Digit Span)
●	●	Working

Math Comprehension

CEC	EEG	Symptom
●	●	Math Comprehension

Verbal Processing

CEC	EEG	Symptom
●	●	Dialogue Organization
●	●	Short Term Verbal
●	●	Tonal Inflection and Comprehension Difficulties
●	●	Tone Sequencing
●	●	Verbal Sequencing

Visual Processing

CEC	EEG	Symptom
●	●	Event Sequencing
●	●	Facial Decoding & Recognition
●	●	Figure Memory
●	●	Short Term Visual Memory
●	●	Spatial Sequence

Reading Comprehension

CEC	EEG	Symptom
●	●	Processing Speed
●	●	Reading Comprehension

Eyes Closed Midline Analysis

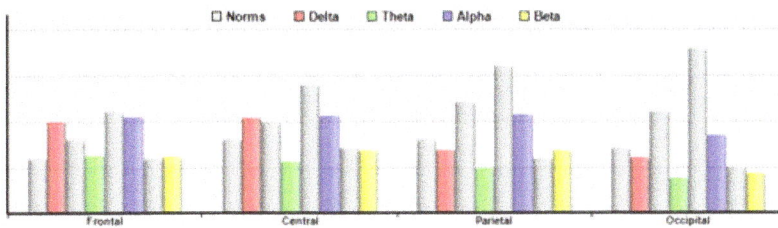

Norms ☐ Delta ■ Theta ☐ Alpha ■ Beta ☐

Frontal   Central   Parietal   Occipital

Eyes Open Midline Analysis

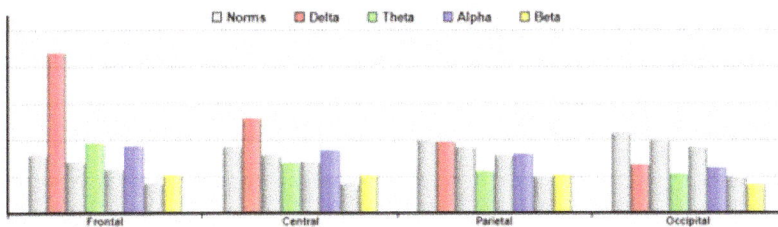

Norms ☐ Delta ■ Theta ☐ Alpha ■ Beta ☐

Frontal   Central   Parietal   Occipital

Soutar & Longo

Brain Map Date: 10/9/2020

Subcomponent Analysis

Lo/Hi Alpha valid only if 'Gamma' filter was set for 8-10hz and 'User' filter was set for 10-12hz when doing map

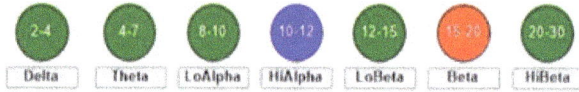

2-4	4-7	8-10	10-12	12-15	15-20	20-30
Delta	Theta	LoAlpha	HiAlpha	LoBeta	Beta	HiBeta

■ = Low   ■ = Ok   ■ = High

Brain Map Date: 10/9/2020

Magnitude

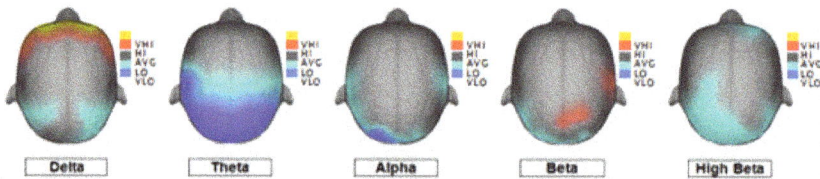

| Delta | Theta | Alpha | Beta | High Beta |

Magnitude Contrast

Down [-2] [-1] [0] [+1] [+2] Up

Dominant Frequency

Overall Dominant Frequency

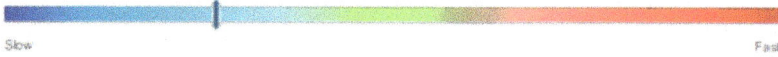

Slow   Fast

Alpha Dominant Frequency

Slow   Fast

Beta Dominant Frequency

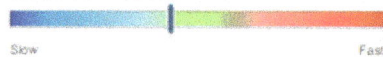

Slow   Fast

⚠ Check Physiology

Inter-Connectivity

Hypo Connectivity

22%

Hypo   Normal

Hyper Connectivity

53%

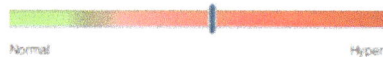

Normal   Hyper

Asymmetry

Normal Alpha Asymmetry

0%

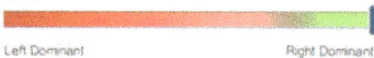

Left Dominant   Right Dominant

Normal Beta Asymmetry

81%

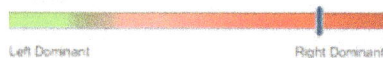

Left Dominant   Right Dominant

104

Brain Map Date: 10/9/2020

Eyes Closed Brain Maps

Magnitude

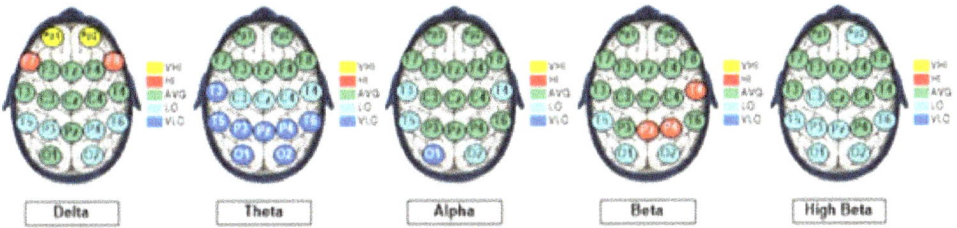

| Delta | Theta | Alpha | Beta | High Beta |

Magnitude Contrast

Down [-2] [-1] [0] [+1] [+2] Up

Dominant Frequency

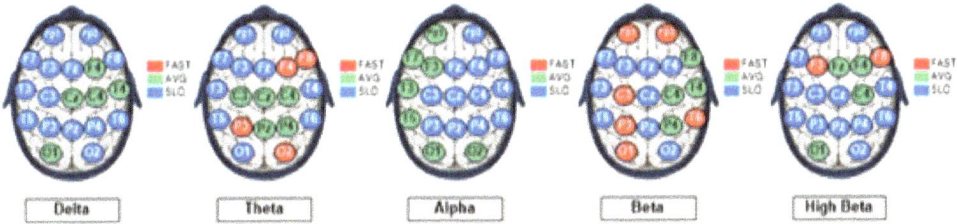

| Delta | Theta | Alpha | Beta | High Beta |

⚠ Check Physiology

Inter-Connectivity

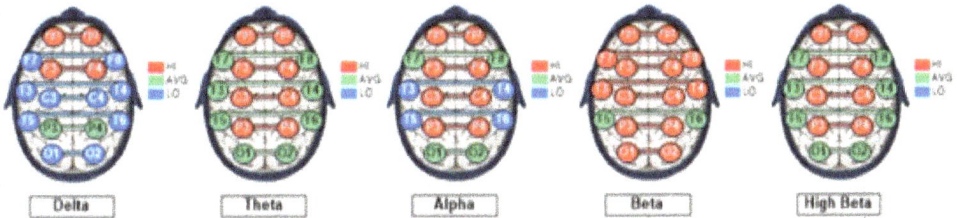

| Delta | Theta | Alpha | Beta | High Beta |

Asymmetry

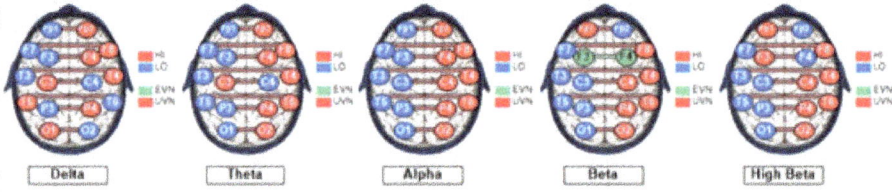

Brain Map Date: 10/9/2020

Magnitude

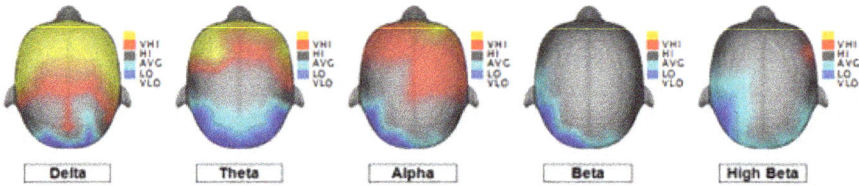

Magnitude Contrast

Down | -2 | -1 | 0 | +1 | +2 | Up

Dominant Frequency

Overall Dominant Frequency

Slow — Fast

Alpha Dominant Frequency

Slow — Fast

Beta Dominant Frequency

Slow — Fast

⚠ Check Physiology

Inter-Connectivity

Hypo Connectivity

19%

Hypo — Normal

Hyper Connectivity

50%

Normal — Hyper

Asymmetry

Normal Alpha Asymmetry

0%

Left Dominant — Right Dominant

Normal Beta Asymmetry

100%

Left Dominant — Right Dominant

Brain Map Date: 10/9/2020

Eyes Open Brain Maps

Magnitude

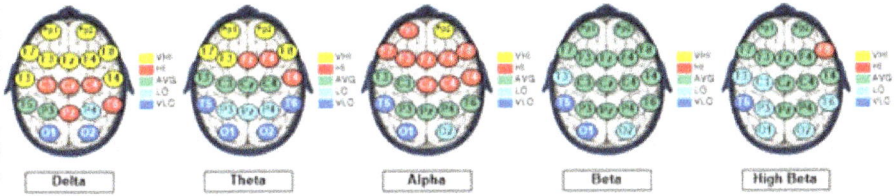

| Delta | Theta | Alpha | Beta | High Beta |

Magnitude Contrast

Down -2 -1 0 +1 +2 Up

Dominant Frequency

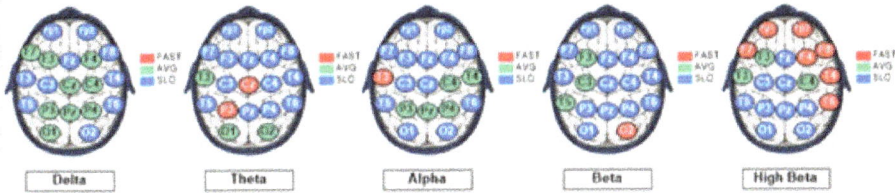

| Delta | Theta | Alpha | Beta | High Beta |

⚠ Check Physiology

Inter-Connectivity

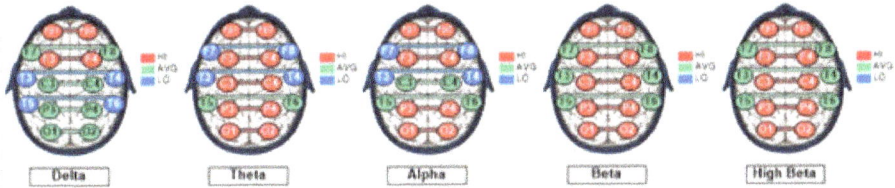

| Delta | Theta | Alpha | Beta | High Beta |

Asymmetry

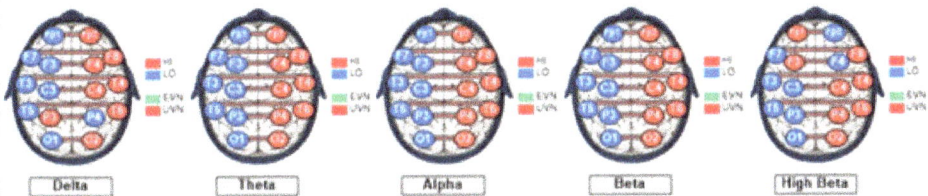

| Delta | Theta | Alpha | Beta | High Beta |

Kirtley Thornton (personal communication), a North Carolina therapist, has spent the last decade developing a clinically-friendly testing procedure involving QEEG and a task-based database to evaluate what he considers the three most critical dimensions of cognitive processing: auditory memory, reading memory, and problem solving. His procedure involves much more than spectral analysis.

Brain Maps and Disorders

Brain maps have become progressively more utilized in diagnosis and training strategies in recent years. Their validity for diagnostic purposes is still hotly debated in the field of neurology, but they have been used for a variety of purposes for many years. One has only to go to PubMed and use the search term QEEG to uncover the thousands of research papers that have used QEEG. However, and as noted earlier in Chapter 3, recent research continues to bring QEEG brain mapping closer to the realm of diagnostic ability.

QEEG brain mapping use in neurofeedback training was hotly debated in the past but today is a common and widespread practice. Since brain mapping is expensive, and not presently covered by all insurance companies, clients may want to initially avoid them but usually become very enthusiastic when they see one and their value is carefully explained. Neurofeedback was initially and successfully done for decades without a brainmap but most practitioners find them very helpful in understanding their clients symptoms and in devising a protocol. As noted above, we strongly encourage their use, especially for clinicians new to the field. The Mini-Q was specifically developed to allow clinicians new to the field to have access to affordable equipment and clinician friendly database report systems but costs have diminished significantly and equipment that can provide a full 19 point map is presently within reach of most practitioners.

Historical Overview of Databases

With few commercially developed databases available, QEEG brain mapping was rarely used in this field before 1996 when the first database was marketed in the form of NxLink. There was also a limited distribution of the Thatcher Lifespan Database through Lexicor, whose NeuroSearch 24 amplifiers pioneered the process. Only 60 NxLink databases were sold worldwide at a cost of around $12,000 each. The NxLink database was at that time the gold standard and it still is considered so by many. Bill Hudspeth was also developing a database system at this time that provided very elegant coherence analysis within 1-Hz bins analysis. Although some differences between the databases existed, there was enough congruence between them to make them useful together. Many were using the Hudspeth system in conjunction with the NxLink system for a more comprehensive analysis.

Around the same time, Barry Sterman and David Kaiser began developing a magnitude database system based on Sterman's work and data from Air Force pilots. It was called the SKIL database. Arguably, this is a Peak performance database, as it measures normal EEG in an elite population of mostly fighter pilots. This database looked primarily at magnitude distribution or average amplitude, and eventually a new dimension of analysis, co-modulation, was added in place of coherence.

Later in the decade, Robert Thatcher began to intensively develop his database system into what is presently the most sophisticated database analysis system available known as Neuroguide. This system provides researchers and clinicians with a huge variety of dimensions for analysis for QEEG. With respect to clinical work in neurofeedback, much of it has limited value. With respect to research, it is a stunning tool that has features for research that have yet to be developed.

The Mini-Q system was co-developed by Richard Soutar and Tom Collura at Brainmaster®. The concept was to provide a data gathering system for entry-level practitioners who could not afford $15,000 to $20,000 for equipment for a cutting-edge technology with limited clinical development and research behind it. The system collected 12 locations of data in homologous pairs in a sequence of 6 one-minute recordings. Brainmaster® provided output data on magnitude, coherence, phase, and other dimensions of analysis, but to date no database system was developed.

Soutar and Demos began developing small reference databases for the Mini-Q concept and began offering them in 2005. Presently, the NewMind Database System, developed by Soutar, evolved into an expert database system that has been cross-validated with the Neuroguide and NxLink databases as well as the SKIL database with respect to normative magnitude (average amplitude) values as well as coherence and phase. Dominant frequency is based on published norms in the EEG literature and asymmetry measures based on a combination of clinical data and the work of Richard Davidson. The clinical data are derived from a decade of subject symptom correlations between QEEG and the Beck Depression Inventory. The database has a discriminant output based on expert rules as well as neurological research and MRI research that matches client symptoms with dysregulated 10-20 locations.. This provides probability levels for a variety of cognitive and emotional problems. In addition, the database system provides output with protocol recommendations based on the published literature and Z-Score location recommendations for Z-Score training. Presently this system provides 19 channel maps with auto-artifacting and automated narrative analysis and report (See Diagram 29: QEEG Brain Map (New Mind Technologies)..

QEEG-guided neurofeedback is likely to be the standard moving forward. Until recently, it has been mistakenly seen primarily as a method for deriving protocols. It has not proven to be the best and only valid method for all neurofeedback cases in a clinical setting. Often the best protocols to be used in any given case may run counter to what appears obvious on a brain map. This is simply because the complexity of brain networks demands extensive analysis with respect to intervention. Although the maps present a complex picture, there may be a simple cause. For instance, sleep deprivation may result in elevated eyes open delta, theta and alpha or simply delta intrusion into the waking EEG. Rather than inhibit delta, theta and alpha in several locations with Z-Score training, it may be more efficient to simply train the client with SMR to improve their sleep quality. Over time and with improve sleep, the elevated component bands will return to more normal levels. In light of examples such as this, it should be apparent that protocols are likely to be developed based on a combination of symptoms, QEEGs, a solid understanding of underlying neurophysiology, and clinical experience. What the QEEG does provide is an invaluable overview of what is going on in the brain and the ability to track changes based on protocol selection. Presently, it is being used in this capacity with other medical and psychological interventions. QEEG provides a roadmap, not the specific directions.

Over the past few years, several groups have formed boards who have developed specialized training programs to become QEEG certified. The class work was recently increased by 12 hours requiring a total of 36 hours of didactic training plus a minimum of 10 contact mentoring hours (see International EEG Certification Board, n.d.). to become QEEG certified. Examples include The International QEEG Certification Board; APED (Applied Psychophysiology Education, n.d.), Stress Therapy Solutions and Stens also offer courses.

For most of us doing neurofeedback today, QEEG is a standard part of the practice and BCIA recognizes this in their Blueprint of Knowledge. Learning QEEG basics is part of learning to become a good neurofeedback practitioner. There are, however, some who feel it should be considered a specialty with boards to oversee testing and certification. This may make sense for those using it as a neurological diagnostic or for medical diagnosis, but it is not employed by neurofeedback practitioners for these purposes. It is our opinion that the present requirements of the BCIA board are sufficient and a QEEG board is an unnecessary redundancy.

QEEG ANALYSIS PROCEDURES

Generally, data are collected from 5 to 19 locations on the scalp using the 10-20 system for electrode placement. Data are collected from all locations simultaneously or in homologous groups. The data are then displayed in the form of standard EEG tracings and artifacts are identified. These artifacts are usually related to eye blinks, eye movement, and electromyography (EMG). The artifacts are manually removed using a computerized artifacting procedure, and the remaining normative samples of EEG are mathematically knitted together. This process provides a high-quality record for analysis.

Minimally, one minute of data is required for a good analysis, but generally two minutes are preferred. In order to achieve this, at least five minutes of recording are required for each condition or task. Recordings to be used for court cases need to be at least 10 minutes in length for each condition. Data are collected separately for eyes-open and eyes-closed analyses and labeled accordingly. It is best to record eyes-closed first to reduce the intrusion of stage one sleep into the record. In the case of Mini-Q, data are collected in sequences of homologous pairs or groups to capture coherence information.

Once a good record has been generated, it can be analyzed and used to generate topographic maps showing the intensity and distribution of the various components and single-Hz EEG band frequency. The primary EEG data are broken down using mathematical analyses with digital filters into component bands of delta, theta, alpha, and beta (and sometimes high beta). Other dimensions of analysis utilize these same component divisions. For instance, they will look at beta coherence and alpha coherence separately.

Various combinations are presented by different database systems. Fairly standard dimensions of analysis are magnitude, power, coherence, phase asymmetry, frequency, and comodulation. These dimensions are studied independently (univariate) and together in combination (multivariate) to determine abnormal patterns that may correlate with various disorders.

Discriminants

Analysis of the various neurometric dimensions together can yield stereotypical patterns that tend to correlate with various disorders. When one is using statistical analysis or expert rules, these dimensions of analysis can yield valuable information for the clinician or researcher. NxLink provided discriminants for a wide variety of disorders. Although their accuracy seemed impressive in a research setting, most of us who use them in a clinical setting find them very misleading and often inaccurate. This situation continues today in most of the research-quality databases.

Jay Gunkelman and many other experts advise against the use of discriminants or at the very least suggest a very cautious consideration of these types of reports. Robert Thatcher emphasizes only using them to confirm an existing diagnosis and only when such a diagnosis is present. He explains that these types of tests are subject to the same potential false positives and false negatives of any lab test and should be used in the same manner.

The NewMind Technologies discriminants have been developed with these issues in mind and represent a different category of discriminant. They represent only a probability level that a certain cognitive or emotional problem may be present (rather than a diagnostic category). They are based on MRI and autopsy research from the neurology literature and not just on statistical correlation with Diagnostic and Statistical Manual of Mental Disorders (DSM) categories. They are used in conjunction with a cognitive-emotional checklist and are, therefore, only confirmatory in nature. The QEEG configurations are grounded in expert clinical observation. The discriminant is used only for neurofeedback purposes and is not designed for medical or psychological diagnosis.

With these features in place, such a discriminant system can be very accurate and useful for neurofeedback purposes. Pioneering such a system has not been easy and has required us to walk a fine line between advocates and critics of the use of discriminants. The system has proven very successful in its preliminary beta test at Old Vineyard Behavioral Health Hospital and in many clinics across the country. Its present users find it extremely accurate. It is now being cross-correlated with the Minnesota Multiphasic Personality Inventory (MMPI) through research at the University of North Carolina and a variety of other psychometrics at the University of St Louis. It is also being correlated with nutritional deficiencies at various clinics around the world. With continued cautious development, discriminant analysis is expected to become the norm in QEEG-guided neurofeedback of the future.

Three factors, in addition to the psychological factors, influence EEG activity:

1. Biological factors,

2. Social /environmental factors, and

3. Equipment.

Taking good baselines and using general protocols that have been developed to deal with various disorders are often adequate. However, difficult cases like head injury, stroke, and some ADD cases may require a brain map. Overall, maps make training much easier because they provide a clear picture of the EEG dynamics at work. The NewMind Maps brain mapping system makes this position clearer and is explained below.

The International Society for Neuroregulation and Research (ISNR) originally published a position paper in the *Journal of Neurotherapy* (Hammond et al., 2004) indicating that although brain maps are not required for neurofeedback, they are preferred. This does not mean they expect everyone to run out and buy $10,000 worth of databases and brain mapping equipment. It does mean, however, that they would prefer qualified practitioners do some form of mapping, if only a Mini-Q. (A Mini-Q is a standard mapping system that maps at 10 sites: F3 & F4, C3 & C4, P3 & P4, T3 &T4, and O1 & O2, whereas a full Q measures at 19 sites: Fz, Cz & Pz, Fp1 & Fp2, F3 & F4, F7 & F8, C3 & C4, T3 & T4, T5 & T6, P3 & P4, and O1 & O2.)

Diagram 30: Early Brain Map from the NxLink Database

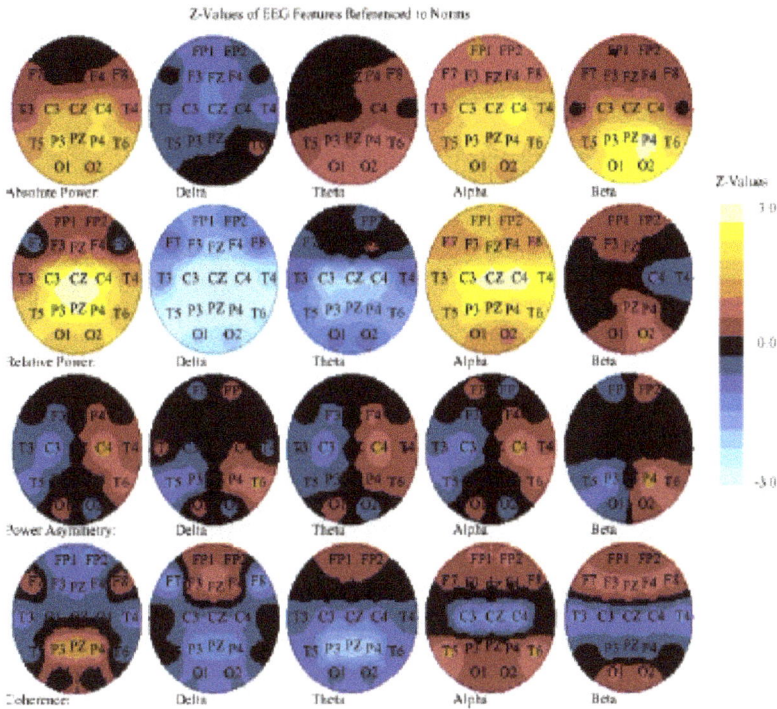

Z-Values of EEG Features Referenced to Norms

Diagram 30: Early Brain Map from the NxLink Database presents a typical early brain map. There are representations for absolute power, relative power, asymmetry, and coherence. In each of these categories there are images representing conventional frequency bands of delta, theta, alpha, and beta. These may not always be optimal for analysis; some databases offer 1-Hertz breakdowns or "one-Hertz bins," as they are often called. In this case, each image, or map, represents only one frequency. The absolute power images represent the electrical power in each band of EEG compared to all other individuals in the database. The color coding represents the intensity of the difference between the subject/client and the normative group. In this example, black is normal, and white represents extremely high amounts of power. Light blue represents extremely low power. This power is measured in Z-Scores, or units of deviations from the average. The scale at the top of the page ranges from one to three in either a positive or negative direction. Power in QEEG is computed when the digital filters decompose the EEG time series into a voltage by frequency spectral graph commonly known as the "power spectrum". Power is approximately the square of the EEG magnitude (average amplitude).

This is different from the standard formula of voltage squared divided by resistance (V^2/R). Consequently, many people involved in the electronics side of this business are uncomfortable with this interpretation. The difference is because we are dealing with AC theory in EEG where certain assumptions are made regarding resistance and capacitance of the brain, dura matter, and skull. During a conversation with Robert Thatcher, he indicated that the resistance of the brain was very low and fairly consistent, perhaps around 8 Ohms.

The relative power images represent the power in one frequency band compared to all other bands. This measurement is then compared to all other similar measurements of other individuals in the database. In many cases this comparison can be more useful as a measurement because the total power of each person's EEG varies so much. It is often more accurate to look at the differences in each frequency band with regard to the person's own EEG. The proportional relationships between each band within the individual's own EEG offer a more accurate picture of how that person differs from others.

Robert Thatcher warns users of his database system to be extremely careful in using relative power because he feels it greatly distorts the general picture. Over the years, however, it has proven to be critical for clinical assessment when individuals have very high or low power globally. Because of the number of individuals encountered with low power EEG, we have become skeptical of the concept that there is only one distribution in the human EEG. We use three different distributions for analysis in the NewMind Database System through a procedure called "shift."

The asymmetry images are developed using information from the absolute power readings. They tell us the difference in power between the left side and the right side of the brain. Although a person may have lower than average alpha, he or she may still have more alpha on the right than the left, which would be normal.

The coherence images show the areas of the brain that are communicating with other areas. A well-functioning brain is very flexible. This flexibility is reflected in a fairly high degree of differentiation between sites pairs showing a Z-Score of –3 would be communicating too little, while pairs showing Z-Scores of +3 would probably be communicating too much. However, too much differentiation (or too little) might mean the areas are not working well together at all. Some databases do a better job than others in communicating this ability in images. Consequently, it is better to rely on the numbers. In fact, the numbers often give a clearer picture of what is happening.

Note: In general, with eyes closed, alpha is dominant, followed by theta, delta, and then beta. With eyes closed, alpha is increased. Beta is decreased with eyes open, delta is dominant, followed by theta, alpha, and then beta. The mean dominant frequency of alpha can predict the entire speed of the brain.

SUBCOMPONENT ANALYSIS

The following quick guide is useful in understanding the subcomponent analysis system of the NewMind Maps brain mapping system (see Diagram 32: Subcomponent Analysis).

- Delta Red is indicative of white matter damage.
- Delta Blue is indicative of too little to no continuity (connectivity).
- Theta Red is indicative of injury to cortex stroke (4–7 Hertz), ADD, or TBI.
- Theta Blue is indicative of lack of emotional connection or lack of memory.
- LoAlpha Red is indicative of metabolic issues, hyperthyroid, or other thyroid problems.
- LoAlpha Blue is indicative of anxiety (in children it can be myelination problems).
- HiAlpha Red is indicative of possible head injury.
- HiAlpha Blue is indicative of anxiety and PTSD.
- LoBeta Red is indicative of anxiety and depression mixed.
- LoBeta Blue is indicative of not blocking information from motor strip, fibromyalgia, or
- overload from sensory input.
- Beta Red is indicative of worry (15–20 Hz) insomnia.
- Beta Blue is indicative of cognitive deficit.
- HiBeta Red is indicative of hypervigilance.
- HiBeta Blue is indicative of under-arousal.

Diagram 31: Subcomponent Analysis

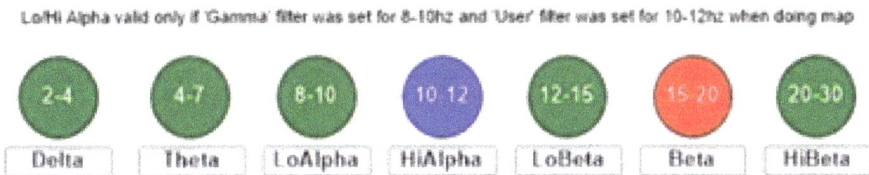

Lo/Hi Alpha valid only if 'Gamma' filter was set for 8-10hz and 'User' filter was set for 10-12hz when doing map

2-4	4-7	8-10	10-12	12-15	15-20	20-30
Delta	Theta	LoAlpha	HiAlpha	LoBeta	Beta	HiBeta

Diagram 32: NewMind Maps Dashboard

Brain Map Date: 10/9/2020

| Underarousal | Inhibited | ISI: 21 | Overarousal |

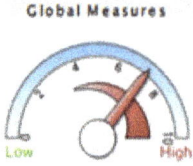
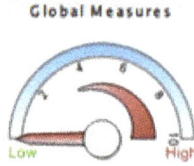
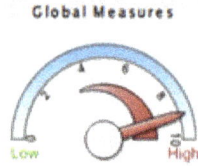

Global Measures · Global Measures · Global Measures

Local Neurogenic

CEC	EEG	Symptom		CEC	EEG	Symptom		CEC	EEG	Symptom
●	●	Impulsive		●	●	Excessive Self-concern		○	●	Worry
○	●	Hyperactive		○	○	Rumination		○	○	Hyper-vigilant
●	●	Easily Distracted		○	○	Anger		○	○	Restless
○	●	Hyper-emotional		○	○	Agitation				
				○	○	Irritability				

Probability Legend
○ Low   ○ Moderate   ● High

Local Psychogenic

CEC	EEG	Symptom		CEC	EEG	Symptom		CEC	EEG	Symptom
○	○	Excessive Speech		○	○	Victim Mentality		●	○	Obsessive Thinking
				○	○	Self-Deprecation		○	○	Dislike of Change/Novelty
				○	○	Passive Aggressive		○	○	Excessive Rationalization
								○	○	Poor Emotional Self-Awareness

Probability Legend
○ Low   ○ Moderate   ● High

Diagram 33: NewMind Maps Midline Analysis

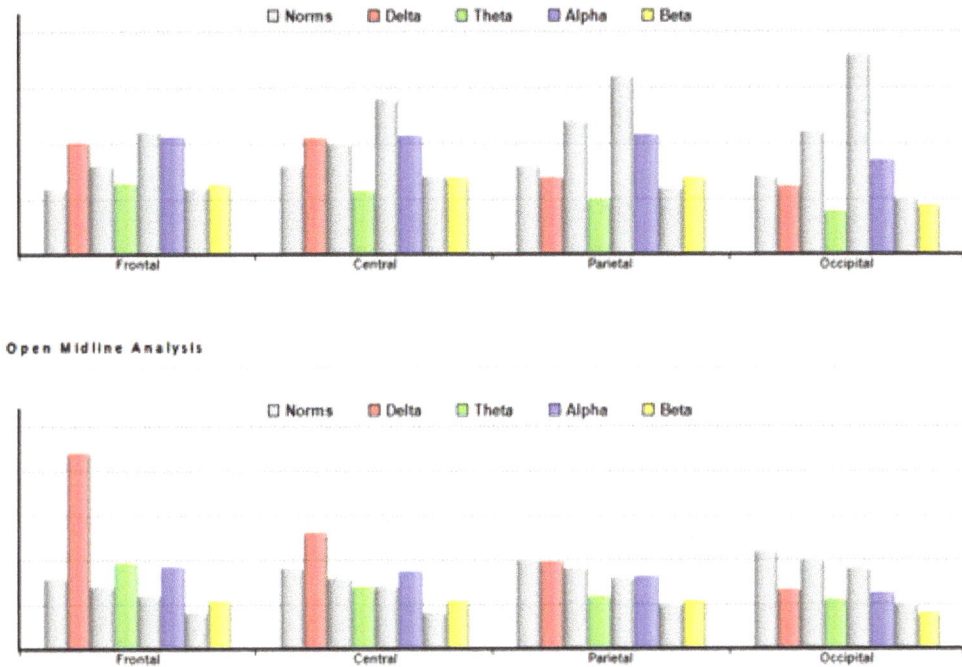

Open Midline Analysis

Learning to use brain maps effectively is an art as well as a science and requires considerable one-on-one training with real cases. It is best to take several workshops on the subject and to develop a relationship with someone who has been reading them for a long time. However, even novices can begin to see the patterns in the relative power and asymmetry measures.

The maps of individuals with bipolar disorder change as they shift from one end of the disorder's continuum to the other. Even though most individuals have very stable maps that do not change over time, certain factors can confound their maps. Too little sleep or drugs such as antihistamines can increase theta. A healthy person can shift his or her alpha asymmetry, so alpha increases in the left hemisphere, by thinking of a very sad event, then shift it back to the right by thinking of a happy event. Elsa Baehr once used a graduate student to demonstrate this in real time at one of her workshops. However, there is a difference between the healthy grad student and a dysregulated client. Through effort, the graduate student can shift asymmetry whereas a client most likely cannot.

A SUMMARY GUIDE TO ASSIST WITH BRAIN MAP INTERPRETATION

A brain mapping system (adapted from NewMind Maps, n.d.) provides the clinician with several parameters of data to best determine potential problem areas and NFB protocols. Brain maps provide the following:

- a summary of data taken from each measured site (magnitude, coherence, phase, dominant frequency, and asymmetry readings for delta, theta, alpha, and beta, Diagram 34: Brain Map NewMind mapping system)
- a subcomponent analysis for delta, theta, lo-alpha, hi-alpha, lo-beta, beta, and hi-beta (Diagram 31: Subcomponent Analysis).
- a discriminant analysis for ADHD, depression, anxiety, and learning disabilities (as shown in Diagram 28: Spectrum Model of Disorders)
- a cognitive analysis with over 20 categories
- an emotional analysis with 20 categories
- a midline analysis chart (Diagram 33)
- suggested supplements
- NFB protocols analysis
- metabolic categories

Diagram 34: Brain Map from NewMind Technologies QEEG Brain Mapping System

Brain Map Date: 10/9/2020

Magnitude

| Delta | Theta | Alpha | Beta | High Beta |

Magnitude Contrast

Down   -2   -1   0   +1   +2   Up

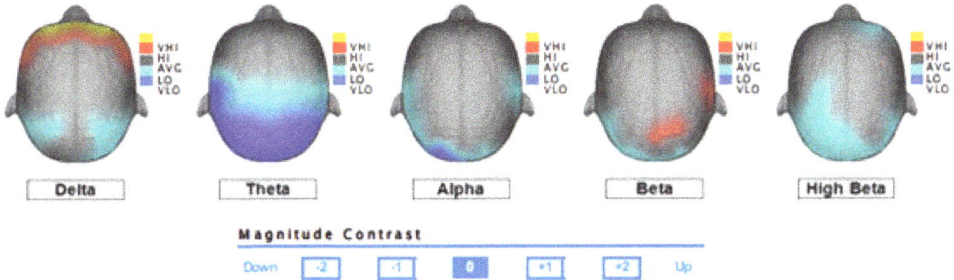

Dominant Frequency

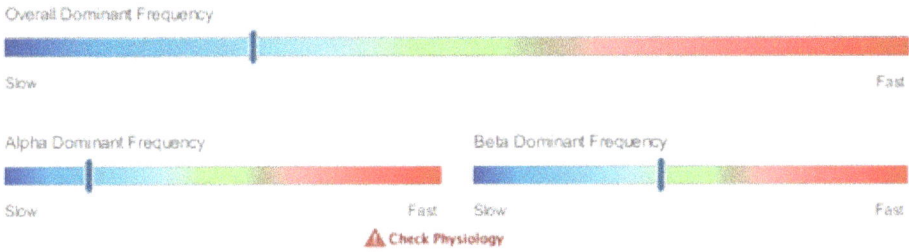

Overall Dominant Frequency

Slow   Fast

Alpha Dominant Frequency

Slow   Fast

Beta Dominant Frequency

Slow   Fast

⚠ Check Physiology

Inter-Connectivity

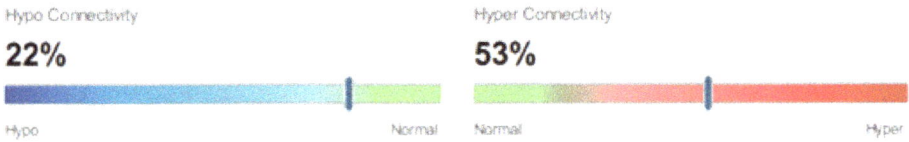

Hypo Connectivity

22%

Hypo   Normal

Hyper Connectivity

53%

Normal   Hyper

Asymmetry

Normal Alpha Asymmetry

0%

Left Dominant   Right Dominant

Normal Beta Asymmetry

81%

Left Dominant   Right Dominant

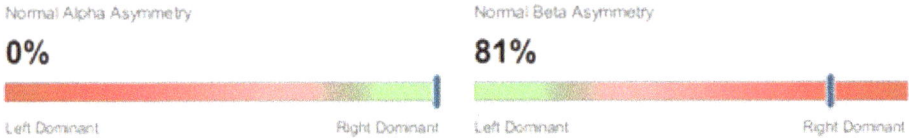

Report intended for exploratory data analysis only and should not be considered a medical diagnosis.   Page 6 of 17

Definitions

The following are definitions to assist with understanding how to read and interpret brain maps.

QEEG

Learning to process and read QEEG reports typically takes years of experience, but Mini-Q systems such as the NewMind Magnitude Analysis System, and those of John Demos and Paul Swingle for example, allow users to obtain a report that is easy to interpret and use, even for those with minimal experience interpreting QEEGs. This allows inexperienced practitioners to immediately begin using QEEG assessment while learning the ins and outs of QEEG-guided neurofeedback: as they grow as neurofeedback providers.

The Magnitude Analysis System provides a reference database system that is tailored specifically for clinicians instead of researchers. Instead of using standard deviations, the maps provide simple output indicating whether EEG is high or low in the various dimensions of analysis (but still based on standard deviations). The cognitive output automatically flags areas of possible problems based on correlations between map output and MRI research. Emotional output information provides similar information based on MRI research, standard neurology texts, and clinical experience. Clinicians can see at a glance the salient issues likely to be present due to the EEG distribution and are provided an appropriate protocol option.

Magnitude

Magnitude is the most important reading since it is a measure of the power of individual brainwaves. Magnitude is used in the NewMind analysis system instead of absolute power because most neurofeedback practitioners work with magnitude; and is also used in the SKIL database (Sterman Kaiser Imaging Labs, Churchville, NY). It is important that practitioners be able to easily refer to their statistics to see the actual microvolt value when an area receives a "high" indication on the map.

Magnitude is the average amplitude over time. The magnitude values in this map are based on a statistical sample in addition to being cross-validated with the major databases. The meaning of high or low magnitudes varies with location and distribution. Learning to interpret their meaning takes considerable experience. The dashboards in this analysis system by NewMind are designed to help practitioners interpret the map information. These dashboards indicate potential problems that may be present when magnitudes are high or low.

Power vs. Magnitude

A digital analysis of EEG uses fast Fourier transforms (FFT) of the digital data to break down the raw wave forms recorded from the brain into component bands or single-Hz bins. The various dimension of analysis used in QEEG are derived mathematically from these transforms.

Power is defined as magnitude squared. This definition has generated some argument in the field as to whether power or magnitude is the best measure of analysis. Barry Sterman has argued for years that power distorts the data significantly enough to be a problem in EEG analysis. However, some database developers disagree with him that magnitude is the best measure of clinical analysis. It is very inconvenient to have maps defined in power when training in magnitude. For this purpose, the NewMind database and the Sterman-Kaiser database provide magnitude as the centerpiece for EEG analysis. Sterman argues that measures of power may inflate the differences between component bands and distort the representation of the EEG landscape. If magnitudes of theta are derived at 6 μV and beta at 2 μV, and then transformed into power, their new values are 36 pW and 4 pW respectively. This mathematical valuation distorts their relationship considerably from 3 to 1 into a relationship of 9 to 1. As long as this type of mistake is not made, however, power is very useful for analysis.

The concern regarding whether there is only one distribution for the human EEG is a major issue that is rarely considered, but should be more carefully researched. E. Roy John (John et al., 1977) addressed this issue through years of research and established that there was only one normative distribution for the human EEG across all cultures. Although this may be true from a purely mathematical perspective, it may not hold up clinically. There is considerable skewness and kurtosis in any given distribution of human EEG (Thatcher, Walker, Biver, North, & Curtin, 2003). This suggests a problem with Gaussianity with respect to the human EEG. Most databases, except NewMind, involve log transforms on some of the neurometric dimensions to provide a more Gaussian distribution to generate robust parametrical analysis. This mathematical sleight of hand is perfectly acceptable with respect to many variables, but it may not be okay with human EEG.

Decades of clinical experience with normative databases have revealed a significant population with globally low EEG who function either normally or exceptionally well within the social order. They are by definition abnormal, according to the normative databases, and should have some correlating behavioral problem. Often, however, they do not have correlating problems (Neidermeyer & Lopes da Silva, 2005). Considerable research suggests that there is a naturally occurring low-power subtype in the population. If this situation is the case, then the database would be invalid with respect to such persons' evaluations, perhaps even unethical. In fact, there is also a high-power subtype as well. These subtypes can be conveniently ignored by treating them as outliers and eliminating them on statistical principle from the Gaussian definition. The NewMind database utilizes three overlapping distributions at present to avoid this problem and may use more in the future.

Phase

Phase is meaningful mostly in relationship to coherence measures. Low phase means the two locations are working in synchrony. High phase means they are out of step. For example, if alpha coherence is high in the frontal region and phase is very low, then it is likely that you will have high-amplitude synchronous alpha that is locked in place. This means the frontal lobes are very much in a state of neutral. This state is commonly found in people meditating.

Phase and coherence may be difficult to understand for individuals just learning about mapping. Their relevance with respect to determining protocols for neurofeedback is still not very clear. Training for coherence and phase are relatively new areas of activity, and little research has been presented on the topic. (If phase is low and coherence is high, then there is a very high level of very synchronous waves; if phase is high and coherence is low, then the brainwaves and the areas they represent are out of synch).

Coherence

Coherence tells us about the brain's efficiency (or lack of efficiency) in adapting to challenges. As challenges increase, the brain increases communication between hemispheres and within hemispheres to compensate (Alstott, 2009). Coherence is especially influential with respect to cognitive function when it occurs between homologous or homotopic sites, i.e., P3 & P4, F3 & F4, etc. One reason for this is that the major Large Scale Networks (LSNs) are homotopic in nature (Menon, 2015). Another is that functional connectivity tends to follow anatomical connectivity (Honey et al., 2007) and the hemispheres are densely connected across the corpus collosum. Consequently, interhemispheric connectivity it turns out, is a good indicator of healthy cortical integration and function (Tiepel, 2009). Loss of general function is closely tied to significant deviance and loss of normal coherence (Gomez, 2009). In a sense, coherence can be more simply described as how much one part of the brain is talking to another part. If areas have high coherence, they are overcommunicating (like a traffic jam). If they have low coherence, they are under-communicating. In both cases plasticity and function suffer. For instance, high or low coherence between F3 and F4 likely indicates a problem in the short-term memory networks of the frontal lobes.

The more disordered the brain, the more extreme its coherence readings. In more technical terms, coherence is how consistent the phase relationship is between two locations. Many maps provide coherence readings between regions with little functional connectivity (Kaiser, 2005). The NewMind mapping system provides coherence readings only between locations that have strong functional connectivity, which is more likely to be clinically meaningful.

When the waxing and waning of the EEG in two locations are compared, there is usually a difference in the timing of the rise and fall of their amplitudes. One signal leads or lags the other with respect to timing. The difference between the two is described through vector analysis and results in comparisons made in terms of degrees. Signals may lead or lag each other by 0 degrees, 90 degrees, or 180 degrees. If they are 180 degrees out of phase, then one signal is at its peak when the other is at its trough. If they consistently lead or lag each other by the same degree over a period of time, they are said to be coherent. This is measure in terms of correlational statistics and may be reported as a Pearson correlation coefficient.

Problems with Coherence

The extensive use of a measurement does not confirm its validity. Often research indicates that a measurement has flaws and should be further developed. This situation have hve been the case with coherence. Coherence has proven to be of limited use clinically and has possibly confounded a great deal of research due to its flaws as a concept and as a unit of measurement. Roberto Pascual-Marqui, who developed LORETA imaging, has characterized coherence as indicating only a statistical relationship and not necessarily a physical relationship. This is partly because a large component of coherence is noise from volume conduction and thalamic input, which may confound its validity as a measure of connectivity. David Kaiser, who developed the SKIL database with Barry Sterman, notes that coherence does have value in conjunction with other measures such as comodulation. Many of the pathways indicated on coherence maps do not exist at the anatomical level, such as between P3 and F4. With this in mind, it is difficult to decide what exactly is being measured other than coincidental correlation. Kaiser and Gunkelman, citing Nunez and other neurophysicists, recommend that coherence is more accurate when first transformed using Laplacian analysis. Robert Thatcher, however, makes strong mathematical arguments to the contrary and presently has broad support from many practitioners and neuroscientists.

The original NxLink database, first developed and marketed by E. Roy John, used homologous sites to generate coherence maps. These were considered the most robust connections with clear clinical relevance. For this reason, and the others cited above, we have continued with that tradition in the NewMind Database. These connections tend to be good proxy measures of general connectivity levels and provide a sufficient sample of coherence for neurofeedback purposes.

There are those who are using coherence measures for the purposes of training coherence with neurofeedback. Many practitioners have noted that coherence training is fraught with peril and many abreactions (Horvath, 2009) and should be approached cautiously with expert guidance. The Z-Score training developed by Mark Smith for Brainmaster® Technologies appears to have diminished this risk to the point where coherence training is safe for almost anyone. The question still remains, however, what exactly clinicians are training when they train coherence. They may be training power with a proxy two-dimensional correlation measure or they may be training with some rudimentary form of connectivity. Still, clinical reports indicate that coherence training is powerful and has impact on clients when other approaches fail. The bottom line is that there are no studies to evaluate it either way.

Functional Versus Effective Connectivity: The Default Mode

It is clear that the value of QEEG is that it records the temporal dynamics of the idling brain. This information is valuable, as recent research indicates this idling state, now known as the default mode, tells a great deal about the functional connectivity of any given brain. "Functional connectivity" is a term emerging in the neuroimaging sciences that describes the healthy functioning of the brain in terms of normal connections. Are all the hubs and nodes of the brain properly connected and operating in normal range? This condition can be best determined by recording brains "at rest." In this state, people are typically engaged in the routine busywork of the brain organized around keeping their autobiographical selves intact and justified. For highly social animals like human beings, this process is critical for survival. Human beings are fundamentally dependent on their social relationships and constantly re-evaluate their status and relationships as if their lives depended on it, because their lives do depend on it. A healthy brain has a characteristic resting pattern; deviations from this pattern suggest that functional problems may exist.

"Effective connectivity," on the other hand, tells how well areas communicate while given some task. This type of dynamic measurement is more reflected in task-based databases that involve reading or math such as the one developed by Kirkley Thornton (2000). This subject has been a more traditional area of interest in fMRI research (Honey et al., 2007). Recently, the research community has recognized that by combining the temporal resolution of QEEG with the spatial resolution of MRI, they can obtain much more comprehensive data.

Unfortunately for clinicians, MRI equipment costs millions to purchase and maintain. However, modern QEEG is an inexpensive modality of neuroimaging that draws evaluative power from its cross-correlation with MRI in the research domain. QEEG, when based on the co-registration studies, is an excellent proxy measure of the BOLD signal (Rosa et al., 2010) and can provide similar information regarding the activation of different areas of the brain. In addition it operates in a high temporal resolution domain that allows it to capture events that the BOLD signal cannot because of its low temporal resolution. As a consequence, sLORETA may provide a more suitable platform in the future for many medical and pharmacological applications.

Dominant Frequency

Dominant frequency is probably the third most important measure. This measure indicates whether the frequency in a specific component band has slowed down or sped up. For instance, alpha in a healthy person should average between 9.5 and 10.5 Hz (Nunez & Srinivasan, 2006). If the dominant alpha frequency drops below 9.5 Hz, then most likely a physiological problem exists. Slowed alpha is often an indicator of depression or physical problems, such as hypothyroid. In this case the modal frequency would be low and show more 8–10 Hz in the subcomponent analysis.

Asymmetry

Asymmetry is second most important in determining if the brain is working properly. For example, increased right frontal theta is indicative of impulsivity, while increased left frontal theta is indicative of disorganization. When delta is predominantly high on the right, it is indicative of emotional issues; when delta is predominantly high on the left, it is indicative of cognitive issues. As mentioned previously, there has been considerable research done over the past two decades regarding EEG asymmetry and its relationship to mood and anxiety. Our own statistical modeling suggests that asymmetry may be one of the best predictors of attentional and physiological problems. Most databases today do not reflect this research very well, but clinicians find it an important source of information.

Our analysis system has been set up so that you can easily read the asymmetries present and compare them to problems your client is reporting. More alpha on the left than the right side usually indicates depression. More beta on the right side than the left usually indicates anxiety. If theta is unusually high and dominates on the left side, it usually indicates a problem with organization. When theta dominates on the right side, it usually indicates a problem with impulsivity.

Comodulation

David Kaiser and Barry Sterman did not have coherence measures in their database system, but saw the need for their own connectivity measures. They have been aware of the many flaws of coherence and have developed an alternative connectivity measure known as comodulation. This measure looks at the covariation of magnitude between two sites and has proven very useful in discriminating clinical problems. It clearly has a valuable future as a dimension of EEG evaluation, but at present is not widely used.

LORETA

This method of EEG analysis was first thought to be the holy grail of QEEG. It soon proved to be another interesting, but flawed, clinical tool for evaluation. Recent improvements resulting in sLORETA have increased its accuracy and value. (Pascual-Marqui, 2002). As soon as we understand connectivity better, it may prove to be one of the best estimates of connectivity available for clinical work. At present, however, connectivity is poorly understood by neuroscience.

Subcomponent Analysis: Single-Hz Bins

The better research quality database systems like Neuroguide usually include a page showing single-Hz bins. This information provides a topographical distribution analysis for each frequency band and assists in identifying exactly which frequency in a component band is most abnormal as well as what location where it is most dominant. It is very useful for setting filter parameters for training. For instance, if alpha is high in magnitude and needs to be trained down, the practitioner needs to know whether it is high-frequency alpha, low-frequency alpha, or the whole component band. Single-Hz bins can provide that information by showing that it is only the 8–10 Hz band that is high and that it is high in the frontal region. Unfortunately, practitioners may find that 8–10 Hz alpha is high frontally, but 10–12 Hz alpha is high in the posterior region. This information results in a picture that is confusing, so that it tends to overwhelm beginners—often, even the more advanced map reader. In addition, single-Hz bins often look different with respect to magnitude and symmetry from the component band analysis.

In the NewMind database system, the single-Hz bin concept is adjusted to make it more clinically friendly. The single-Hz bins are grouped into small component bands that have proven consistently to be correlated with various disorders or behavioral and cognitive features. The distinctions are then based not on some arbitrary mathematical determinant, but on extensive clinical experience. The dominant frequency is presented as the most salient with respect to overall distribution and the key frequency in a given single-Hz range. The result is an easy-to-understand bird's-eye view of the general lay of the land with respect to frequency distribution.

SUMMARY OF KEY POINTS IN READING BRAIN MAPS

Delta

Delta is generated from the brain stem resonances and the cerebellum. Delta measures do not give clear indications for diagnostics. Parietal delta (P4) affects association and cortex/processing. A delta deficit is indicative of problems with working memory. Arrhythmic delta is normal, while rhythmic delta may indicate pathology. A high delta/beta ratio may indicate slowing (for example eyes-closed delta is 15 and eyes-closed beta is 5). Increased global delta may indicate cognitive decline with age (delta, theta, and alpha start to slow). Table 4 shows delta wave indicators below.

Table 4: Delta Wave Indicators

Area	Indicator	Indicator	Indicator	Indicator	Indicator
Frontal	TBI	LD	Dementia	Parkinson's	Decreased delta may indicate short-term memory problems
Temporal	TBI	Language, processing problems			Short-term memory problems
Global	TBI				Emotional processing problems/ ADHD/ list acquistion problems
Posterior		LD			

Theta

Key theta generators in the limbic system communicate with the cortex through two major pathways, one frontal through the anterior cingulate and one posterior (Mitchell et al., 2008) Theta has a high frequency component and a low frequency component such that the higher frequencies tend to be involved with memory searching and the lower frequencies tend to be involved with emotional valence (Kirk & Mackay, 2003). Theta emerges from the hippocampal loop (the septal hippocampal circuits/limbic system). Theta issues may develop from input from the anterior cingulate into the cortex or may indicate focal activation problems in the cortex. Generally, when there is increased theta, there may be increases in delta and alpha (all slower waves). Having increased theta and beta is like driving with the brakes on (the brain does not run smoothly).

A theta/beta ratio greater than 3:1 constitutes a slow-wave disorder. The normal theta/beta ratio is 2:1 (i.e., theta 8.7 over beta 11.07 = .79 or too much beta). The largest theta/beta ratios are found at Cz or Fz; the smallest theta/beta ratios are found in the temporal lobes. The normal theta/beta ratio at Cz is 1.6:1, and at Fpz is 1.5:1. A high theta/beta ratio is a signature of ADHD (i.e., 2.5:1). Children with ADHD often show a 3:1 ratio. Table 5 shows theta wave indicators.

Table 5: Theta Wave Indicators

Area	Indicator	Indicator	Indicator	Indicator	Indicator
Frontal	ADHD ADD Anxiety	Impulsiveness/ Impulse control D/O / lack of inhibitory control (When theta is higher on the right front and right hemisphere)	Foggy headed /LD (Unable to grasp concepts, ideas, information	Emotional: PTSD / Depression/ Overwhelmed / Emotions shut down.	Disorganization (when theta is higher in the left front and Left hemisphere).
Temporal			Language processing problems Short-term memory problems	Emotional processing problems	
Global		Decreased delta globally may indicate a person is low energy (especially when alpha is high)		Emotional processing problems	Trouble with accessing emotional information. Retrieval problems.
Posterior	Pain and anxiety. Decreased theta may indicate attentional problems.	OCD / Perseveration (hard time letting go).	LD Reading Comprehension-problems.		

Alpha

Alpha is generated from resonance between the thalamus and the cortex. The brain idles in alpha, and constantly shifts up into beta and down into theta. The traumatized brain idles too fast (in the beta direction), or too slowly (in the theta direction). If excessive alpha coherence is present, the brain may be locked up in alpha and be hard to speed up or slow down. Low amplitude alpha may be indicative of anxiety, and may be involved in PTSD, or short-term memory impairment. (Low alpha results from chronic effects of cortisol on the brain, which affects the hippocampus and thus short-term memory). Alpha should be higher in the right hemisphere than in the left hemisphere. Alpha asymmetry and regionally increased alpha are indicative of depression. With an eyes-closed map, the normal dominant frequency should be alpha. When the dominant frequency is at 11–12 Hz, it is faster than normal; it is slower than normal from 8–9 Hz, and considered normal when 9.5–10.5 Hz. Slow (or low) alpha can be indicative of metabolic problems, toxin-related issues, bipolar disorder/depression, and substance abuse (i.e., marijuana use/abuse). Increased fast alpha in the posterior may indicate emotional rumination. Table 6 shows alpha wave indicators.

Table 6: Alpha Wave Indicators

Area	Indicator	Indicator	Indicator	Indicator
Frontal	Depression (alpha asymmetry with more alpha on the left than on the right). Lack of motivation.	Decreased alpha is indicative of impulsivity, being controlled by anxiety, feeling overwhelmed, and impulsivity with explosiveness.	ADD Attentional problems.	Pain and anxiety.
Global	Increased alpha on the left may indicate emotional shutdown.	Depression Metabolic issues Substance abuse.	Parkinson's may include alpha slowing.	Person's energy level is low (especially when delta is low).
Posterior	Depression, passivity, and avoidant personality.	Trauma PTSD.		Fibromyalgia (decreased alpha).

Beta

Beta is generated from resonances within the cortex. Beta should be higher on the left than on the right. Increased beta asymmetry in the right hemisphere is indicative of anxiety. Global elevated beta on the right hemisphere is generally indicative of anxiety (look at magnitude and asymmetry). Increased beta in the left frontal area blocks amygdala input. Beta hyper-coherence may indicate anxiety, panic attacks, and test anxiety. Panic attacks can look like full-body seizures especially when there are sensory integration problems.

Faster than normal dominant frequency beta may indicate that there is excess norepinephrine. Increased beta alone is often indicative of withdrawal from social interaction or inhibited behavior responses (when theta and alpha are lower). Increased beta at Fp2 and F3 simultaneously can be indicative of the patient hiding all feelings and emotions (flat affect may be seen). Increased beta and decreased alpha in frontalis is indicative of agitation, being controlled by anxiety, feeling overwhelmed, and impulsivity with explosiveness. Table 7 shows beta wave indicators.

Table 7: Beta Wave Indicators

Area	Indicator	Indicator	Indicator	Indicator	Indicator
Frontal	Anxiety Impulsivity (being controlled by anxiety and feeling over-whelmed), and impulsivity with explosiveness. Mood shifts.	Pain	Emotional Hyper-vigilance and controlling, passive, and/or avoidant personality Insomnia Person hides all feelings and emotions (flat affect may be seen).	Fear (increased frontal beta) Aggression (decreased frontal beta)	Increased beta in frontal areas and in the right hemisphere (the brain is running too fast) may indicate anxiety, OCD, mania, and worry.
Temporal	TBI			Anger Irritability	
Global	Anxiety ADD Insomnia (insomnia often reveals LoBeta/Beta at 5.1/4.5).	Insomnia Muscle tension Head-aches	Self-regulation problems		OCD
Posterior	Anxiety disorder(s) Rumination.	Fibromy-algia	Rumination Trauma.		OCD Rumination.

EEG Correlates of Disorders

QEEG is not considered a diagnostic tool at this time; however, the QEEG may indicate and or validate a particular disorder or concern. Certain QEEG profiles may be indicative of one or more disorders.

Table 8: QEEG Interpretation Chart

GLOBAL	
Low Power Fast or Slow	metabolic resource depletion, cellular degeneration, alcoholism
Low Alpha	stress, adrenal fatigue, confusion, reduced cognitive stamina
High Alpha	hypothyroid, initial inflammatory process, chronic anxiety, sleep deficit, and depression
Low Beta	reduced cognitive efficiency, chronic hyperarousal phase 2 (Stress)

High Beta	worry, chronic hyperarousal Phase 1 (Hyperarousal is a specific cluster of post-traumatic stress disorder symptoms that some people with PTSD experience; and/or is the consequence of heightened (hyper) anxiety and altered arousal responses and includes symptoms such as: having a difficult time falling or staying asleep), and hypermentation
Low Theta	memory deficits, reduced emotional awareness
High Theta	ADHD symptoms, executive deficits, low cortical perfusion
Low Delta	TBI, low dopamine, white matter damage, chronic drug use, poor functional integration
High Delta	TBI, inflammation, insomnia, food sensitivity, chronic emotional trauma, white matter inflammation, low acetylcholine, heavy metals
High Power	allergies, asthma, toxin exposure, food sensitivities
High Theta and Beta	oppositional, impulsive
High Delta and Theta	mild to severe cognitive decline
REGIONAL	
High Frontal Alpha	low motivation
Low Frontal Alpha	excess worry
High Posterior Alpha	perseverance, positive rumination, bargaining, sleep problems
Low Posterior Alpha	confusion, slowed processing
High Frontal Beta	excess worry- anticipatory, hypervigilance
Low Frontal Beta	executive processing deficits
High Posterior Beta	emotional instability and negative rumination
Low Posterior Beta	attention deficit
High Frontal Theta	impulse control and attention deficits
Low Frontal Theta	working memory deficits, low emotional self-awareness

High Posterior Theta	sensory integration issues, and confusion
Low Posterior Theta	short term and sequential memory deficits which generate poor attention
High Frontal Delta	general cognitive and social accuracy deficits, attention deficits, impulse control deficits
Low Frontal Delta	poor working memory
High Posterior Delta	poor short term and sequential memory, sensory integration deficits, facial decoding deficits
Low Posterior Delta	short term and sequential memory deficits
LOCAL: See Brodmann 10-20 Function-Location Chart. Use Only As General Guides.	

Anger, Fear, Irritability, and Aggression

Right hemisphere frontal activity is often associated with the amygdala's response to fear. Aggressive patients have excessive slow waves in the frontal area; they cannot control the fear, so they act out. ADD and anxiety may indicate that the patient can be explosive. Patients with irritability and anger usually have temporal lobe problems. The patient may be over-aroused.

Anxiety

Anxiety results from elevated amygdala action. The activity travels to the thalamus and inputs into the medial frontal cortex. The hypothalamus controls hunger, thirst, sex drive, and body temperature. Anxiety is the brain's first line of defense. Anxiety is associated with too much fastwave (beta) activity in the right frontal area. Anxiety can have a global impact through the amygdala and RAS enhancement of norepinephrine. Increased activity in the amygdala often displays as increased beta at Fp1 and Fp2. Increased beta activity in the frontal area blocks worry and anxiety. Anxiety problems lead to memory and retention problems.

ADD/ADHD

Often, ADD presents as slowing of the brain's electrical activity. ADHD shows increased frontal theta in the left and right hemispheres (short-term memory). Learning disabilities and ADHD may indicate white matter problems.

Bipolar Disorder

Bipolar disorder usually reveals increased beta in the right hemisphere and frontal beta (during the manic phase). During the depressive cycle, there is usually low frequency alpha in the frontal area.

Cognitive Concerns

Temporal lobe theta may indicate language and memory processing problems. Temporal lobe delta may also indicate language and memory processing problems, or if it is coming from the insula just above the temporal lobes, it may indicate integration problems between the cortex and the peripheral nervous system. Emotional valence is also affected by abnormalities of the temporal lobes.

Depression

When patients become depressed, they have exhausted their systems through being anxious all the time. The left frontal area slows down and depression sets in. Depression usually reveals increased alpha on the left side and may often be displayed as increased global alpha, especially in the midbrain (emotion). Depression can look exactly like ADHD in children. When patients are angry, bargain, whine, and are hyperactive, it may be depression, not ADHD.

Physical Pain

High amplitude non-rhythmic theta and delta bursts are often seen with migraine headaches. They are usually combined with excessive beta in the cingulate, as is high blood pressure. Pain is often associated with excessive activity in the cingulate, especially the anterior cingulate. Other authors (Hassan et al., 2015; Jensen et al., 2013) have also identified a region around the insula, which is often especially active in pain, that can often be trained to assist in pain reduction.

Trauma and PTSD

The patterns associated with PTSD vary and a precise distribution has not emerged. However, many key features are often present. PTSD often manifests as increased posterior beta with an alpha deficit, and high frontal coherence. When a patient experiences fear, right-side beta increases to shut down panic. The patient will pull back more. PTSD often reveals increased 16–19 Hz beta globally. The frontal area lights up with beta and looks like severe insomnia. When patients are in a chronic state of hyperarousal, the brain exhausts or depletes the neurotransmitters and omega 3 (60% of the brain is fat, of which 25% is omega 3), which means the brain is often overloaded with omega 6 and omega 9. The amygdala is blocked when there is excessive beta activity. Increased 13–15 Hz beta in the frontal lobes blocks emotional information (emotions are kept at bay).

The "Normative Problem"

A well-known editor for some of the major texts on neurofeedback confessed a serious concern about the concept of "normalcy." E. Roy John and Leslie Prichep addressed this issue in their original research, but many experts in sociology and psychology are not satisfied with their treatment.

A whole book could be written on this topic, but we will attempt to be concise here. To make things worse, the preliminary screening test data for NxLink has never actually been published. Testing for other databases is quite flawed as well. Much of the screening for the existing databases has provided valuable data and has narrowed the population in the direction of psychological "normalcy," but may prove to be very insufficient in the long term. Taking a large population sample, randomly selecting from it, and then cross-correlating the EEG distributions with known psychological and sociological measures is proposed. This process would be a more honest appraisal of the total potential variance in the EEG of the human population. It is for these purposes that an internet-based QEEG system for NewMind has been set up. Presently, several universities are participating in the project. No doubt political and economic issues will drive many critical arguments—thinly veiled as scientific—against the project, but then again, science has always been highly political and economically driven.

Miscellaneous Differential Diagnostics

- Lack of blood flow to the brain increases delta and theta waves, and to a lesser degree alpha waves
- Damage to focal areas results in stereotypical deficits that have been consistently noted in neurology. Slow-wave activity in these areas may have similar effects
- Focal damage to the central parietal region in the area of the posterior cingulate (Pz) typically results in perseveration
- Frontal circuits include three basic executive circuits. Increased frontal (Fz) beta indicates the brain being overactive, which affects attention and decision making. Excessive delta and theta have a slowing effect, and the brain is underactive
- The anterior cingulate (Fz) is the gateway to dorsal lateral circuits. The anterior cingulate processes attention and decision making
- At Cz with eyes-closed and along the other midline sites (Fpz, Fz, Pz, Oz) the norm is that alpha is dominant at approximately 14 µV, theta 10 µV, delta 8 µV, and beta 7 µV

LESION RESEARCH

Below are listed behavioral correlates of focal lesions from the neurological literature. High levels of theta in the regions listed often have a similar impact.

Left Hemisphere

Fp1   Orbitofrontal circuit-socially cavalier

F3   Dorsolateral circuit-depression, short-term memory difficulty, word retrieval problems, and problem-solving difficulty (Wisconsin Card Sort)

F7   Word retrieval problems, recall difficulties, difficulty filtering environment, and irritability

Temporal

T3   Self-deprecation, episodic memory problems, especially event sequencing, difficulties with verbal-emotional understanding, reading difficulties

T5   Difficulty making sense of events, problems understanding meaning, problems understanding what is read

Parietal

P3   Memory, organization, digit span problems

Beta Correlates

The same research indicates behavioral correlates of excess beta activity in the areas listed below.

Fp1   Dislike novelty, over-focus on structure and predictability

F3   Obsessional thinking

T3   Cortical irritability

T5   Constant confusion/questioning

P3   Excessive thinking and worrying

Right Hemisphere

Fp2   Emotional impulsivity, poor social awareness, socially inappropriate behavior, edginess and anxiety, over-talkativeness

F4   Poor organization of dialogue, poor use of analogy and irony, impolite discourse

F8   Too little prosody

Temporal

T4   Anger, sadness, aggression, emotional tonality problems, voice tonality problems

REVIEW QUESTIONS

1. What are the some of the impacts of trauma on the brain?

2. What are the differences between "brain too slow" and "brain too fast?"

3. Is QEEG widely accepted within the fields of NFB or neurology? Why or why not?

4. How are asymmetry measures useful to the clinician?

5. What is magnitude and how does it differ from power?

6. What is coherence and what are some of the problems associated with its interpretation?

7. What are single-Hz bins?

8. What are the four basic brainwave frequency ranges? What are two indicators of disorders that might be apparent from each range?

CHAPTER 5: BASELINES & ASSESSMENTS

Often new practitioners buy equipment and take workshops on how to use it, but find they are lost when they return to their own practices. Before hooking up clients, it is crucial to thoroughly learn how the equipment works and to train with a clinician/mentor who has experience with the same equipment. The nuances of the equipment and how it performs in a clinical setting will emerge. Our new book, *Mentoring for Neurofeedback Certification: A Guide for Mentors and Mentees*, provides more information about the mentoring process. We would recommend that you begin with equipment that provides you the opportunity to do basic 1, 2, and 4 channel traditional neurofeedback as well as the ability and software to assess client/patients with a full 19point QEEG.

At the very least, you should begin practicing on yourself. This method is a good way to explore the equipment and try different protocols to see how they feel subjectively. This experience is immensely helpful in understanding how clients respond to training and to help identify progress indicators.

The following contains the information practitioners should minimally understand.

BASIC ELECTRONICS THEORY

Most practitioners coming into the field know little about electronics theory. Since NFB deals with electromagnetic activity issuing from the brain and uses electronic equipment to evaluate it, practitioners must know some of this basic theory to save time, confusion, and frustration.

Voltage (Volts): The amount of electrical potential between two locations with different electrical charges is measured in Volts. Usually the difference is measured between ground and active electrodes. EEG is read in microVolts (μV). It is the most common unit discussed in neurofeedback. For example, when a client's alpha is 30 μV, the alpha is very high and needs to be trained down.

Amperage (Amps): The flow of electrical energy is usually defined in terms of fluid dynamics. The stream of electricity flowing between two locations has a rate of flow. The material/energy flowing is electrons. The rate of flow of electrons determines the current, which is measured in terms of amperage or Amps. This term is not frequently discussed in EEG.

Resistance (Ohms): This is the resistance to the flow of current. Some elements conduct electricity more readily than others. Those that have few free electrons, such as the scalp, conduct electricity less readily than, for instance, copper wire. Resistance is measured using a unit of measurement called Ohms. The input to

EEG equipment at the ends of the electrode is measured in a form of resistance known as impedance. Equipment with very high impedance levels usually gets a better EEG signal with less prep work on the scalp.

Ohm's Law (E = I x R), where resistance (Ohms) is resistance to the flow of energy (Amps). Ohm's Law is also depicted as:

$$V = R \times I$$

$$I = V / R$$

$$\text{and } R = V / I$$

These are all ways that the formula for voltage is computed using resistance and current, as is shown in Table 9, below.

Table 9: Electronics Terms

Quantity	Symbol	Unit	Sign
Voltage	V or E (energy)	Volt	V (amplitude in EEG)
Current	I	Ampere (Amp)	A
Resistance	R	Ohm	O
Power	P	Watt	W

RESISTANCE TO AC = IMPEDANCE; RESISTANCE TO DC = RESISTANCE

Power (Watts)

Power refers to the actual amount of energy available in the electrical current. This energy may have been originally in the form of waterpower, diesel fuel, or chemical energy such as batteries or cells. Such energy is transformed into electrical energy through various processes.

Power can be represented mathematically:

$$P = V^2 / R$$

where P is power, V is voltage, and R is resistance.

The brain puts out about 30 Watts of power and burns about 50% of the body's glucose to do this. Brain maps usually report EEG in terms of power rather than microVolts, which is confusing because most of the statistics on neurofeedback are reported in microVolts. Fortunately, some QEEG database makers are beginning to provide information in microVolts.

Current

There are two kinds of current: direct current (DC) and alternating current (AC). DC flows continuously in one direction. AC flows first in one direction and then in the opposite direction. AC current is the kind you find in the household socket. EEG is originated by DC current in neurons; but emerges as AC current. The EEG microvolt readings obtained on equipment are usually based on peak-to-peak current changes.

Impedance

AC current behaves differently than DC current and requires a special unit of resistance called impedance. Impedance in AC is a unit of resistance to the flow of AC. High impedance is desired for equipment input in the megaOhm range. Resistance between the scalp and the electrode should be low—10 kOhms or less. To accomplish this, we buy expensive equipment and scrub the scalp with an abrasive preparation such as Nuprep®.

Capacitance (microFarads, mfd)

 A capacitor is a component that stores electricity and allows only AC current to pass through it. It is basically two conductors with a resistance in between. It is a relationship that occurs naturally in the world quite frequently. Cell walls act like capacitors and so do electrical wires that are used to hook up clients. Frequently you have to touch wires to drain off an electrical charge that builds up in the wires and distorts your readings. Some clients, during cold dry weather, will give practitioners a mild electrostatic shock when touched, which will end troublesome readings.

Phase

Phase is about the relationship between two AC currents or two electromagnetic wave forms. EEG waves are electromagnetic waveforms that move from positive to negative voltage. Two waveforms may resonate or cancel based on how much they shift from positive to negative at the same time. If two wave forms shift from positive to negative at exactly the same rate, they are in phase. Two wave forms that shift at the opposite rate are out of phase. Diagram 35: Phase Waves, shows examples of in-phase and out-of-phase signals. Areas of the brain that emit consistently in-phase signals are doing so because they are communicating and processing the same information. Consequently, they are referred to as coupled.

Diagram 35: Phase Waves

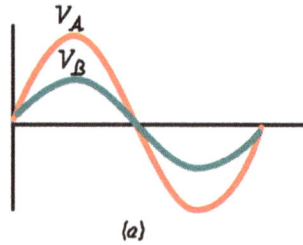

In-Phase waves

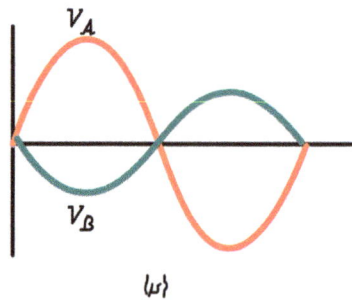

Out-of-Phase waves

Common Mode Rejection

The common-mode rejection ratio (CMRR) of a differential amplifier (or other device) measures the tendency of the device to reject input signals common to both input leads. A high CMRR is important in applications where the signal of interest is represented by a small voltage fluctuation superimposed on a (possibly large) voltage offset (voltage offset may have no meaning to most people), or when relevant information is contained in the voltage difference between two signals. This important feature of the differential amplifier makes it very useful when recording the weak signal of the EEG. We usually anchor one side of the amplifier to the ear lobe which has very little voltage and the other side to the location of interest. This results in a very clean signal reflecting primarily activity from that specific location while rejecting information from other locations.

Another important way this feature is used in neurofeedback is to place both the active and reference lead (both sides of the input to the differential amplifier) on different areas of the brain in order to do what is referred to as "bipolar training." More on this topic in the chapter on protocols.

CMRR is often important in reducing noise in many applications in electronics. In the case of EEG, artifact may occur from a variety of sources: EMG, blinking, outside electrical interference, etc. For example, when measuring, make it a common-mode voltage signal. The CMRR of the measurement instrument determines the attenuation (reduction of background noise) applied to the offset or noise. In short, common mode rejection does the following:

1. detects the difference between the active and reference electrode, then

2. subtracts the difference between active and reference, then

3. rejects unwanted signals common to both amplifier inputs.

Fast Fourier Transform

The fast Fourier transform (FFT) is the mathematical method of calculating the frequency composition of a wave. A good metaphor for this is the prism. When held up to sunlight, a prism breaks light down into a rainbow spectrum of colored light bands. These are the light frequencies that, when combined, make up white light. Like a prism, FFT analysis breaks up the composite EEG into its individual frequency components, decoding the raw wave forms into individual frequencies.

HOW NFB AMPLIFIERS AND EEG EQUIPMENT WORKS

Electrodes attached to the head must pick up an electrical signal (waveforms) that is highly attenuated. Voltages at the cortical surface are in the millivolt (mV) range, but voltages at the surface of the scalp are in the microvolt range (µV; see Diagram 36: Microvolt Ranges and Wavelengths). This is because the skull has a great deal of resistance and is not a good conductor of electricity. To help make a good connection with the scalp, apply electrode paste so that electrons can flow easily from scalp to electrode. If they do not, then the waveforms are distorted.

Diagram 36: Microvolt Ranges and Wavelengths

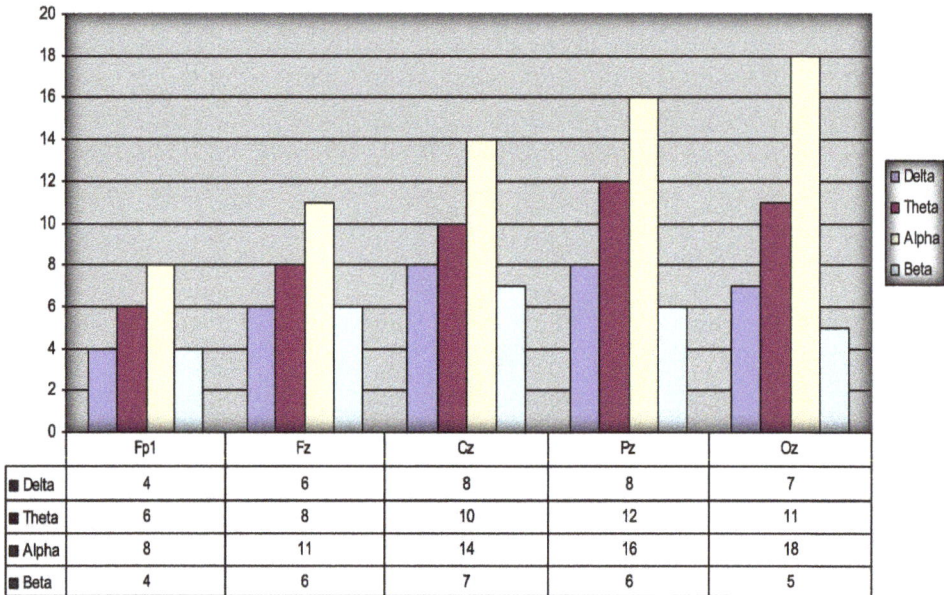

	Fp1	Fz	Cz	Pz	Oz
■ Delta	4	6	8	8	7
■ Theta	6	8	10	12	11
■ Alpha	8	11	14	16	18
■ Beta	4	6	7	6	5

Since microVolts are too small to measure easily, a special type of amplifier is used to help increase the amplitude of the waveform so the computer can use it. This amplifier is also able to reject undesired electrical signals. When picking up a signal in microVolts, it is also easy to pick up tiny signals from other sources since electricity is everywhere at this voltage level. As previously mentioned, a device known as a differential amplifier employing common mode rejection is used. Diagram 37: Differential Amplifier, shows a diagram of such a device. It has two inputs for EEG signals and a third reference input. Any signals that are out of phase with the EEG signals are cancelled and only the EEG signals pass through the amplifier. They are made larger in amplitude through an initial stage of pre-amplification so that other stages of amplifiers can increase them more. Eventually, they are large enough to be digitized and passed on to the computer to use for neurofeedback.

Before the amplified EEG signals reach the screen, they are often broken down into their respective frequency ranges. This way, the raw EEG or a filtered version that shows delta, theta, alpha, and beta (lo-beta, beta, and hi-beta) can be viewed. The filters used for this process are either physical components called analogue filters, or virtual components called fast Fourier transforms.

The analogue filters give real-time results, while there is a very slight delay in fast Fourier. This delay happens because the equipment must do ongoing calculations with the signal information in order to break it down into fundamental components and reconstruct it into frequency bands. There are arguments regarding the effects of such a delay. The use of "digital" filters has enhanced the speed of almost all modern equipment. In fact, Margaret Ayers marketed equipment that theoretically has no digital delay.

Diagram 37: Differential Amplifier

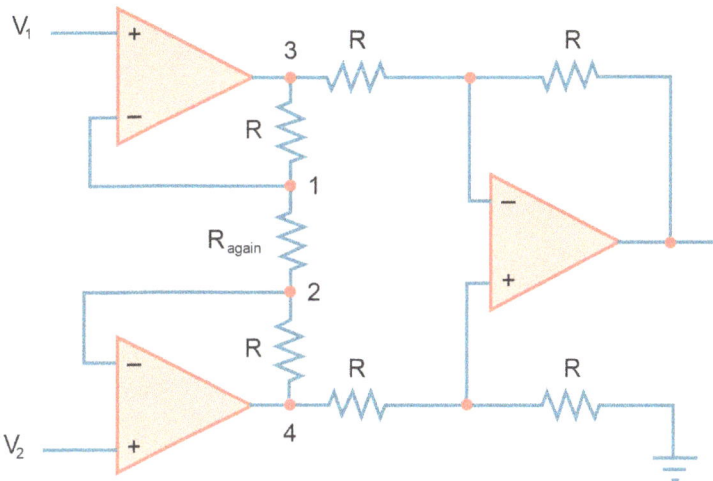

With EEG, there are various filters that can or may be applied. Most commonly we hear about low-pass filters and high-pass filters.

Low-pass Filter

A low-pass filter is a filter that allows lower frequency signals to pass but attenuates (reduces the amplitude of) signals with frequencies higher than the designated cutoff frequency. The actual amount of attenuation for each frequency varies from filter to filter. When used in audio applications, such a filter is sometimes called a high-cut filter or treble-cut filter.

The concept of a low-pass filter exists in many different forms, including electronic circuits (like a hiss filter used in audio). Low-pass filters play the same role in signal processing that moving averages do in some other fields, such as finance. Both tools provide a smoother form of a signal by removing the short-term oscillations, leaving only the long-term trend. Low-pass filters can be used to block out artifact from muscle tension (EMG) and 60 Hz noise from a poor ground.

High-pass Filter

High-pass filters decrease artifact. A high-pass filter is a filter that passes high frequencies well; but attenuates (reduces the amplitude of) frequencies lower than the cutoff frequency. The actual amount of attenuation for each frequency varies from filter to filter. Such a filter is sometimes called a low-cut filter; the terms bass-cut filter or rumble filter are also used in audio applications. A high-pass filter is the opposite of a low-pass filter. High-pass filters can be used to block out eye blink, eye movement, and other low frequency artifacts. A band-pass filter is a combination high-pass and low-pass filter.

DIFFERENCES IN EQUIPMENT

EEG instruments are designed differently. Some instruments have two reference leads and a ground and others have only one reference lead and a ground. Some instruments have two or four EEG amplifiers or channels and others have only one. With four amplifiers, four EEGs can be run at once and train or monitor several locations at once. This method can have tremendous advantages. More recently 19 channel amplifiers have become popular for recording brainmaps and even doing 19 channel training.

Today, there is equipment that has 20 plus channels and the clinician can do full "cap" training; often used with sLORETA, which is used to target specific Brodmann areas of the brain.

Some equipment has raw EEG trace displays and other equipment does not. Since brainwave morphology can supply important information, the latter can be a serious drawback. Some equipment supplies only dichotomous feedback while other devices supply continuous or proportional feedback or both. Some have good graphics and others have limited but higher quality graphics.

How and what information is displayed is crucial. It is often nice to have a dominant frequency display, but this is not available on most equipment. Some displays provide only theta-to-beta ratio information while others can be programmed to give information in any desired format. Session averaging information and statistical report information are especially important. However, these reports are often very poorly designed. A quality report will allow the practitioner to take a baseline of any length using any frequency configuration and have instant averaging in a readable format. These reports are not easy to find.

Most equipment is designed for one way of doing neurofeedback. If practitioners want to learn a new approach, they may be forced to buy new equipment in order to operationalize a protocol. One advantage of a simple program based on one approach to neurofeedback is that it is easier to learn. However, its narrow approach can be quite limiting. On the other hand, sophisticated programs that offer greater flexibility can be very difficult to learn and easily overwhelm and confuse beginners.

Some manufacturers make a good profit from selling a long series of costly workshops to learn their equipment. We recommend you buy an inexpensive and simple piece of equipment such as those developed by NewMind Technologies or Brainmaster®. You may want to first utilize a basic neurofeedback system, then upgrade to the fancier equipment as you learn more about what you want to do. Later, you can use the simple equipment for backup or as a home trainer. You need to be sure that your equipment complies with federal regulations if you plan to use it for clinical work and collect insurance. This step is extremely important depending on your clinical setting, for example, a hospital setting in which all medical equipment must meet FDA requirements.

At least two amplifiers are required to do complex bilateral training typical of most asymmetry protocols. NeuroCare Pro utilizes two channel training combined with a non-linear adaptive strategy integrated into the software. NewMind also utilizes two channel homtopic training extensively in conjunction with QEEG. Multiple tones that sound nice together are important. The ability to program custom tones is an important feature. For example, advanced peak performance training involving synchrony often requires a four-channel system. Adam Crane at American Biotech was the first to develop a four-channel synchrony program specifically designed for synchrony training. Presently most training. In addition, lead configuration is important, and most equipment can be adapted for bipolar and monopolar montages. NewMind Technologies has recently come out with this type of equipment.

Knowing what type of voltage values are utilized on the equipment, that is, peak-to-peak or root mean square (RMS) is essential. Peak-to peak amplitude is the measure of the change between peak and trough. Peak-to-peak amplitudes can be measured by meters with appropriate circuitry, or by viewing the waveform on an oscilloscope. Peak-to-peak is a straightforward measurement to make on an oscilloscope, the peaks of the waveform being easily identified and measured against the graticule. It remains a common way of specifying amplitude but sometimes other measures of amplitude are more appropriate (Amplitude, n.d.). Root mean square (RMS) amplitude is used especially in electrical engineering. The RMS is defined as the square root of the mean over time of the square of the vertical distance of the graph from the rest state. When dealing with alternating current electrical power, it is universal to specify RMS values of a sinusoidal waveform. The peak-to-peak voltage of a sine wave is nearly 3 times the RMS value, but is a rarely used measure in this field (Amplitude, n.d.).

The voltage readings between machines vary a great deal. If you want to compare your voltage readings to others, you need to know each format, so you can adjust for differences. This step is especially important if you are using two different machines or if you want to interpret research.

While no standards exist in the field, more and more machines are using peak to-peak.

$$RMS = .707 \times peak\ value$$

Other methods are used for calculation of voltage values including average value and peak value.

$$Peak\text{-}to\text{-}Peak = 2 \times peak\ value.$$

$$2.828 \times RMS = Peak\text{-}to\text{-}Peak.$$

Most machines today have such high input impedance that even if the technique is not great, good readings are still possible. Still, connections should be less than 35 Ohms maximum. Conventionally, the standard is 5 Ohms but this is an antiquated convention base on 20th century amplifier technology. Often you will have to settle for 10 Ohms. On some equipment there are impedance lights informing you of the connection quality. After some practice, you will usually be able to tell from the signal trace quality if the client was prepared properly. When beginning, it is a good idea to get a device to check the impedance of the leads. In this situation, live supervision can help you a great deal and teach you good techniques.

Hooking It Up

Reference areas are slightly controversial, but the most common location for reference electrodes is the ear lobes. Some practitioners claim that this location is the only viable placement, but the explanations are not very well documented. Nunez (1995) indicates that there are many equally good locations for ground and reference. For example, many practitioners utilize mastoid references, the boney area behind the ears, with good results. QEEG databases use the ear lobes (linked ears) so it would be best to do so for conformity's sake.

Either one active electrode and one reference electrode with a ground electrode (called monopolar montage) or two active electrodes and a ground electrode (called bipolar montage) is required. The monopolar montage can be utilized with either linked ears or individual ears. The monopolar montage provides specific local information about a given site. A bipolar montage provides more general regional information. The ground can be anywhere on the scalp, but many clinicians use Cz as the ground site unless they are training at Cz in which case any location will work for the ground.

The term linked ears refers to a condition in which each electrode connected to an ear lobe is linked to the other ear electrode, thus the ears are linked together. The rationale behind linking ears is that it should produce the same magnitude readings as a linked-ears database. In addition, the linked-ears electrode arrangement has an added advantage in that it will give more specifically accurate readings at each site; if the clinician relocates the so-called "active" electrode to other areas of the head, he will get more consistently accurate readings. Since amplitude should theoretically vary with the distance from the reference electrode, having two reference electrodes, one on each side of the head linked together, should compensate for voltage variations in the readings that are due primarily to electrode location.

The ground is another issue of controversy. Some suggested locations are the ear, the forehead, the nose, the side of the neck, and the back of the neck. Paul Nunez (2006) indicates there is no theoretically superior placement for the ground. Generally, practitioners agree that placement anywhere above the shoulders is good, otherwise cardiac artifact becomes a problem. Using the back of the neck on a bony prominence, the ear lobe, or forehead provides great success. However, note, most people do not like wires and electrodes on their faces. Therefore, as noted above, many clinicians use a single site on the scalp such as Cz.

Bipolar montages go in and out of fashion frequently. The common term, according to Jay Gunkelman (personal communication), is serial montage. Most equipment can be adapted to support this montage. One problem with the serial montage is that recorded EEG amplitudes are frequently lower if the electrodes are placed too closely. Some clinicians can be confused by this phenomenon. They may mistakenly compare serial montage baselines with their monopolar baselines and believe that they are getting poor results or that their equipment is malfunctioning. Equipment sensitivity, if not adjustable, may also prove a problem and small readings may be difficult to work with. Training may become almost impossible because amplitude variations are so small. Most modern equipment, however, can compensate for this problem.

In the bipolar, or serial, montage, both reference and active electrodes are placed on the scalp. For instance, one might place one electrode halfway between Fz and Cz and the other halfway between Cz and Pz (Lubar, 1995). This placement was often popular for training ADHD in the 1990s. Interestingly, both of these locations have direct connections with the basal ganglia and directly influence the mesolimbic dopamine system. Margret Ayers often placed one electrode at T3 and another at T4 to increase overall EEG amplitude. She indicated that this placement is dangerous for individuals with family histories of seizure disorder because it increases activity across the corpus callosum. The Othmers have used this montage extensively with a very complex set of inhibits and enhancements.

THE 10-20 SYSTEM

The standardized system for electrode placement is known as the international 10-20 system (see Chapter Three). Diagram 13: 10-20 International System shows the format of this system. It is not necessary to put electrodes only at these placements. The system provides a method of describing where the electrodes are placed when you write notes and/or conduct research. Research indicates that considerable variation occurs between individuals with regard to the association between these locations and underlying brain structures (Homan, Herman, & Purdy, 1987). Consequently, it is not necessary to be too precise with electrode placements unless the brain map indicates a very focal abnormality. If placement is within an area slightly larger than the size of a quarter over a particular site, the 10-20 site will be targeted. In the 10-20 system uses the letters and numbers for purposes of identifying specific areas on the scalp. The letters stand for the specific lobe of the brain; F= Frontal, Fp=Pre-Frontal, C=Central, T= Temporal, P= Parietal, and O= Occipital. The numbers indicate specific areas of each lobe where odd numbers indicate the left hemisphere, and even numbers indicate the right hemisphere.

In some cases, you may want to train in different areas besides the 10-20 locations. You should not be afraid to do this with sufficient understanding of the underlying brain anatomy and how it relates to function. Research shows that there can be much variance between the 10-20 system and the underlying structures (Homans, 1987). So, it can be valuable to move the electrode around the area by 5–10% (again, about the diameter of a quarter) during each session.

There is also the matter of individual variation in brain structure. No two brains are alike and there are notable differences and variations of brain structure as the photo below illustrates.

Diagram 38: This MRI scan shows how brain structure varies within individuals.

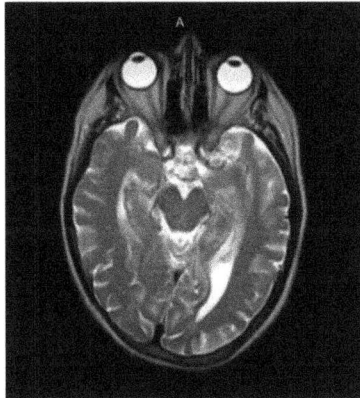

Photo: Courtesy of Dr. Adam Breiner (2017)

Many people entering the field focus excessively on being precise about electrode placement, but research contradicts this approach. There are, however, some clinicians presently doing coherence training. In this instance, accuracy may be important because the locations on the brain maps are the actual locations on the client's scalp; however, an error of 3-6 cm is still probably acceptable. The locations have been determined by how the 10-20 system interfaces with that individual's head and are not based on anatomy. The coherence is measured between locations defined by the 10-20 system.

Artifact

Artifact may at first seem a boring subject of unnecessary detail; however, often a session cannot begin until a troublesome artifact is resolved. When confronted with a client and a time limitation, not being able to determine what is interfering with the readings can be one of the most embarrassing moments in practice. Many novice neurofeedback providers go into a panic when this happens.

Poor connections are usually the source of artifact, which is why there is so much emphasis on good clinical technique. Good technique actually comes from practice more than anything else.

Steps for Electrode Preparation and Placement

1. Use an alcohol pad and/or abrasive preparation such as Nuprep® to thoroughly wipe the scalp (see Diagram 40)

2. Part the hair and hold it down, so that the scalp site is clearly exposed.

3. Maintain control of the hair over the site (this can be difficult) as you try to place the electrode and paste with the other hand. Some practitioners place a cotton ball over the electrode to help keep it in place.

4. Many clinicians use a 1"x1" non-sterile cotton gauze or a cotton ball placed over each attached electrode in order to keep the electrode in place and to absorb excess paste. This helps the clinician place a little extra pressure on the electrode to make sure it is a good tight connection and prevents paste from getting on the clinician's fingers.

Diagram 39: Electrode Placement with guaze covering

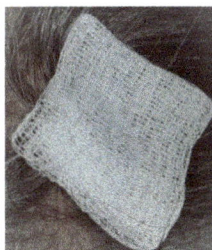

Photo of gauze over ground and bipolar electrode placement.

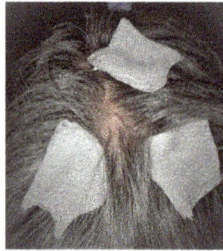

Photo of gauze over ear clip.

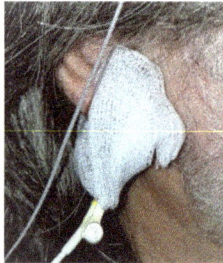

Note: Make sure there is a pea size dab of paste on the electrode first then ask the client to hold it while you do other things.

Diagram 40: Scalp preparation, electrode preparation, and placement.

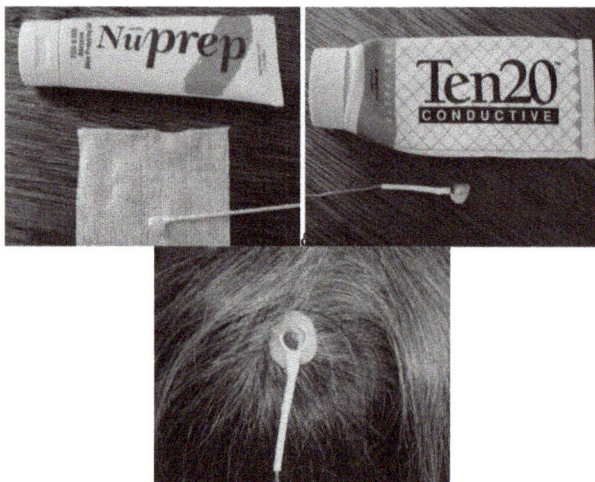

Some novices try to use as little paste as possible to please the client and appease their complaints about how troublesome the glob of paste is in their hair. You need to be firm and remind all involved that this is a clinical procedure and not entertainment. Too little paste is often a major source of trouble. Very short hair will especially prove this point. The bristle of the hair pushes the electrode away from the scalp more so than long hair. Bald heads often require considerable preparation and may need scrubbing with a mild abrasive (i.e., Nuprep) at the site. Special abrasive pads/skin wipes (see Appendix A) can also be used for this procedure.

Poor connections can result in too much amplitude in some component bands and too little in others. For example:

- A poor ground connection can result in very high measures and wild swings in EEG amplitudes.
- A poor reference electrode connection usually looks like there is too little amplitude, as does a poor active electrode connection. There also often appears to be a highly elevated beta with a poor active electrode or reference electrode.
- Eye blinks frequently cause large excursions of the EEG, especially in the low frequency domain.
- Some individuals will register eye blinks as far back on their scalp as Cz. Some individuals move their eyes around a lot as well. This movement looks like smaller hills in the EEG.
- Too much heat coming off the scalp causes excursions that look like hills in the raw EEG.
- Beware of gum chewers and those who grit their teeth when they focus intently, as this will increase general amplitude.

With some children, it is necessary to put an EMG electrode on their jaw muscles to make sure they are not producing what looks like wonderful results by clenching the jaw. Some people generate deviations in EEG when they swallow; this motion also shows up especially well in low frequencies. Diagram 41 shows EEG artifact due to physical movement. To become acquainted with all of them, you should hook the equipment up to yourself. It is well worth the time and effort.

In addition, variation due to head structure and scalp tension exists. Too much scalp tension generates elevated beta frequency that can be very deceptive. Often, when people are training, they will unknowingly tense up their scalp muscles and appear to produce incredible amplitudes of beta. Sometimes the effect is so subtle that it is difficult to tell if beta increases are artifact or scalp tension. If the high beta frequencies are elevated above 8uv at the same time as the beta frequencies are elevated, then it is very likely you are getting contaminated with EMG. Placing an EMG electrode on the scalp can also help identify the difference (if there is a difference). Some equipment has built-in scalp tension sensors that automatically invalidate any data that is tainted. By watching the parallel activity in the beta range and the EMG range, practitioners can roughly assess how much of the signal is EMG. A helpful approach is to work on relaxing the scalp and see how low clients can get their EMG. Over several trials, the clinician can get a sense of what component of the beta is scalp tension and coach clients to stay relaxed during training.

Posture while sitting in the training chair can also create scalp and muscle tension. Make sure the client is relaxed, feet on the ground, legs not crossed, feet not crossed, arms not crossed and on lap or arm rests. A person chewing on their lip or inside of their cheek can create artifact as will a neck that is not well supported.

Diagram 41: EEG Artifact Due to Physical Movement

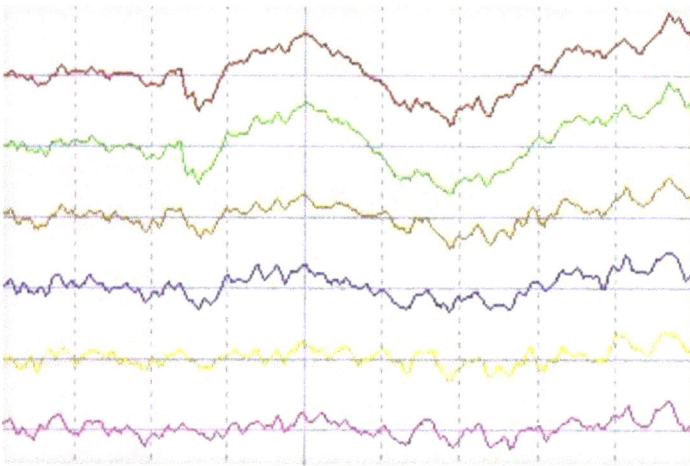

The Sudden Rise and Fall of Waves is Indicative of Movement

It is interesting to note that some clinicians are not convinced that people can learn to appreciably increase beta amplitudes and suspect that perhaps practitioners are just conditioning scalp muscles. Both Barry Sterman and Marvin Sams (personal communication) are convinced that beta is very unreliable and not to be trusted. When training at NewMind, we focus on observing theta reduction even though we may be telling the client to increase beta. We note that during efforts to increase beta, they usually decrease theta first. In fact, Margaret Ayers and Barry Sterman (personal communication) focus more on theta reduction techniques rather than beta enhancement. Many clients can learn to decrease their EEG just as easily, or more easily, than they can learn to increase it. In many cases, this action is preferable. Overall, it is easier to work with slow waves, even though much of the general artifact shows up in these ranges. It is important to watch the client and check to see if the artifact is an eye blink or body movement, being careful because most clients get very uncomfortable when observed too intently.

Feedback usually occurs within 500 ms, based on equipment response times. Considerable training occurs between eye blinks and other periodic artifacts. Our clinical experience shows that good results still ensue.

Clinicians using Z-Score training may have more varied results. Just how much artifact interferes with Z-Score training is not yet clear. In the meantime, it is best to avoid frontal lead artifact as much as possible. One of the best ways to do this is to keep impedances low through good electrode contact.

Some clients register a heartbeat in their EEG. This can be difficult to eliminate but moving the ground to a location higher up the neck or onto the forehead or nose can reduce it considerably. Increasing the time constant or sample rate (also called averaging or damping) of the equipment can help filter out the rhythmic changes in the EEG enough for training purposes. Some individuals, such as those with chronic headache, have such high EMG that on many occasions their EEG is impossible to record or train. They often average upper body EMGs in the range of 25 µV or higher.

For example, one client completely scrambled our signal almost every session. We frequently concluded that our equipment was faulty because all of our connections were perfect. We checked and rechecked everything and were about to give up training her when she informed us that the right side of her face frequently went numb. Like so many other clients, she never told us this important fact—it was not on the intake form. One day, she came in complaining of this condition. We put the EMG electrode on that side of her face. The EMG showed that all her muscles were in spasm, so we trained her to gain control of those muscles and relax them. Once that was done, we were able to get a good EEG signal.

Another example was a seven-year-old boy being trained at Fp1 and Fp2. His Hi-Beta readings were often in excess of 40 µV. A referral to a physical therapist revealed he had postural deficits causing the muscle tension to go up his back, neck, and then scalp to his forehead!

Since then, we have found that some clients come in with so much EMG that their EEG cannot be trained until relaxation training is successful. Once they get more control over their EMG, this situation ceases to be a problem. This is another reason why we like to begin clients with a few sessions of HRV training. They learn to relax in the office chair and produce fewer artifacts. Thus, in some cases, relaxation training may be indicated before a patient is started in neurofeedback.

Sometimes individuals may come in with contact lens problems and/or allergy problems that cause them to blink and swallow a lot. and you will be forced to move your electrode to more posterior areas of the scalp or have the client train with eyes closed. There is some indication that training with eyes open and eyes closed affects the brain differently. However, there is not enough research to verify this. It is worthwhile to look for individual differences in this area in order to compensate, if necessary. We generally train adolescents with eyes open. With adults, we may ask a preference, and when possible, accommodate them.

Don't Panic

Novice neurofeedback trainers often panic as the hour goes by and they cannot isolate the problem with their equipment. They often look less than competent in the new client's eyes. However, the more aroused they become, the poorer problem solvers they become, and they overlook important details. Instead, they need to go through the connections methodically starting with the most common problems and then considering the more rare ones. It is helpful to put the client on audio visual entrainment (AVE) when these problems occur. Less time is wasted, and it does not interfere with the problem-solving efforts. Under these conditions, it is even possible to make a phone call to the manufacturer and ask questions without losing client confidence. In addition, obtaining one-on-one troubleshooting training and drilling is a good idea.

TAKING BASELINES

Baselines are controversial. Some clinicians only take baselines at the outset of treatment and after long intervals of training. Others say that they are almost useless; still others demand a QEEG every 10 sessions. The Othmers have a huge database on baselines before and after training and have noticed very little change in many individual baselines despite dramatic changes in behavior. So, what is actually changing, if this is the case?

The argument has often been made that mostly responsivity, or plasticity, is changing under cognitive load. That is to say, the way the EEG looks when the brain is performing a task is changing. Therefore, a better measure of change is training performance. To deal with this controversy, Lubar (1995) averages baseline and training averages together. The results appear useful, but the reasoning may not hold up under close scrutiny. One of the major problems with training any one neurometric dimension such as amplitude is that the major changes occurring may be in one of the other four neurometric dimensions such as asymmetry which you may not be tracking. In addition, the changes occurring may be at other nodes or hubs associated with the location(s) you are training rather than a major change occurring at the location you are actively training. In this case a map looking at all five neurometric dimensions in all locations is more likely to capture change. For this reason, we tend to measure percent of change across all locations and neurometric dimensions with the assumption that we are training the brain as a highly integrated system.

With this method we can also review what percent of the change is in the normative direction and what percent is moving away from the norm as the brain reorganizes. Our archival analysis of thousands of brainmaps from the NewMind database indicates a change of approximately 28-30%% is typically common with neurofeedback. We therefore recommend that clinicians remap every 15 to 20 sessions and compare the percent change in the map with the percent changes in the symptom tracker. Ultimately, what really counts, is the clients experience of change.

Without a map you can often estimate the changes you might expect from remapping if you have years of experience but those starting out would be better advised to use a pre-post map evaluation. Nevertheless, significant findings can occur just using a single or two channel baseline.

Diagram 42: One Month Cycle

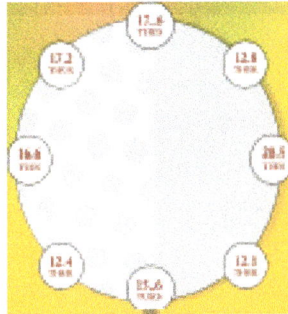

Diagram 42. One-month cycle: alpha (7–10 Hz) baselines in microVolts. This figure shows how the baseline varied in one client. In her case, the baseline EEG shifted as much as 8 µV from session to session within the same week. The figure shows only the variation in the alpha amplitudes, but other frequency component bands shifted similarly. It is interesting to note that the client's frontal alpha was consistently high on Tuesday and low on Thursday. Overall, the baseline amplitude decreased over the month, possibly due to the training. As mentioned before, this is not always the case, but in this instance, the baseline correlated with symptom improvement. The chart below shows the baseline blood pressure drop as the baseline alpha dropped.

Hz	T	Th		T		Th	T	Th
	4/22	4/24 4/29		5/8 5/13		5/15	5/20	5/22
4–6	7.1	6.1	7.2	6.5	9.6	6.3	6.9	6.9
7–10	17.6	12.8	20.5	12.1 15.6		12.4	16.6	17.2
15–30	14.9	14.0 14.7		14.1 19.0		13.6	15.3	14.9
BP	----	---- 17	190/1	---	---	163/107	---	158/106

The client's depression shifted into the normal range as well. If a baseline had not been taken at each session and instead the alpha threshold had been set consistently at 15 µV, one would have the impression that she was doing a better job of training her alpha down on Thursdays than on Tuesdays. This could have led to making the training too difficult on Tuesdays and she would have not trained as well (due to ratio strain).

In the past, many clinicians have taken a baseline at just Cz alone. Michael Tansey, an early pioneer in the clinical use of neurofeedback (Lubar Workshop) obtained tremendous results doing eyes closed SMR training at Cz alone. The Othmers originally used to take their baselines at C3, Cz, and C4. This process is arguably a limited picture of the brain's EEG activity and perhaps explains why QEEG specialists see changes others do not. They may be seeing more subtle shifts due to the resolution of their database. In spite of rumors to the contrary, those of us using QEEG do see changes and usually in the expected direction. These changes are not as dramatic as was once expected early in the development of the field, but research has shown that the brain does not get rid of old networks, it builds new networks (Turner et al., 2011). The changes are going to be more subtle in many cases rather than dramatically returning to some theoretical norm.

In our experience, we have often seen greater changes in asymmetry or coherence than in spectral distribution and amplitude. Either way, it is the client's subjective perspective that counts most in the end. If the client feels better and symptoms are diminishing, then the brain is changing. When doing research, it is clearly best to use QEEGs. However, many clinicians do fine with monopolar analysis.

Monopolar Analysis: The Mini Q

Monopolar exploration can be used almost as effectively as QEEG. If the norm for Cz is known, you can almost predict what the brain map is going to show generally, due to volume conduction, by taking five or six readings at different basic sites. Careful monopolar exploration around other areas of the scalp can further confirm initial observations of possible emerging patterns. This approach, however, works best with the right kind of EEG equipment, a good working knowledge of neurophysiology, and considerable prior experience or training in what to look for.

Diagram 43: EEG Distribution

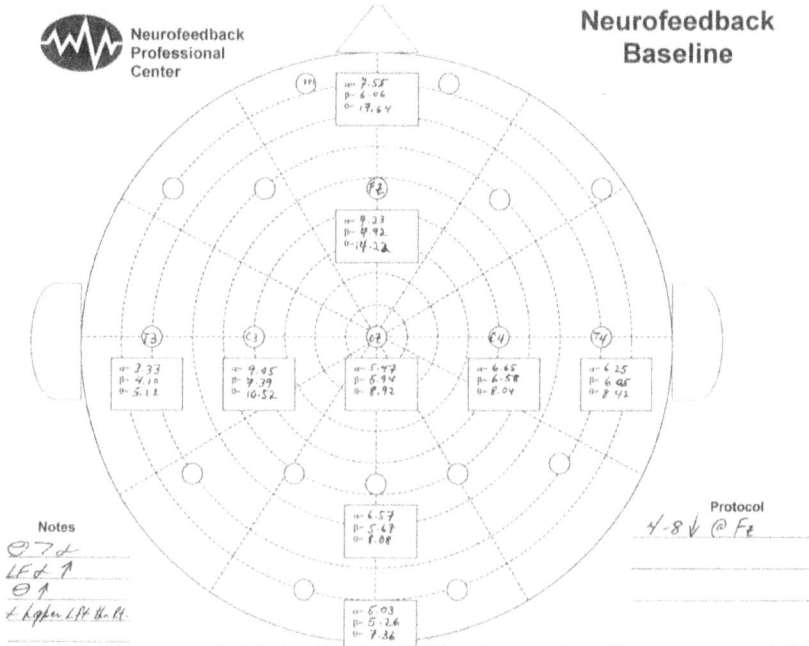

Diagram 43. EEG distributions on a sample single-electrode eyes-closed brain map. When starting with Cz, it is apparent that alpha is lower than beta or theta, which is less than optimal for the eyes-closed condition. In terms of anterior to posterior amplitude (i.e., in front of and behind the sensorimotor strip, theta clearly decreases in the posterior direction and increases as you move frontally from 8.92 to 17.64 by the time you reach Fpz. This individual is clearly ADHD with too much frontal theta. Beta at Fz is 4.92 while it is 5.67 at Pz, which is also abnormal.

Because of this tremendous variation, the neurology community was initially skeptical of the value of QEEG, and still is today. E. Roy John (1988), however, has demonstrated a strong consistency in EEGs across cultures and age groups for normal individuals and has found a method to calculate a useful database. Hershel Toomim (personal communication) has long been a champion of looking at beta-to-theta ratios to offset this problem in another way. By calculating the ratios among all standard frequency ranges (component bands) in normative individuals, those ratios can be used as an indicator of EEG deviance by comparing them with ratios of other individuals.

Diagram 44: Estimated Standard Deviations of Magnitude at Cz

Estimated Standard Deviations Of Magnitude At Cz

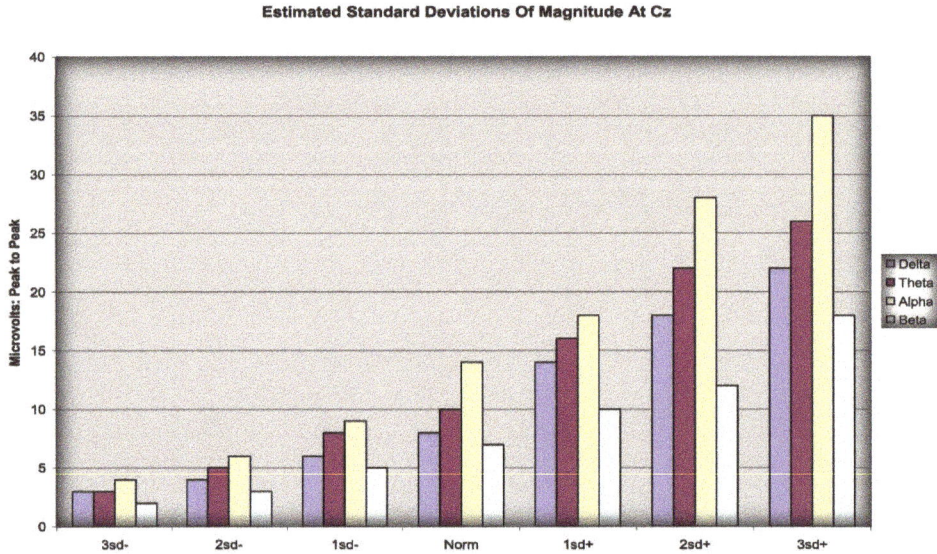

REVIEW

It is often useful to look at the brain in terms of activity in the front versus activity in the back and left versus right. The brain should be running faster in the front and slower in the back. It should also be running faster on the left side than on the right. At Cz, research indicates that with eyes closed, alpha should be highest with theta about 2/3 of alpha and beta 1/2 to 1/3 of alpha (Montgomery, 1998). Brain maps indicate that the ratio should shift slightly as you move forward toward Fpz with beta becoming progressively higher and alpha and theta becoming progressively lower. The ratio should also shift backwards with beta and theta diminishing and alpha increasing. By taking a baseline at Fz, and perhaps Fpz, you can watch for a trend in the spectral or component band distribution. If theta is increasing, then ADHD may be present. If alpha is increasing, then depression may be present. If beta increases dramatically, then anxiety is possible. By taking a baseline at Pz, you can look for similar trends. If theta increases dramatically in the component band distribution, then repressed trauma is possible. If beta increases, intense emotionality related to anxiety is possible. When moving toward the occipital cortex, alpha should increase. This type of analysis is known as midline analysis and can be found in the NewMind map report (see Diagram 45: Midline Analysis).

Diagram 45: Midline Analysis

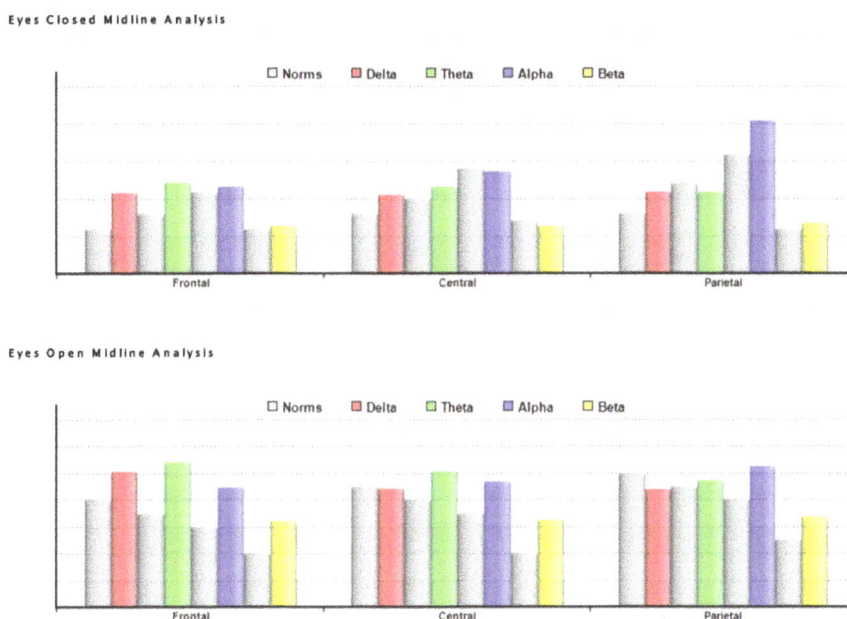

Eyes Closed Midline Analysis

Eyes Open Midline Analysis

Taking bilateral readings simultaneously at C3 and C4, on the other hand, allows you to compare differences and determine hemispheric symmetry, based upon magnitude differences. Anxiety, depression, and ADHD have definite bilateral signatures. Anxiety and especially mania, tend to push beta to the right. As previously mentioned in the other chapters depression usually shows as alpha higher on the left side than the right. Bob Gurnee at the ADD Clinic in Scottsdale Arizona (personal communication) was one of the first clinicians to use QEEG and believe that high alpha in the right frontal area is associated with a subtype of ADHD. Other research relates high frontal theta or alpha to OCD in some cases (see Chapter 3).

Eyes-open frontal theta or alpha can also indicate ADHD or depression. If you ask a client to perform backward serial 7s, that is, count backward from 100 by 7s, and the client's alpha or theta increases, then you are likely dealing with ADHD. Clients can read or do a computerized performance test and show the same phenomenon. Alpha waves can be further broken down into low 8-10 Hz alpha and high 10-12 Hz alpha. Many individuals with depression have very high eyes-open alpha, but very normal eyes-closed alpha. When brain maps are evaluated, this alpha is often found in the 8–9 Hz range. Alpha in these ranges is also found in cases of damage to the frontal area due to toxic exposure or excess use of amphetamines or cocaine derivatives. It frequently looks like ADHD on the testing and this frequency has been found dominant in one case with drug-related psychosis. We have seen elevated SMR in over a dozen cases of mycotoxin exposure along with a great deal of global slowing with very low amplitudes in the beta range. (Aflatoxins are naturally occurring mycotoxins that are produced by many species of Aspergillus, a fungus. Aflatoxins are toxic and among the most carcinogenic substances known; Aflatoxin, n.d.). We have seen a similar pattern in some seizure disorders. Interestingly, coherence was not relevantly abnormal in these cases.

If the equipment allows you to look at frequency in some form of spectral display, you will find that anxiety varies in appearance between excess 16–20 Hz to excess 23–30 Hz. The lower 16–20 Hz range is referred to as the "beta ridge" by the Lubars (personal communication). It often shows up in individuals who are very controlling and argumentative. In addition, they often have a lot of physical symptoms, especially severe sleep problems. The 23–30 Hz range tends to show up more as a hyper-vigilant type of anxiety. At this point in the evolution of our technology we can see that these beta issues are actually the subtle results of EMG bracing.

Focal areas of high theta or delta are often related to local tissue damage (Knyazev, 2012). The theta appears to be more related to the reduced perfusion that accompanies lesions (Caltagirone, Guido, Menghini, Pasini, Spalleta, 2001).

These baselines provide clear indicators of where to train. Although not as accurate as a QEEG, they closely predict what the maps will show with respect to amplitude or magnitude. The most difficult frequency to assess in this manner is beta. Beta typically changes very little in amplitude and small deviations in beta with respect to the norms can be meaningful, but hard to recognize. The beta-to-theta ratio is often a good alternative indicator of the strength of the beta level.

The baselines can be checked regularly as clients are treated without sacrificing a great deal of time and expense. Dramatic changes can be seen in bilateral baselines and performance averages. Large global changes, on the other hand, tend to occur very slowly over time. Sometimes they are not visible for a year or so.

Research finds correlations between intense emotions, rumination and posterior beta (Engles et al., 2007). Many clinicians report posterior beta present in anxiety as well. In this case, you will see that beta is higher in the right temporal or parietal area than in the left, which suggests anxiety.

If you check the asymmetry between left and right hemispheres in Diagram 43, you will see that the alpha is 6.65 on the right and 9.05 on the left. Clearly, alpha is highest on the left, which is consistent with depression. Theta is much higher on the left as well. The left hemisphere is under-activated.

In this example, we decided to start with theta suppression at Fz. If such a client does not respond well to this protocol, we might try dealing with the depression first by up-training alpha in the right hemisphere or beta in the left hemisphere or both at the same time. Every client varies in his or her response to a protocol, which is why neurofeedback is not a cut-and-dried process.

Basic QEEG Preparation

The more popular alternative these days to the above assessment approach is the QEEG. When planning to conduct a QEEG (a full 19 point assessment), on patients, there are a few basic instructions to follow. QEEGs are best conducted in the morning versus afternoon, that is, between the hours of 9:00 a.m. and 1:00 p.m. Many experts insist on avoiding caffeine, but many people are habituated to caffeine, with associated neurophysiological changes. Avoiding it may actually distort their "usual" record. With no caffeine, more drowsiness and slowing may be present in the record, whereas with the caffeine, they may demonstrate a more normal record because of their habituation. On the other hand, too much caffeine may also distort the record with excessive fast-wave activity. In this case, moderation is likely to give the most accurate record.

If the patient is taking stimulant medication (i.e., ADHD medication), it is preferable to do the QEEG after the patient has not taken the medication for 48 hours. The patient MUST check with his/her prescribing physician to determine if it is possible to stop taking the stimulants 48 hours prior to the QEEG. If a break of 48 hours is not advisable, a break of 24 hours is the next preferred length, and a break of 12–24 hours is the next preferred length after that. Do not make changes in any other medication (unless authorized by the patient's physician). Follow these steps:

1. If the patient is sick, instruct him or her to call to reschedule, even if he or she only has a cold.

2. The patient should not drink the usual amount of coffee, tea, Red Bull, caffeinated soft drinks, or any other substance with caffeine for at least 15 hours prior to the QEEG. A small amount is preferable.

Note: If the patient drinks coffee or caffeinated beverages in the morning, then stopping caffeine may affect the outcome of the QEEG. Over time, individuals may habituate to a mild stimulus such as regular coffee and develop a physiological adaptation. For instance, not drinking the usual amount of coffee may result in headaches and fogginess that generate an abnormal EEG pattern with increased alpha slowing and/or increased scalp EMG. This may accentuate the EEG abnormalities more than the coffee. More research needs to be done in this area to clarify these kinds of confounds.

3. Patients should avoid taking any over-the-counter medication or supplements for 3 to 4 days prior to the QEEG.

4. The patient should be instructed to wash his or her hair the night

before the QEEG by doing the following:

- Wash hair three times with a pH neutral cleansing/clarifying shampoo, such as Neutrogena non-residue shampoo.
- Do not use creme rinse or any other hair product prior to the QEEG appointment.
- Do not wash hair again in the morning of the appointment.
- Make sure hair is completely dry before coming for the QEEG.

5. The patient should be instructed to get a good night's sleep before the QEEG (let the practitioner know if there are any sleep problems or disturbances); 6 or more hours of sleep are preferred.

The day of the QEEG, the patient should:

6. Eat a high-protein breakfast.

7. Drink plenty of water.

8. Use the restroom just prior to the start of the QEEG.

9. When conducting a QEEG, you should always begin with eyes-closed measures.

Testing

Testing is not always necessary, since clients frequently arrive with a diagnosis. However, it can be very helpful for a variety of reasons. Clients often arrive with a diagnosis that may or may not be accurate. Often, they self-diagnose and present their diagnosis as if it were professionally derived. On the other hand, diagnostic categories do not always correlate with EEG patterns. One protocol does not always work best with a specific disorder. Because of these problems, it is not a good idea to rely too much on diagnostic categories for treatment plans.

For neurofeedback, an EEG analysis is more important. Since symptoms are usually being treated, it is more important to have a list of specific symptoms and problem behaviors. The symptom and behavioral changes guide the practitioner. Using a symptom tracking system is helpful to track changes over time.

Monitoring session progress helps show changes to the client, so clients can see their progress. Often the changes are very subtle for the first 10 sessions. Some clients may not even be aware of the changes taking place until 20 or 30 sessions. Even then, they may not recognize that changes have been happening until they have changed a great deal. In fact, others around them often notice the changes first. For this reason, it is important to involve those who are close to the client to observe the changes and make comments and use a symptom tracker of some kind to keep a record of the client's self-report.

The tests we have used in the past were the Test of Variables of Attention (TOVA) or the IVA, which very similar but shorter, the Beck Depression Inventory, the Interactive Self Inventory (ISI) or Personality Assessment Inventory (PAI), and MicroCog. Recently, we have (NewMind Technologies) developed a subjective questionnaire that generates a predictive brain map called the the Cognitive Emotional Checklist (CEC). It can be accessed on our website at www.newmindmaps.com. This questionnaire can help clinicians determine which locations should be reviewed with the greatest scrutiny on the actual brain map with respect to symptomology. In addition, we have the NewMind Computerized Performance Tests to assess progress with respect to attention, short term and working memory and filtering. CNS Vital Signs is also a very popular computerized cognitive battery. These tests are not especially long or expensive. They cover basic areas of change such as mood, cognitive functioning, and personality.

The clinician determines the frequency and administration of all these tests. To demonstrate change, some individuals require more objective measures than others, depending on how much self-awareness they have in the beginning. Others may require the tests for review by other professionals, such as medical doctors or lawyers. We have especially relied on the TOVA and Beck Depression Inventory in the past. The Interactive Self Inventory, which we developed, provides us with much of this information in one package, including information on personal interaction style that can confound training outside of the office environment.

The Othmers should also be commended for developing a short TOVA-like test, the Quick Test. This test can be conducted at the end of each session for session-to-session evaluation. With these new emerging tests designed especially for the neurofeedback practitioner, the clinician should find his or her job much easier in today's clinical environment.

Diagram 46: Example of targets used in the Test of Variables of Attention (TOVA)

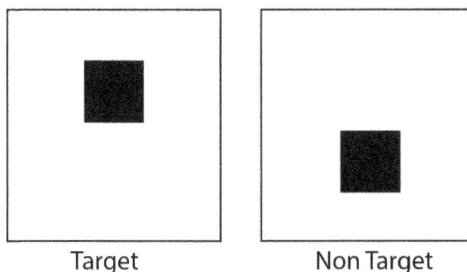

Target   Non Target

Test of Variables of Attention

In the TOVA (Diagram 46), targets flash on the computer screen in a relatively random pattern. Clients must click on a button, which they hold in one hand, when the target appears and avoid clicking when the non-target appears. The test is nonverbal in nature and lasts 22 minutes.

The test records the following:

- missed targets (omissions)
- clicked non-targets (commissions)
- consistency and response time

This test provides a very good measure of attention and is sensitive to how it is impacted by ADD, depression, and anxiety. Since it is normed, relatively quick, and inexpensive, it is a good objective measure of progress in neurofeedback training. The IVA is a similar test that integrates auditory testing with the visual test and is also available to neurofeedback clinicians.

Using Tests Together

One client came to us with problems of memory, concentration, and complaints that she might be less than intelligent. This client had trouble getting motivated. Her EEG showed very high amplitude eyes-closed low frequency alpha. We often find that this situation is an indicator of depression or ADD. In order to distinguish between the two disorders, we gave her the above combination of tests.

Before testing, we made sure there was no history of head injury. Her TOVA showed a mild attentional difficulty, but not ADHD. The MicroCog indicated normal intelligence, but poor short term memory function. The Beck Depression Inventory confirmed problems with anxiety and some mild depression. We showed her the tests and explained that the short-term memory deficit was likely a result of chronic anxiety leading to depression. The prolonged over-arousal of her sympathetic nervous system had generated so much cortisol that it had degraded function in her hippocampus. We then began training her for the depression that likely developed as a result of chronic anxiety. (Beta training at C3 often works well, and in more recent times we typically combine it alpha asymmetry training as well.)

We have had other clients who were only interested in a reduction of symptoms and did not see the value of the tests. One option in dealing with this kind of client, is to use a subjective symptom checklist that the client fills out at the beginning of each session. Through self-reporting, clients easily see progressive changes. This process sensitizes them to their own changes and provides us with a way to go back and show them what they themselves have observed in the course of their own training. In fact we have found it very effective to use such a checklist on a regular basis with all clients. It aids significantly in helping clients recognize important changes which they might otherwise experience and simply habituate to without acknowledgement. This acknowledgement of progress is often very valuable with respect to client retention and compliance. A sample of this type of checklist can be found in Appendix D: Forms.

Clinical Etiquette

Most clinicians are familiar with the rules of clinical etiquette; however, issues arise unique to neurofeedback that should be discussed.

Creating the Environment

Managing the environment so that it is a relaxed and predictable atmosphere is important. When clients are alpha training or engaged in Alpha-Theta training, it is important to keep the room quiet and avoid all distractions. Eliminating ringing phones or other intrusions is critical. Making sure the client's chair is comfortable and adequate and maintaining a comfortable room temperature are important. Having a fan present can help some clients avoid getting overheated which can lead to artifacts and poor training. For example, when clients get too hot, the electrode paste tends to melt, distorting signals as electrodes come loose and fall off. A blanket for individuals with low core temperature or poor peripheral vascularity may also be helpful with getting them to relax and let go. On the other hand, during beta or SMR uptraining, distractions are actually helpful challenges to client training.

Developing Routines

Practitioners should develop a set routine to avoid upsetting sensitive clients. Explaining each step of the routine before it is performed helps clients remain calm and comfortable until they are familiar with the protocol. This is especially important with anxious adults and children and children with ASD, including filling out progress reports, electrode placement on the scalp, and general preparation for a neurofeedback session.

Explaining Neurofeedback

Because of the nature of neurofeedback training, many practitioners find clients complaining that they don't understand what they are doing, or asking, "How am I doing this?" Clients may often say, "I still don't get how this works." Although clients would never question a pill or the mechanisms of anesthetics, the neurofeedback environment is so novel and alien to their way of thinking that it is difficult for them to accept what is going on until they experience a dramatic change.

It is a good idea to develop a series of well-rehearsed short answers that can become more complex as the knowledge of the client grows. Clients frequently want something to read regarding neurofeedback and its efficacy. At NewMind, we often give them scientific research, which they happily accept even though most of them do not have the training to interpret the research. Providing client friendly brochures may be more helpful. Rob Longo (2018) has written a book specifically for this purpose which we handout to every client. It is presently available on Amazon. The internet can also be a good tool because clients can access detailed explanations from your own site and/or other sites at any time.

Having printed information available to clients/patients can also help with understanding of QEEG mapping and the neurofeedback process (Longo, 2018).

Recognizing Changes

To help clients recognize changes, you should discuss expected changes before training begins. Clients are very likely to attribute changes to other factors at first. Changes in response to stressors and sleep patterns are among the first that they notice. Asking about symptoms at each session will help keep track of changes, so you can support client observations and assist them in arriving at their own conclusions based on their own observations. It often takes an extended period before they realize that the changes are permanent and likely due to the neurofeedback.

Having clients/patients chart weekly progress on symptoms for they would like to see improvement can be beneficial in demonstrating overall progress with neurofeedback and illustrated below.

Diagram 47: Example of Progress Tracker

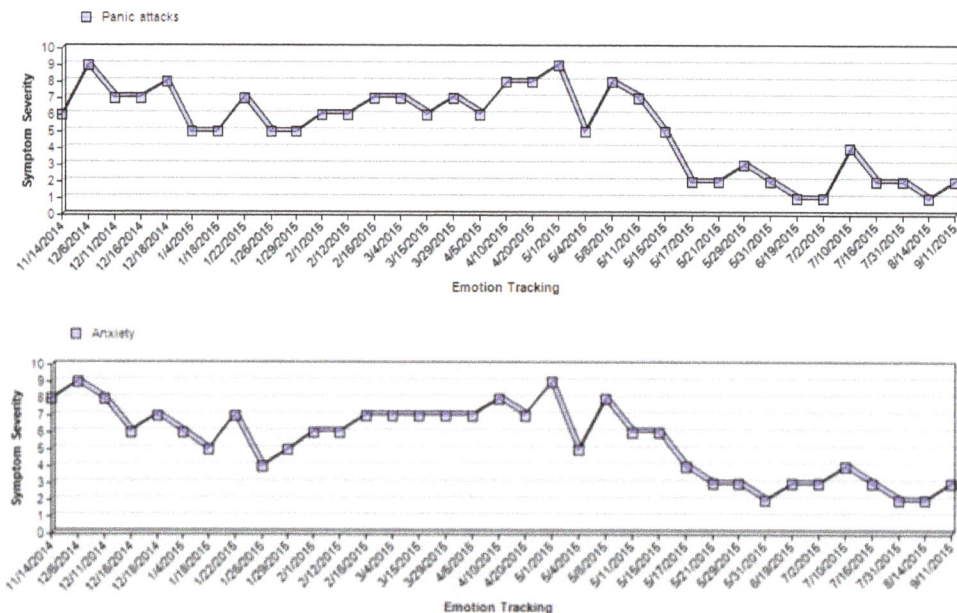

Note: problems may arise if expected changes are emphasized too much, because many clients will believe that change is due to the placebo effect.

Audio visual entrainment or AVE is a tremendous help for managing clients. When they come in overtired and falling asleep during training, a 10-minute AVE session can refresh them and get them working effectively at training again. When they look for something dramatic during the first few sessions, AVE provides them with the stimulation they seek. They are often more willing to accept the efficacy of AVE at the outset because it is so dramatic. Interestingly, in our experience, clients ask fewer questions regarding it.

Results from AVE are usually short lived but dramatic, and clients are excited about the training. This helps them focus on the NFB more. Eventually they realize on their own that the effects of the NFB are more profound and longer lasting. Clients then shift their enthusiasm over to NFB with fewer questions and complaints. Consequently, our approach has evolved to the point where we combine neurofeedback with the photic stimulation component of AVE throughout the entire course of training, with the exception of Alpha-Theta training. The two work so well synergistically that several vendors have evolved their equipment to encompass both technologies.

Problem Clients

Occasionally clients are confrontational and suspicious and their questions reflect this. This situation often happens with individuals with personality disorders or with severely depressed clients who harbor considerable anger. Until clients experience dramatic changes in their conditions, this needs to be delicately managed, which requires more patience on the part of the clinician than with other clients. Patient and consistent responses with firm reassurances are often necessary and most effective.

For example, should you be challenged by a client at every session in a way that undermines your confidence, it is possible that the client has borderline personality disorder. These individuals require a practitioner with considerable clinical skill. It is best to refer them to someone who has this expertise Importantly, these clients may be prone to legal action. Personality tests at the outset can be a great help in identifying this type of client.

Clients who are highly sensitive to environmental conditions may also be hypersensitive to neurofeedback. When working with this population it is a good idea to start them out with a 3 to 5 minute session of SMR training at Cz and wait overnight to assess their response. If they have a strong abreaction then they are likely a poor candidate for neurofeedback training and should do biofeedback training such as HRV training first to stabilize their system more before again trying neurofeedback.

Note: do not engage in argument with clients. Refer to more experienced clinicians if necessary.

Under What Conditions is Neurofeedback Less Effective in Achieving Optimal Results?

In our experience, we have found three circumstances in which clients/patients may show low or minimal progress while participating in neurofeedback (Longo, 2018).

1. When patients taking multiple medications for mental health disorders, such as anxiety, depression, ADHD, insomnia, etc., are not working with their health care prescriber to adjust their medications. This includes appropriately discontinuing medication in response to their progress with their neurofeedback program. In no case should a client use illicit street drugs, e.g., cocaine, marijuana, etc., as they also interfere with neurofeedback training.

2. When persons who experience ongoing stressors during most of their day, e.g., job related stress, or stressful relationships avoid addressing these stressors through mental health counseling and/or other mental health interventions.

3. When persons who have certain serious physical health problems, i.e., serious GI problems, untreated thyroid conditions, heavy metal toxicity, chemical imbalances (i.e., excessive copper); these problems can lead to significant sleep disturbances.

Drug Effects on EEG

A fair amount of literature is available on this topic. It is important to know this information to better assess the baseline analysis of clients. Table 10: Drug Effects on EEG, lists the drugs most frequently encountered that have a significant effect on EEG. Overall, at typical doses they do not make dramatic changes in the EEG to the point where they interfere with the QEEG and training process. At high doses they can have a significant effect on both.

In most cases our goal is to reduce our clients' reliance on pharmaceuticals as much as possible if not get them off of drugs entirely. If clients do not reduce their dose levels after approximately eight sessions they will typically begin to feel the side effects of the drugs and often attribute the side effects to the neurofeedback rather than realize they are improving due to the neurofeedback and therefore require less medication. Clients should be made aware of this potential predicament before they begin training.

Recently, it has come to our attention that benzodiazepines can confound training with NFB—especially Alpha-Theta training. Many people using these drugs are either addicted to them or experiencing a long withdrawal and recovery period. Some psychiatrists even refuse to work with them. Typically, training someone who is on SSRIs or methylphenidate derivatives does not retard training results, but some newer drugs appear to have this capacity.

Table 10: Drug Effects on EEG

Family	Drugs	Purpose	EEG Impact
Neuroleptics	Haldol, Prolixin, Thorazine, Mellaril	sedative	increase delta, theta and beta above 20 Hz and decrease alpha and beta below 20 Hz.
Neuroleptics	Seroquel, Risperdal, Geodon	non-sedative and antipsychotic medications	decrease alpha and increase beta in general.
Anxiolytics	Valium, Halcion, Librium, Dalmane	anxiety relief	decrease alpha and increase beta, especially 13–20 Hz beta
Benzodiazepines	Valium, Xanax, and Ativan	anxiety, panic relief	decrease alpha and increase 20–30 Hz beta
SSRIs	Prozac, Paxil, and Zoloft	a class of antidepressants used in the treatment of depression, anxiety disorders, and some personality disorders.	decrease in frontal alpha and a mild increase in 18–25 Hz beta.
MAO Inhibitors	Marplan, Parnate, Eldepryl	antidepressant	tendency to increase 20–30 Hz beta while decreasing all other frequencies
Tricyclic antidepressants	Imipramine and Amitriptyline	useful in depressed patients with insomnia, restlessness, and nervousness	increase delta and theta while decreasing alpha; increase beta 25 Hz and up Beta Band
Antipsychotics	Lithium	used for the treatment of manic/depressive (bipolar) and depressive disorders	increases theta, mildly decreases alpha and increases beta
Amphetamines	Adderall, Vyvanse, and Dexedrine	a group of drugs that act by increasing levels of norepinephrine, serotonin, and dopamine in the brain	decrease slow-wave activity and increase beta in the 12–26 Hz range
Marijuana		recreational and Medicinal	increases frontal low frequency alpha; affects EEG for 3 days

Opiates	Opium, hydromorphone, oxymorphone, heroin, morphine, oxycodone, Talwin, codeine, methadone, meperidine, hydrocodone, Vicodin	pain relief	generate high amplitude slow alpha in the 8 Hz range
Barbiturates	Brevital, thiamylal (Surital), thiopental (Pentothal), amobarbital, Amytal, pentobarbital, Nembutal, secobarbital, Seconal, Tuinal, Phenobarbital, Luminal, mephobarbital, Mebaral	produce a wide spectrum of central nervous system depression, from mild sedation to coma, and have been used as sedatives, hypnotics, anesthetics, and anticonvulsants	increase beta at 25–35 Hz amplitude
Caffeine		Increases alertness	increases beta and decreases slower waves

REVIEW QUESTIONS

1. What is Ohm's law?
2. What is impedance?
3. What are $E = I \times R$; $V = R \times I$; $I = V / R$; and $R = V / I$?
4. What effect do barbiturates have on the brain?
5. What is common mode rejection?
6. What are the differences between a low-pass filter and a high-pass filter?
7. What is a fast Fourier transform?
8. What effects are seen from opiates?
9. What is a standard deviation from Cz?

Chapter 6: Protocols and Training

LEARNING THEORY AND EEG TRAINING

Neurofeedback training is a form of operant conditioning and to some degree classical conditioning as well. It is important to know the basics regarding these two subjects and a basic psychology text can refresh your memory. See also Sherlin et al. (2011) for a review. The discussion that follows is based on a review of that article and several related articles.

The literature on operant conditioning and classical conditioning is vast and reaches back to its birth in the early 20th century. Discussions on this topic could fill volumes and its relationship to neurofeedback could easily fill a book. It requires considerable training and studying just to understand the intricacies of operant conditioning schedules and their implications. There is considerable disagreement within the field of neurofeedback on how the principles of operant and classical conditioning should be interpreted and applied as well as what procedures are most effective. Within the field of neurofeedback Sherlin et al. (2011) attempted to lay the basic theoretical groundwork, which was a good start. However, their overview did not articulate caveats noted by other authors. We will attempt to review the issues in terms of how they inform the practice of neurofeedback and will avoid detailing the theoretical disagreements.

Frederick (2016) observes that in 1962 Kamiya initially engaged in experiments where subjects learned to identify a state associated with alpha and then could produce that state and alpha at will. This ability to discriminate the alpha state is very similar to the practice of "Neuromonitoring" as taught by Anna Wise (1997) and based on the research of Maxwell Cade (1987). In her workshops she would guide individuals through exercises and monitor their EEG pattern in order to teach them to recognize subjective states associated with each component band. In this manner they appeared to learn to produce the states at will. She did not publish experimental results, but her success could easily be observed in the workshop settings. In a sense she was guiding them or sensitizing them to interoceptive sensations that indicated they were successful. This approach involved both awareness and discrimination. There is a response plan involving an anticipated effect and a response effect. A comparison and a reward occurs (actual state achievement) or does not occur.

Kamiya wanted to see if conscious discrimination was required to produce alpha and then trained subjects by rewarding them whenever alpha occurred. He found this also worked well and Frederick notes this was how the field neurofeedback was born. Neurofeedback was adopted by behaviorists and the phenomenological side of subjective state awareness was jettisoned- except for Anna Wise. Nonetheless Frederick notes that both types are a form of operant conditioning and suggests we may find value in exploring the EEG discriminative training in more detail.

Sterman (1963), following a long history of classical and operant conditioning of the alpha blocking investigations going back to 1935 began experimenting with classical and operant conditioning of the EEG in cats as it relates to sleep. In 1968 he demonstrated it was possible to use operant conditioning of SMR in cats. After decades of replicated studies, Sterman has proven that brainwave training in humans through operant conditioning is not only possible but also has outlined the basic principles involved (Sherlin et al., 2011).

Sherlin et al. (2011), whose authors included Sterman and a who's who in the field of neurofeedback, was published in 2011 in an effort to define the basic principles underlying the operant conditioning of the EEG and articulate how they should be adhered to in the clinical setting. The investigations of other authors such as Luft (2014), however, suggest there is more to be considered then the publication offered. This agrees with our observation that a large majority of practitioners and vendors in the field have ignored several of these principles or their proposed method of implementation and have produced excellent results at the clinical level. What appears true in a lab may not necessarily generalize to the clinical setting. With the existing paucity of research at this point on this topic and an abundance of theoretical admonishments, it is probably best to understand the basics and utilize them as a tentative guide. You will likely be able to innovate clinically in a more effective manner to aid your clients if you understand these basics. Although most are achieving excellent outcomes, some of the disregarded aspects, such as post reinforcement synchronization (PRS) and the innovations around maligned abundant use of auto-thresholding may lead to new clinical insights and improvements.

These challenges regarding the principles of neurofeedback training will become more problematic over time as the field continues to grow, and more companies and developers produce an increasing number of devices on the market claiming to do neurofeedback with a phone app.

Let's begin with classical conditioning. As we have said, research in this area lead to operant conditioning research but the role it plays in neurofeedback is still not well defined. Classical conditioning involves pairing a natural reflex (potential or unconditioned response) with a neutral stimulus (that otherwise would not produce the response) such that the stimulus elicits the same response every time. The neutral stimulus becomes the conditioned stimulus. Pavlov found that a dog salivates when he hears footsteps associated with food in his bowl. Salivation, which is an unconditioned response to food (a natural reflex) becomes transformed, when it is constantly paired with footsteps plus food, into a conditioned response. It is conditioned to the footsteps. Footsteps become transformed into the conditioned stimulus as it has gained status in the dog world by hanging about the food all the time. It is a food associate. Footsteps now call forth salivation instead of just food alone. The dog has learned a new association.

Frederick (2016) argues that repeated pairing of subjective correlates of the physiological state with the feedback signal is a key component of neurofeedback and allows response effort and response effectiveness to be perceived by the organism. Identifying that such a relationship exists and bringing it to the foreground of attention is a key initial phase in order that operant conditioning can occur. But is EEG a reflex in the classical sense, an inborn reflex that is an unconditioned response? We would argue it is more an unseen operant, a freely emitted but unseen behavior- Skinner's black box is not so opaque. Earlier researchers in the 30s and 40s, however, considered alpha blocking, that is the reduction of alpha waves that occurs when a light appears in a dark room (they believed this was a reflexive response to light) as an unconditioned response. They used it to see if they could classically condition brainwaves. Soon this led to more questions and they began pairing alpha blocking with different stimuli. Arguments followed that it was not a reflex, but the unconditioned response was to an anticipatory response or "cortical state" that mediated and resulted in the alpha blocking. This led to using other stimuli as they realized alpha blocking was not exclusively tied to light. Further studies resulted in not resolving the issue whether blocking was due to classical conditioning or simply sensitization. We have learned that alpha blocking represents a response to any novel stimulus to be processed- it is not a true reflex.

In learning theory, the terms positive and negative do not mean good and bad. Instead positive means you are adding something (a stimulus) and negative means you are taking something (a stimulus) away. Reinforcement is meant to increase a behavior by adding a stimulus or taking a stimulus away. Punishment, on the other hand, can be used to decrease a behavior but it is not the preferred method of altering behavior because it can produce unanticipated and undesirable consequences. Consequently, neurofeedback methods focus on reinforcement and present a stimulus.

An operant is any freely emitted behavior and not a reflex (reflexes are related more to classical conditioning theory). Brainwaves do appear to be abundant and freely emitted as well as tied to behavior if not a behavior in their own right. For instance, imagining a behavior causes specific EEG activity in specific motor areas that correlate with the activity imagined. Operant conditioning can increase a preferred behavior (pattern of brainwaves) or "response" by introducing a rewarding stimulus or taking away an annoying stimulus. But we cannot see or feel a brainwave, so how do we condition it? Enter cybernetic interface. We can connect the brain to a computer and observe brainwave behavior. We can then select a brainwave pattern that we would like to increase or decrease and provide a rewarding stimulus to encourage it to be repeated.

This might be a pleasing tone, points in a game or increased ability to view something we desire to see.

The reinforcer is a reward that "effectively" increases the likelihood of the response, like increased SMR waves which are now the operant. Of course, we can have positive or negative reinforcers. An neurofeedback tone can be meant to be a reinforcer, but it may be a tone that the client doesn't like or it may take too long to manifest and therefore will not be effective as a reinforcer. If they don't like the tone at all it may become a punishment. Remove the tone and it becomes a negative reinforcer bringing relief.

So, there are positive and negative reinforcers. *Positive:* Give a dog a treat every time they do it right. *Negative:* Give someone an Advil to take away their headache. *Positive:* Play a soft pleasing music when a child is reading well or *Negative:* Take away a loud unpleasing sound when the child is reading well. A client's definition of what is pleasing will alter the nature of the reinforcer. Some people love violin music and some people hate it. It is important to take into account your client's preferences.

Another variation on reinforcement are the concepts of *Intermittent Reinforcement* and *Continuous Reinforcement.* Intermittent Reinforcement involves providing a reinforcing stimulus only when a specific criterion is met. This is often referred to a dichotomous training. The client hears a pleasing tone only when they increase a component band, such as beta, above a specific predefine amplitude threshold. Their average amplitude of beta is 4uv and they increase it to 6uv and consequently hear a pleasing tone. Most neurofeedback software reinforces every correct response if it lasts 500 ms or longer. At times some individuals may perform better at 1-second reinforcement intervals. Continuous reinforcement is often referred to as proportional training. In this the clinicians rapidly reinforces every change in response that moves in the desired direction. For instance, a client may hear a tone move up in pitch as he or she increases their beta amplitude in the desired direction. It may also move down in pitch as their amplitude decreases. In this manner the pitch changes continuously in direct proportion to the amplitude as it moves up and down. The same effect can be achieved with increasing and decreasing brightness of the screen when viewing a video. In fact, visual reinforcement is superior to auditory according to investigations to date (Hinterberger et al., 2004; Strehl, 2014).

Transfer of the skill learned in neurofeedback trials to any situation in life where it is needed is often referred to as generalization in behaviorism paradigms. In successful transfer, context is often considered a crucial component. If there are cues from the novel situation that are similar to the old context where the task was learned, then transfer of the skill is more likely as there are greater chances of receiving a reward for the behavior learned. For this reason, it may be that training clients with instructional videos that relate to their predicament may be of importance. For instance, if office videos involve learning new concepts and reinforce paying attention and activation during this process, the skill is more likely to transfer to a similar environment where learning new concepts is important and rewarded such as the classroom. This would suggest that avoiding purely entertaining videos may be of value, although practitioners are still documenting improvements in pre post maps and symptom tracking with videos of a mostly entertaining nature. Strehl (2014) would go one step further and simulate classroom situations to maximize transfer. This may be true, but it is clinically very difficult to achieve and there are not studies to confirm this idea.

Conscious strategies to enhance feedback performance and efficiency are not likely to enhance training and may in fact interfere (Kober et al., 2013). This is likely because the video screen becomes an extension of the motor system through the feedback loop itself. In this case the CNS quickly adapts to the feedback loop and adjusts its function accordingly to maximize viewing pleasure.

Both auditory and visual reinforcements may not always have a desired effect. For example, many practitioners permit trainees to select items they would enjoy watching from movie streaming via YouTube, Netflix, and other movie/video streaming sources. When clients/patients are given such choices, their selections may include visual stimuli that will elicit a particular thought or emotion. Horror movies often generate fear reactions, dramas and action films can often generate anxiety while romances and biographies might result in a depressed reaction. Music is known to generate emotional memories and reactions; especially when the music is a well-known or popular song with accompanying lyrics. Popular songs are often attached to specific memories and/or emotions. Neutral educational shows and less "popular" music without lyrics do not generate memories and emotions as often as well-known music and movies.

Habituation occurs when an individual decreases their response to a stimulus because it ceases to be novel or of interest. This occurs when you are continuously exposed to the same stimuli. This can occur if you are listening repeatedly to the same boring tone during neurofeedback and your attention drifts. It can also occur if the child or teenager you are training is presented primitive video games that have no novelty compared to the video games they have become accustomed to playing. Humans, on the other hand, can find more extended interest in tones if they believe they are of value or producing good results. Training a child to a boring stimulus may thus counterproductive while convincing an adult of the value of the tones they hear my result in ongoing interest and a sense of novelty. Hence the use of video to simplify these contingencies!

Sensitization occurs when a stimulus becomes irritating or fearful in nature. Again, country music may be nice to one person but to the same person rap music may be very irritating. Some percepts may actually trigger a fearful response that undermines reinforcement. Selection of appropriate sounds, music or video may be critical factor in successful training. The same principles apply to visual stimuli.

Frequency of sessions is another issue. Behaviorism theory indicates spaced practice works better than massed practice (Hull, 1943). Based on those findings, early practitioners encouraged clinicians to do two or three sessions a week. Albert et al. (1974) found that spacing practice with a 24-hour period in between was superior to continued practice with only a minute or two in between. Strehl (2014) argues that more than one session per day does not seem practical but many clinicians have reported successfully training twice a day. Scott et al. (2005) trained twice a day for 14 consecutive days with over 50 addicts and showed consistent normalization of TOVA protocols demonstrating that multiple daily sessions are possible. So, this indicates spacing between sessions can be shorter than theory would suggest to many theoreticians. Arnold et al. (2013) compared clients trained twice weekly with those trained three times a week and found no major difference in outcomes but clients did prefer three times weekly. It seems clear from the literature on operant conditioning that learning varies greatly with respect to individuals, the issues they confront, the task difficulty etc. Our experience shows that clients tend to improve dramatically in the first eight to 10 sessions, degrade in performance for five or 10 sessions and then continue to improve. Those with complex trauma tend to consistently backslide for an extended time and usually respond best to Alpha-Theta training after 20–25 sessions.

Dichotomous (percent time reinforcement) vs proportional (amplitude-integration reinforcement) has been an ongoing controversy since Hardt & Kamiya (1976) brought it up to explain experiments that failed to show operant conditioning of the EEG. This is a complex argument at the research level, but it seems to boil down to something more concrete at the clinical level. With dichotomous training the client must clearly exceed a set threshold to be reinforced and will not be reinforced for partial achievement. With proportional reinforcement, the client is constantly given feedback regarding the degree of their success. Travis et al. (1974) and then Kisil & Birbaumer (1992) seemed to have resolved the issue for many concluding proportional works best. Kisil and Birbaumer (1992) comment that feedback should be as immediate as possible as well, and if shaping toward a goal is indeed part of the process than ongoing and immediate proportional makes sense to use.

This led us into post reinforcement synchronization or PRS and fixed verses auto-updated thresholds.

Let's review auto thresholding first. Lubar & Lubar (1999) employed fixed thresholds in his experiments at the University of Tennessee with children with ADHD. He and many others argue that based on the principles of operant conditioning, this is the only reasonable approach. The problem is that auto-thresholding has been widely used for over 20 years very effectively and many of us reverted to it out of experience, as we did with the use of videos during training.

There is an important concept in learning theory called "shaping" that comes into play at this point in the discussion. Shaping involves reinforcing small increments of behavior until a final larger or more complex final "goal" behavior is achieved. Shaping should be incrementally and consistently moving in the same direction. Sherlin et al. (2011) argue that shaping plays an important role in training and auto-thresholding can confound the shaping process. The concern is that the client will be rewarded not for achieving their goal but for a goal that is less than and therefore in the opposite direction from the goal, that is, shaping in the wrong direction. If the threshold shifts down and it becomes easier to obtain a reward, then the client will be shaped in the wrong direction. After watching and adjusting thousands of sessions over 25 years, this does agree with our clinical observation. For example, let's say the clinician is uptraining alpha. The client's baseline is 10 µV. The client begins training well and exceeding threshold but begins to fall below threshold due to disinterest, fatigue, drowsiness, pain, dissociation etc., and eventually there are longer and longer lulls with fewer and fewer reinforcement tones. As time passes there is no reward. The client becomes restless, concerned and alpha decreases even more. More time passes. Eventually extinction begins to occur. We have what is known in operant scheduling theory as ratio-strain. It becomes obvious that clients must have enough reinforcement to keep them motivated but not too much reinforcement.

Based on clinical experience, most clinicians find that the optimal reinforcement rate can vary between 60–90% depending on the individual. Depressed individuals may need more reinforcement since they have lower motivation levels. The same applies to those who are anxious with low frustration tolerances. Peak performance may engage high achievers that thrive on less reinforcement and enjoy the challenge.

Without auto-thresholding and as time passes and reinforcement diminishes, an observant clinician begins to sense the feedback failure and the client's concern and slightly lowers the threshold, so a reinforcing tone again occurs. The clinician notes suddenly progressively more tones and higher alpha amplitude again occurring. He raises the threshold and more tones and higher amplitude occur (shaping). He raises the threshold above the baseline and finds even higher amplitudes and more tones. Suddenly the alpha drops way down and the process begins again (the brain activity is non-linear cyclical). Comparing this procedure to a fixed threshold the clinician observes that the client's performance is enhanced compared to the fixed threshold. They achieve higher amplitudes of alpha although the grand average is approximately the same. Is the grand average the best measure of performance? Unfortunately, there appears to be very little correlation between session grand averages and improved symptomology. Most of us in neurofeedback discovered that long ago the hard way.

Post Reinforcement Synchronization (PRS)

PRS is similar to auto-thresholding in that most clinicians have ignored it and have experienced splendid results anyway. Clemente, Sterman, and Wyrwicka (1964) reported this parieto-occipital alpha they termed PRS in animals after being reinforced. But it was contingent upon the operant response, that is, the lever press. Other investigators concluded that PRS could enhance learning in animals and people. PRS could possibly increase the speed of learning. The proponents argue that neurofeedback should involve discrete "episodes" or learning events with a tone or light resulting and space between the events allowing for the PRS. This seems to contradict the findings regarding proportional training which is continuous and without discrete training events. They PRS advocates argue that the client should be consciously aware of the whether the response was wrong or right. This appears to contradict Birbaumer et al.,'s (2013) findings that neurofeedback is fundamentally an involuntary learning process. Advocates also argue against using games and videos and claim that the client will associate the reinforcement with the stimulus rather than the brain behavior response. Although this is theoretically a valid consideration, it appears to be hairsplitting at the clinical level. There is voluntary biofeedback and involuntary biofeedback, Birbaumer et al. (2013), Strehl (2014). Frederick (2016) notes that awareness is not necessary for learning but in some cases it may improve learning involving task performance where interoceptive awareness of motor or sensory activity is available. Once a task is learned it can interfere with performance and we see this with individuals who try to develop conscious strategies to enhance their neurofeedback session performance. There are no receptors in the brain to note changes as there are in peripheral biofeedback to identify successful change and interoceptive correlates are not typically clearly identified. Luft (2013) identifies feedback as "an outcome of actions captured by the senses." But there is no interoceptive mechanism for launching a brainwave. Luft reports that there are also other electrophysiological signatures besides PRS that attend successful reinforcement. Theta power in the midfrontal regions increases after an error or lack of reinforcement, while 20–30 Hz beta increases in the posterior region in response to positive feedback. The author distinguishes between finely-graded error-based learning and reinforcement learning involving rewards and punishment that appear to utilize somewhat different but related pathways in the brain. The error-based learning in this paradigm would be more similar to involuntary video feedback. It is associated with implicit and procedural learning involving acquisition of skills. Birbaumer et al., (2013) observe that skill learning, or implicit learning, usually follows a positive exponential function. They review investigations that demonstrate that this type of learning does not require any instruction or strategy. Categorical feedback involving volition only informs if the response was correct or not. The selection of which pathway will dominate appears to be based on how much information is in the feedback. Birbaumer et al. (2013) argue that the evidence points to the basal ganglia as playing a major role but volitional reward-based learning involves additional higher level networks. This suggests there may be many features of involuntary learning that have yet to be distinguished with respect to neurofeedback that make it different than the usual task-based trials of traditional operant conditioning. As Strehl (2014) emphasizes, feedback itself is reinforcing. Maintaining your balance on a bicycle is a continuous reward in itself once the basic motor skills have been acquired. PRS may be in fact the ongoing experience of alpha from a brain that has successfully learned a task to the point where it is the effortlessness of the task that is enjoyed as in juggling etc. The learning is based on a response plan (Birbaumer et al., 2013) where anticipated effect and actual effect are consciously compared. It usually involves a motivational function. One of the difficulties of training adults is that they often surreptitiously attempt to formulate a strategy based on volitional reward-based criteria. Birbaumer et al. (2013) notes this results in considerable variability in task acquisition. Initial instructions to the client play an important role. The human brain can significantly delay gratification and individuals can create their own criteria of success and consequently alter reinforcement schedules by their definition of the situation. The fact remains that thousands of clinics are using video-based feedback with high rates of success. Sherlin et al. (2011) note "To date, no studies could be found empirically testing the efficacy of continuous feedback, such as a game or video presentation, to applications with a discrete feedback of game or video presentations" (p. 298).

There is experimental support for both sides but the non-PRS camp wins on the side of practicality. If PRS is a significant factor, then a very new innovative method will be required to make it amenable to the modern neurofeedback context. In addition, some drugs appear to block the PRS and many of the individuals we train are on at least one drug. In the meantime, most of us are doing quite well with video, auto-thresholding and both dichotomous and proportional feedback. We arrived there through 25 years of hard in the trenches experience and learning.

Clinicians use a variety and often a mix of traditional and non-traditional methods to enhance client training effects. With eyes closed, some use a single tone while others use relaxing music as a background with the tone as the reinforcement. With eyes open, some use videos with both sound and visual fading while others use just visual fading and a tone in the background instead of audio fading. Still others have had a client read a book while using a tone as the reinforcement. Each of these methods has proven to be effective in neurofeedback training.

Strehl (2014) remarks that she is concerned that picking up artifacts like eye movement or muscle activity will learn those behaviors even more. Again, on the surface this looks theoretically correct but in the clinical setting fails to hold true. We have trained hundreds of kids with autism at Fp1-Fp2 who initially produce massive amounts of artifact but gradually calm down and produce progressively less while demonstrating improved EEG sessions along with improved behavior. We had been informed by the theoreticians that operant conditioning would be impossible with this level of artifact and yet we have the data to show that this is not true.

Falling asleep during a session may be due to sleep disorder, which is highly common in children diagnosed with attentional disorders, but it may also occur if the reinforcement level is too low. In classical conditioning, Pavlov found that there was a point before extinction when the pairing took so long the dogs would abruptly fall asleep.

The truth of the matter, is that with eyes-opened training, the clients falling asleep may result in a less or ineffective session, however, if the protocol is established to use specifically during eyes-closed training and the client falls asleep, they train equally effectively.

Applying Learning Theory To The Clinical Setting

Most instructions suggest setting thresholds so that enhancement reinforcement rates are at 75% and inhibition rates at 25%. However, we use several different brands of EEG equipment and have not found these settings to be appropriate for all of them or for our clients either. In fact, our databases confirm our observations. Setting thresholds so that reinforcement rates are in the range of 80% to 90% can often result in much better performance depending on the individual. Inhibition amplitudes are better if reinforcement is around 10% to 20% in the positive direction or an inhibition reward of 80% to 90%. In other words, most equipment will read 20% on the inhibitory filter. This means the client will be reinforced for being below threshold 80% of the time. This is where equipment that allows the clinician to use either auto thresholding or manual thresholding during a neurofeedback session can be very helpful in maximizing session benefits.

Whether or not to use auto-thresholding versus manual thresholding continues to be controversial within the field. In our clinical experience we have found both to result in client/patient progress and improvement in a variety of disorders.

If practitioners deviate very far from these settings, ratio strain occurs. This means that the reinforcement rate is too low to be rewarding to clients, and they do not make as good an effort. So, it isn't worth the time. This situation has very little to do with conscious motivation of the client. Even the most motivated client does not do as well when ratio strain occurs, proving once again the validity of behavioristic research.

Note: reinforcement rates have to be adjusted differently for the same person on different pieces of equipment. For instance, individuals who perform best at 75% on Thought Technology® equipment perform best at 60% on the BrainMaster® equipment. For example, the NewMind Trainer has a default setting of 75%, however, with some clients/patients, this needs to be adjusted up to 80 - 85% when starting neurofeedback and then slowly adjusted back down of the case of several sessions.

Types of Reinforcement

As mentioned previously, dichotomous reinforcement occurs when clients receive feedback in the form of a sound, image, or both, when they exceed a given threshold. In some cases, they may receive reinforcement only when they stay above or below a given threshold. Clients either meet the criteria or they do not. There is also equipment on the market that provides constant but variable reinforcement of images and sound. It is constant and ongoing because it informs clients of their performance through pitch variance or image changes. This method is called proportional feedback. Joe Kamiya's (personal communication) research on reinforcement and training indicates that constant proportional reinforcement is superior to dichotomous.

With proportional reinforcement, it is usually better not to set a threshold at all-just tell the client to do the best he or she can. We have also found that the range of pitch of the tone being used for reinforcement is crucial. Lower pitched tones reduce performance. Humans respond better to higher pitched tones when trying to increase their amplitudes. In addition, when 120 training with eyes open, providing training graphs with wave forms displayed near the top of the graph increases reinforcement. With dichotomous reinforcement, such factors do not play a crucial role; however, a pleasing tone increases reinforcement more than a harsh tone.

Optimal Training

This brings us to optimal reinforcement in particular. In more recent times most of the clinicians we encounter have converted to training using video contrast or games. The video contrast shifts the screen darker if threshold criteria is not met and brighter if it is met. Prior to this technological innovation most practitioners were training clients using several short trails during each session watching a simple image on the screen in addition to a reward tone. This older and more conservative approach was derived from the theoretical considerations reviewed above as well as the work of the Othmer's and Travis. Travis et al., (1974) had found that 10-minute intervals were optimal for training alpha and that one could run three 10-minute intervals in one sitting; proportional or non-dichotomous training was most effective. We had found it true as well and also included beta in that category. On the other hand, optimal training times for theta appear to be 20–30 minutes. It was routine for us to do most of our training in the form of 3- to 7-minute trials (7 minutes is the average attention span of an adult). Pushing clients beyond these considerations appears counterproductive when we evaluate the performance data post session. It is important to provide clients with a rest between trials. Data indicates they usually become tired and begin performing more poorly after the third trial.

With advances in neurofeedback equipment and software over the past decade, we have found that running 30 minute sessions without a pause or break can be beneficial to most clients/patients regardless of the protocol being used and bandwidths being trained.

Many neurotherapists find that there is no limit to the frequency of training sessions. Research published by Bill Scott et al., (2005) showed empirically that training individuals twice a day every day for 14 days could normalize a TOVA. This method is great for a client with unlimited funds flying in from out of town who wants to get the job done right away. However, realistically, most individuals respond well to a twice-a-week schedule. Longo & Hefland (2016) demonstrated this in a single case study training a post chemotherapy patient 2-3 times per day every day for a total of 30 sessions over a two week period.

However, given the costs and time commitments many individuals/families do not have the time and/or financial resources to have sessions more than once per week. Thus, we have found that even one session per week can result in symptom improvement as would be the case with multiple sessions per week, however, the process takes longer before significant improvements are noticed.

Physiological changes take place between sessions and neural growth takes time and cannot be pushed beyond a reasonable limit. Individuals also need time to adjust their lives to the changes taking place in their brains. Dysfunctional networks take years to grow and it will probably take a year or two to undo the damage even if training takes only several weeks or 3 months. The match between these two factors has not been adequately researched. However, we find that people continue to experience profound changes even a year after training, which supports theories regarding initial conditions from a chaotic systems perspective. One of the characteristic features of a non-linear dynamical system is that small initial changes in such a system can iterate into larger extended effects over time without any further reinforcement.

In spite of all our innovation and efforts to try out everybody's protocols, we still find that most people require at least 30–40 sessions (even with Z-Score training) to solidify their gains, even if they experience dramatic gains in the first 15 sessions. Once initial gains are made in the first 10–20 sessions, frequency of visits can be reduced. Our records indicate that progress is slowed considerably if clients only come once a week at the outset.

Another valuable tool is audio-visual entrainment (AVE), also known as photic stimulation. Chapter 9 explains how to use AVE. If used in conjunction with neurofeedback, AVE enhances performance dramatically. By using it in between neurofeedback trials, practitioners can provide clients time to rest while their brains are passively trained to do the task. An analogy often used is that AVE is to EEG as training wheels are to a bike when learning to ride. After AVE, clients begin the next trial refreshed and usually perform much better. Sometimes the difference is dramatic. They also find the training sessions more enjoyable and look forward to them more. On occasion, when they are sleep deprived, AVE provides them with the opportunity to catnap while also getting entrained. This method also enhances performance on the next trial and provides a good training session that otherwise might have been wasted trying to keep clients awake.

Protocol Determination

Neurofeedback Complexity

Unfortunately, neurofeedback deals with a complex structure and system. Protocol selection is one of the greatest mysteries of neurofeedback and also one of the most intimidating areas for those practitioners just starting out. People entering the field want clear guidelines to assure they are doing the right thing. Many practitioners are frustrated and impatient with the complexity and vagueness of this topic. Trying to generate subtle shifts in that system is a daunting task. However, there is the "Church of the 14 Hz" as Julian Issacs has called it (personal communication).

The neurofeedback pioneer Michael Tansey (Lubar Workshop) found that he could treat almost any disorder effectively if he up-trained a person at 14 Hz at Cz long enough. Although this is not always true, in many cases it is an effective approach. On the other hand, it could cause serious problems if the individual had too much 14 Hz to begin with. Nevertheless, the idea of a few simple protocols that can be used systematically is very appealing to clinicians. This is one reason why the Othmers' initial approach to neurofeedback was so popular. It is very simple and systematic, even if they have not always been sure of why it worked or why practitioners should ignore other alternatives, such as QEEG or Val Brown's approach. Sue Othmer has completely changed her method and protocols over the years and now she is doing "Infra-low" neurofeedback which involves training frequencies below one hertz that are technically shifts in DC currents rather than EEG AC electrical activity.

Of course, there are a dozen other high-profile figures in the field claiming that their methods are the best, and we have experimented with most only to find that all the methods work pretty well. Many newcomers to the field shake their heads and say "How can this be that so many different approaches work? The effects of neurofeedback must be due to the placebo effect." To understand that this is not the case, that neurofeedback outcomes are not due to placebo effect, it is necessary to go back and read the research of Barry Sterman. Sterman carried out experiments using control group designs with animals that are not susceptible to placebo effect. These replicated designs consistently demonstrated that the EEG can be trained using operant conditioning and were originally based on research going back to 1935 (Sherlin et al., 2011). Even more remarkable is his research wherein he trained cats to produce SMR resulting in their robust resistance to the toxic effects of hydrazine fuel.

Many clinicians in the past preferred to begin at the motor strip and the Othmers initially trained exclusively there because their method was originally derived from Sterman's research. They have moved on to another method with different protocols done at many locations just as many in the field have gravitated toward QEEG guided neurofeedback. Margaret Ayers (personal communication) believed that it was the best place to start and then frequently moved to the temporal lobes or another area in the posterior depending on the problem. The Othmers (personal communication in several workshops) argued that the largest and oldest pyramidal cells are in the motor strip area, so it is easiest to influence thalamic oscillators from this area. They even began with their next generation of protocols largely from this same starting point. Lubar (personal communication) did a lot of his training with a bipolar montage that extends from Fz back to Pz. Some of his research at the time suggested that training in one area can influence quite a wide region of the brain. Valdeane Brown's protocols (personal communication in several workshops) are usually done along the motor strip as well, C3 and C4, although he has begun to expand this repertoire. Bill Scott relies heavily on C3-C4 in his paradigm using Brain Paint software. Another reason for the popularity of this area is that it is relatively artifact free. It can be very difficult to train in front of the motor strip with eyes open because this region is often contaminated by eye blink and muscle artifact. New advances in auto-artifacting are now making it possible to remove this artifact on the fly while training.

None of the above trainers relied especially on brain maps when they first began using neurofeedback. Some of them still do not use them. So, moving training locations was not an especially important consideration for them. Bill Scott (personal communication) differs from many people in that he trains with one electrode at C3 and the other at Fpz with eyes open and ignores the entire artifact. He claims that his clients still train well. At NewMind, we have tried it, and he is right. For more on this procedure, see the sample QEEG report in Chapter 4.

Early in the development of the field, most practitioners were using common protocols that seemed to work well with different disorders. New protocols were continually developed. An example is the Peniston protocol for treating alcoholism and addictions (see Martins-Mourao & Kerson, 2017). The exact nature of the protocol was never clearly reported, but those who I have spoken to who also have spoken to Peniston personally indicate that they only up-trained 8–12 Hz at O1. Their equipment, at that time, did not have a means of training theta. Later, they added 8–12 Hz up with 4–7 Hz up. The exact thresholds are unclear to this day. These latter sessions with PTSD used O2.

In the beginning, neurofeedback involved a small group of practitioners at the ISNR and Futurehealth, Inc. It was very exciting to compare notes and discuss case histories. Neurofeedback is now larger, more complex and sophisticated. The use of QEEG is common and the technology behind expert systems like Val Brown's is very esoteric. The Othmer methodology has grown very complex as well. The addition of LENS and the fantastic claims regarding Z-Score training confuse the picture even more. Coben et al. (2018) have reviewed some of these alternative paradigms, including Z-Score training and found very little research support.

Over the past decade a growing number of devices have been introduced into the field of neurofeedback. It is for this reason, among others that we encourage consumers to do their homework BEFORE purchasing equipment. Many devices claim to be doing neurofeedback but are not actual neurofeedback devices. The term neuromodulation has begun to increase in popularity because many of the newer devices effect the brain and brain function but are not truly neurofeedback devices by definition. Infrared light devices and magnetic devices such as microtesla are two examples.

Toolbox Approach

In spite of the lack of research report, many of these methods, such as Z-Score training, appear to be effective based on clinical observation and provide important pieces of the puzzle. That is why we promote the idea of the clinical toolbox. The question new practitioners entering the field need to answer is, "Which protocols work best for me and my clients?" There is no replicated research to date that clearly indicates one method as being better than another. Practitioners may find that they have to buy a couple pieces of equipment and try out a couple of methods before they discover what works best for them and helps them feel confident in their clinical applications of the technology. Attending just one workshop or reading one book will not launch a practitioner confidently into a career in neurofeedback. That being said, Joel Lubar (personal communication) has put together a valuable list of standard neurofeedback protocols found in the existing research literature that he has found to be effective. Table 11: Protocols supported by Peer Reviewed Journal Articles, shows these protocol guidelines. This list is integrated into the protocol suggestion section of the NewMind Maps report system.

The Othmers initially developed a system in which they take baselines at C4, Cz, and C3 and the based upon symptoms, they determine how to train each side of the brain. They developed a sophisticated decision tree based on their extensive clinical experience and the findings of their affiliate clinics. In the simplest terms, they tend to speed up the left side or slow down the right side of the brain or do a little of both at each session. Consequently, for someone with depression they would most likely do beta training on the left side at C3. For anxiety they would more likely do SMR training at C4. This approach is still widely used and has been expanded by many trainers and clinicians.

Sue Othmer abandoned this approach in the late 1990's for a new bipolar montage method that involves a comprehensive EEG inhibit with a select moving window of enhancement. This then evolved evolved into training frequencies below 1 Hz, sometimes down as far as .01 Hz and even lower. This method is sometimes called sub-delta training or Infra-low Frequency training. In parallel with the Othmers, Mark Smith has developed a similar approach known as Infra-slow Fluctuation neurofeedback. Practitioners definitely need to take several of her workshops or Mark's workshops in order to master this approach as it involves some special training in observational skills because the approach is very interactive.

Mark Smith, a clinician in New York, a developer of ISF neurofeedback, was the first to grasp the advantage of using a DC coupled amplifier for Infra-slow training. Smith notes, "Infraslow Fluctuation or ISF neurofeedback is a unique brain training method that targets the infraslow frequencies (meaning below 0.1 Hertz) occurring throughout the brain. Clinical research shows that these slow oscillations determine the overall excitability of the cortex. In addition, these slow frequencies coordinate processes in the body with processes in the central nervous system. From a neurofeedback perspective, this means that they offer a highly valuable target for reinforcement. In fact, shifts (or fluctuations) in these infraslow frequencies directly affect the brain's internal regulation of the autonomic nervous system, including our fight-flight-freeze stress response as well as our rest-and-digest state. By providing real-time auditory feedback regarding small shifts in infraslow frequencies, the brain learns to optimize its ability to self-regulate, readjusting baseline levels of activity in various regions. Given that the root cause for dysregulated brain states and mental illness is often hyper- or hypo-excitability, ISF neurofeedback offers an unparalleled form of neurotherapy for many suffering from anxiety, trauma, depression, and much more."[1]

---

1   https://neurofeedbackservicesny.com/types-of-neurofeedback/

Table 11: Protocols Supported by Peer Reviewed Journal Articles

(from Joel Lubar—2001 ISNR Workshop)

Disorder	10-20 Site	Number of Sessions	Protocol (Hz) Enhance	Inhibit
ADD	Pz age 7–9	30–50	16–20	4–8
	Cz age 10–15	30–50	16–20	6–10
	Fz age 16–25	30–50	16–22	6–10
	Fz age 26–50	30–50	16–24	6–10
ADHD	Cz or C3	20–30	12–15 Or 6–9	4–8
Seizure disorder	Cz or C3	30+	12–15 Or 6–9	4–8
Dyseidetic dyslexia	P3 or PS	30+	beta Or 6–10	4–8
Dysphonetic dyslexia	F3 or FS	30+	beta Or 6–10	4–8
Tourette's syndrome Tic disorders	Cz or C3	30+	SMR	4–8
Anxiety disorders	P4 or O2	Varies	Alpha 8–12	beta 15–24
Depression	F3 & F4	20+	alpha F4 Or train ratio of alpha F4 to F3	alpha F3
OCD	F4 or P4, P6	20+	Alpha 8–12	beta 15–24
Insomnia (sleep onset)	Cz or Fz	Varies	theta 4–7	beta 15–24

In Table 12: Early Othmer Protocols, locate the symptom and find the protocol to use listed at the top of the column. Sue Othmer would usually inhibit 2–7 Hz and 23–38 Hz or some similar high and low range in addition to up-training one of the frequencies below. For instance, "C3 Beta Up" might include 2–7 Hz inhibit, 16–19 Hz enhancement, 23–38 Hz inhibit.

Valdeane Brown began in a very similar way. Val, however, began training both sides at the same time: beta on the left and SMR on the right. In addition, he would suppress both the low frequencies and high frequencies, which he usually found to be a source of problems. He saw this method as a sort of remedial work to stabilize the brain and normalize circadian cycles. Once this was accomplished, his next step or "period" of training involved something very similar to Alpha-Theta training. Finally, he finished up with a protocol that focused on two specific frequency ranges that he found especially valuable in enhancing transcendent insight and spiritual awareness.

Unlike many other clinicians, Val included an explicit spiritual component in his model of training. This situation is not surprising, since most of clients seem to wrestle with spiritual issues toward the end of their training cycles—even when the topic isn't mentioned. According to the literature, many psychologists and counselors find themselves forced to deal with this dimension with their clients in the later stages of psychotherapy. Clearly, it is an emerging trend and is further discussed in the section on Alpha-Theta training.

Table 12: Early Othmer Protocols

C3 Beta Up Theta Down Turning Up the CNS	Cz Beta	Cz SMR	C4 SMR Up Theta Down Turning Down the CNS
Inattentive	Bruxism	Anxiety	Impulsivity
Difficulty staying asleep	Night terrors	Panic	Bipolar
Social anxiety	Narcolepsy	OCD	Restless leg
Depression		Tics	Sleep apnea
Eating disorders		Onset insomnia	Poor social skills
Poor word fluency		Restless sleep	Migraine
Poor reading comprehension		Seizure	Aggressive and manipulative
Math problems		TBI	Rushes through work
PMS		Spasticity	
Memory problems			
Explosive rage			

- Val had multiple tones going at the same time and feeding back to his clients. He maintained that this is not a problem because neurofeedback is not an especially conscious process. We also may use as many as three tones at the same time, but we find that we must follow certain rules with this procedure. For instance, the tones should at the very least harmonize with each other, as dissonance tends to be a punishment rather than reinforcement for most people (Z-score training presently uses one tone, scale of tones, or image to train 240 variables over four channels in the domains of phase, coherence, symmetry, and power). Each of the stages or periods of training are done one at a time in sequence.

- Bilaterally suppress 3–5 Hz, 8–13 Hz and 23–38 Hz. Simultaneously, augment C4 SMR and C3 beta. Symptom resolution through re-establishing circadian cycles.

- Bilaterally suppress 3–5 Hz and 23–38 Hz. Bilaterally augment alpha. Self-integration through profound relaxation.

- Bilaterally suppress 3–5 Hz, 8–13 Hz and 23–38 Hz. Cycle between bilaterally augmenting 19-23 Hz and bilaterally augmenting 38-42 Hz. Spiritual transformation through transcending multi-focal awareness and deconstructive presence.

Table 13: The Period 3 Approach (Val Brown) shows this.

- Bilaterally suppress 3–5 Hz, 8–13 Hz and 23–38 Hz. Simultaneously, augment C4 SMR and C3 beta. Symptom resolution through re-establishing circadian cycles.

- Bilaterally suppress 3–5 Hz and 23–38 Hz. Bilaterally augment alpha. Self-integration through profound relaxation.

- Bilaterally suppress 3–5 Hz, 8–13 Hz and 23–38 Hz. Cycle between bilaterally augmenting 19–23 Hz and bilaterally augmenting 38–42 Hz. Spiritual transformation through transcending multi-focal awareness and deconstructive presence.

Table 13: The Period 3 Approach (Val Brown)

C4	C3	Purpose
3–5 down 8–13 down 23 38 down 13 15 (SMR) up	3–5 down 8–13 down 23–38 down 20–30 up	Symptom resolution through reestablishing circadian cycles
3–5 down 23–38 down 9–11 up	3–5 down 23–38 down 9–11 up	Self-integration through profound relaxation
3–5 down 8–13 down 23–38 down Cycle between: 19–23 up & 38–42 up	3–5 down 8–13 down 23–38 down Cycle between: 19–23 up & 38–42 up	Spiritual transformation through transcending multi-focal awareness and deconstructive presence

NeuroCARE Pro, now better known as NeuroOptimal is the updated version of Val's work. It is a proprietary neurofeedback method that has minimal published material available to explain in detail what is taking place. In fairness it must be noted that this is not unusual in the field and other vendors such as Brainmaster® have proprietary Z-Score techniques or other techniques as well. The NeuroOptimal approach began with a training strategy that looked like a combination of the early Othmer protocols and Alpha-Theta Training as described in his Five Phase Model (1995). Val Brown, embracing Non-Linear

Dynamical Theory, saw neural processes as reflecting a non-linear dynamical system and evolved his initial methods of training into what he called the Period Three Approach. The Period Three approach utilized two channel training of both hemispheres at the same time using areas C3 and C4. This approach was defined in traditional filtering and thresholding terms using Thought Technology software. Val was eventually able to bring investors together to generate his own software designed to more specifically accomplish the goals that were growing more difficult to achieve with standard neurofeedback software. Rather than fixed thresholds Val developed box targets to define regions of frequency activity of interest to select for feedback to the brain. This was in an effort to use a Synchronization through Chaos model of non-linear dynamical theory in which the brain would be guided toward a more flexible and resilient state and away from rigid attractor states. For Val the brain was an intelligent self-organizing dynamical system. Training from the key central locations of C3-C4, the intent was to influence the entire system through this special type of feedback.

From the NeuroOptimal perspective an inefficient or unstable brain arises from traumatizing challenges resulting in rigid attractor states, limiting brain resources, and showing up as too much or too little amplitude variability in up to 16 groups of frequency bands ranging up to 62Hz. The software provide two spectral arrays showing each of these groups and the proprietary thresholding activity involved. Excess variability especially shows up in the .1-2 and 2.5-5.5 Hz frequency ranges and one key goal is to reduce the variability in these ranges below 3Hz which he identified as a key problematic frequency with respect to disorder in his Five Phase Model Brown (1995). As these lower frequencies reduces it variance, energy is made more available for other higher frequencies to re-organize toward more balanced and efficient activity, especially 7 Hz. Val saw this frequency range as key to client's gaining insight. Reducing the lower frequencies around 3 Hz was also seen as a way to avoid elicitation of old traumas and unwanted side effects. The CNS is seen as a system which is always seeking to optimize itself and will readily adopt feedback toward that end in an intelligent manner not requiring conscious awareness. Following Pareto's law, feedback is provided at a rate of 80% percent of the training time. Providing the accurate information of the correct type will maximize the brains effort at re-organization. No other special mapping or diagnostic procedure is required in order to implement the software and the method. Clinicians are not viewed as necessary to implement this technology and it is widely marketed for home use.

Table 14: Single-Channel Monopolar and Bipolar Protocols (Earlobe References)

Disorder Protocol	10-20 Site	Number of Sessions	Protocol (Hz) Enhance	Inhibit
Alpha training	P4 or Cz	20–40	9–11	4–7
				20–30
Alpha-Theta	Pz	30+	5–8	1–5
			8–11	13–30
Seizure	Cz	30–40+	13–15	1–4
				20–30

Table 15: Two Channel Monopolar and Bipolar Protocols

Disorder	10-20 Site Channel 1, 2	Number of Sessions	Protocol (Hz) Enhance	Inhibit
General	C3 Fz	30–40	15–20	2–7
	C4 Pz		9–11	12–15
General	F3	30 40	15–20	2–7
	C4 Pz		9–11	12–15

Table 16: NewMind Protocols (Eyes Closed)

Purpose	10-20 Site	Number of Sessions	Protocol (Hz) Enhance	Inhibit
Relaxation	Pz	Alpha-Theta	5–8	2–5
			8–11	15–30
Relaxation	Pz		8–12 70%	8–12 20%
Relaxation				
Relaxation	Pz	Hi amp alpha	8–10	10–12
		10–12	13–15	8–10
		Hi amp alpha		
		8–10		
Relaxation	P4		9–11	
Relaxation	P4		9–11	2–7
				20–30
Relaxation	P4		9–11	15–30
Relaxation	P4		8–10	
Depression	F3		8–12	8–12
	F4			

192

Table 17: NewMind Protocols (Eyes Open)

10-20 Site		Conditions	Protocol Enhance	Inhibit
C3	Fpz	Attentional	15–20 20–30	2–7
C3	Fpz		15–20	20–30
C3	Fpz		15–20	8–12 20–30
C3	F3		15–20	20–30
Fz			15–30	2–7
F3			15–30	8–12
C4	Pz	Relaxation	9–11	
C4	Pz	Anxiety	9–11	15–30
C4	Pz		9–11	20–30
C4	Pz		13–15 (SMR)	2–7 20–30
C4	Pz		13–15	8–12 20–30
Pz		Relaxation	13–15	2–7
Pz		Anxiety	13–15	20–30
Pz		Hi amp alpha is 10–12 Hz	13–15	8–10
Pz		Hi amp alpha is 8–10 Hz	9–11	12–15

Table 18: Additional Protocols

Purpose	10-20 Site	Number of Sessions	Protocol Enhance	Inhibit
Seizure	Cz	30–40+	13–15 20–30	2–7
Pain	T3T4	30–40	13–15	
TBI	T3T4	30–40+	12–15	1–3

Training by Quadrant

For many years, we have been talking about quadrant training rules and what training is possible in each quadrant. John Demos (personal communication) has found this a valuable teaching concept as well. When you try to choose a protocol for training, the choice will often be limited by rules governing each quadrant. Suppose a client has too little alpha and you want to up train it. The quadrant rules say you cannot train alpha in the left front; it is not a great idea for the left back quadrant either. You would be better off training alpha on the right side and in most cases the right posterior is best. Beta, on the contrary, is best trained up in the left frontal quadrant.

Dagram 48: Training Quadrants, is a chart that if you do a Mini-Q assessment you have something to guide you in protocol selection. For instance, you can train alpha down in quadrant A, but not alpha up. You can train beta up, but not beta down. If beta is too high in the left front, you might want to train alpha up on the right instead of beta down.

Diagram 48: Training Quadrants

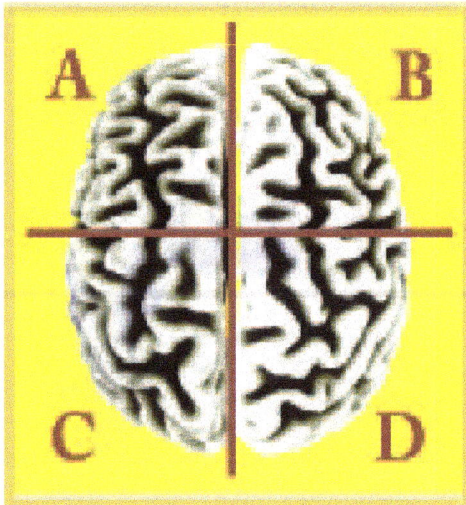

A: Alpha down, beta up, theta down, delta down

B: Alpha up, beta down, theta down, delta down

C: Theta down, delta down

D: Alpha up, beta down, delta down

THE PROTOCOL DECISION TREE

After doing a Mini-Q assessment or QEEG, both of which are fairly common methods of assessment these days, you will find that there are several possible protocols you could try to remedy the abnormal features of the EEG distribution uncovered by the assessment. (see Peter van Deusen, John Demos, EEG Spectrum, Jon Anderson, Bob Gurnee, or Richard Soutar workshops for assistance.)

When difficulties arise, you need to decide the best protocol to begin with and how long you should try it until you change it. To help with these decisions, we developed the Protocol Decision Tree. The rationale behind the Protocol Decision Tree evolved out of Richard Soutar's staff meetings at NewMind clinics over a decade. So, it came from "in-the-trenches experience" working with brain maps and a very wide variety of disorders and ethnic populations. NewMind Center has had offices in Phoenix, Shreveport, Atlanta, and Jacksonville, so the client population has been quite varied. NewMind Center records even show that there is a demographic difference in the types of depression that typically show up in a neurofeedback office in the west coast versus the east coast.

The Protocol Decision Tree also provides clear steps to take once you have decided on the beginning protocol. If you can't make up your mind which protocol is best, then call for a consultation with someone with more experience. Once you start, you'll find that the method guides you quite clearly. Generally, you begin in one location and try different component bands. Then you move to a nearby site to train off site. If you are still not getting good results, try the next best location and frequency.

For example, if you have too much beta in the posterior region, you may initially try to train it down at Pz. If the beta does not train down easily, but the alpha goes up or the client becomes more anxious from the beta down-training, you may want to try and train the alpha up (the brain gave you a hint about what it might be willing to do). If you train alpha up and things go well, but beta does not go down, you might consider moving to P4 nearby, as that is an area that usually responds well to alpha up-training (see Diagram 48: Training Quadrants). When you train at P4, you might see alpha going up, beta corning down on its own, and the client feeling much better in the next session.

People often ask how long to try a protocol before they should switch to another. Our experience has been that some kind of change in client symptoms should occur within five sessions. Obviously, exceptions exist. If a client has a bad reaction, you should stop using that protocol right away.

The Common Thread

We find that a common thread exists between all these approaches. Rather than encourage just one or the other, we try to establish some basic principles to guide protocol development and implementation. Since NewMind Center has access to multiple databases, which we use on all of our clients, we have been able to watch for patterns of disorder and implement different protocol approaches developed by various experts to see what difference in effectiveness they might have.

We have found them all fairly equivalent in results. Some, however, do seem to work better with certain individuals than others. It will clearly take years of research to determine exactly why. Unfortunately, there is still little research published that can provide objective comment all of this in a formal manner.

During a brain map analysis of the E. Roy John databases (personal experience and observation derived from a decade of teaching others), it is easy to be misled if you don't look closely at the numbers and morphology. Jay Gunkelman (personal observation) also exhorts everyone to focus on this information in all of his workshops. This process can inadvertantly lead to a sort of electronic phrenology[2]. It is very important to analyze exactly what specific frequencies are deviant/off norm. The advent of the Thatcher and Hudspeth (personal observation) databases made this analysis appear easier at first with the development of 1-Hz bins. These tools allow us to look at each frequency band individually, see how it is distributed across the scalp, and determine whether it is outside the normal expected range. With the passage of time, however, this addition of analysis ended up providing more confusion than new and useful information. This has often been the case with databases and software designed with research in mind, or love of gadgetry, rather than with the complexities of the clinical context. This clinical context requires simple and efficient and reliable software that focuses on the most important and salient issues based on clinical research that may be of most value to address rather than every analysis dimension imaginable. To some extent the same can be said true for sLORETA.

We have found that a pattern exists in many of the disorders wherein the spectral analysis shows that higher frequencies need to be enhanced and the mid-frequencies suppressed. Other variations may be a suppression of lower frequencies or a suppression of higher frequencies. The goal is to train in a manner toward normalizing the spectral distribution. Jay Gunkelman (in workshops and multiple discussions at every ISNR meeting from 2000–2008) calls this process "shaping the EEG." Interestingly enough, Valdeane Brown's protocols appear to do just that in a general shotgun manner. Adam Crane's general theory of neurofeedback, we are really moving the brain out of the wrong parking place (Crane & Soutar, 2000) also fits roughly into this category. The Othmers (personal communication) were also originally inhibiting higher and lower frequencies and up-training the middle frequencies. In fact, it appears that most practitioners are doing a version of this method because it reflects how the brain works. Once you take your baselines, you should look for patterns that deviate from the normal distributions. If there is a trend in which alpha increases at C3 so that it is higher than at C4, we need to either down-train alpha on the left or increase it on the right.

One last item to keep in mind as you are training: if you are reviewing the session as it progresses on the trend screen, the normal distribution or layering of the component bands would appear as having (with eyes closed) alpha highest in amplitude, then theta, then delta, and finally beta. Beta would be approximately half the power of alpha. With eyes-open training, the review or trend screen should show delta highest in amplitude, then theta, then alpha, then beta. Again

---

2   *Phrenology is a defunct field of study, once considered a science, in which the personality traits of a person were determined by "reading" bumps and fissures in the skull (Phrenology, n.d.).*

beta should be 40-50% lower than the other component bands.

Note: With NewMind Technologies and BrainMaster® you can create a review screen and monitor separate waves as the session progresses.

Side Effects of Neurofeedback

As with many treatments, whether drug or otherwise, neurofeedback also has the potential to create side effects during or after a session. The source of these effects appears to be the result of moving the client faster than they are prepared to change. This is particularly true in sensitive areas such as the temporal or parietal lobes. Below are a few areas to remember:

- Watch out for anxiety, irritability, increased physiological activity/vitals, sleep disturbance, agitation, nausea, headaches, mood elevations, general discomfort.
- Alpha-Theta training can trigger trauma episodes and dissociation.
- Training beta down in the posterior may create anxiety.
- Training alpha down on the right may create anxiety.
- Sensitivity to drugs can also create reactions to neurofeedback.
- Doing neurofeedback can also result in iatrogenic effects.

Additionally, it should be noted that training with neurofeedback can occasionally result in adverse response(s) that temporarily increases symptoms which are typically associated with relaxation and calming of the central nervous system such as fatigue, headaches, lightheadedness, dizziness, irritability, moodiness, weeping, insomnia, agitation, and difficulties with focus and anxiety. These reactions, if they occur, are temporary and typically only last 24-48 hours. Once clients/patients become more relaxed and aware, they tend to integrate past emotional issues and these symptoms subside.

The terms iatrogenesis and iatrogenic artifact refer to inadvertent adverse effects or complications caused by or resulting from medical treatment or advice. In addition to harmful consequences of actions by physicians, iatrogenesis can also refer to actions by other healthcare professionals, such as psychologists, therapists, pharmacists, nurses, dentists, and others. Iatrogenesis is not restricted to conventional medicine and can also result from complementary and alternative medicine treatment. Hammond and Kirk (2008) addressed iatrogenic effects from neurofeedback.

Since the first edition of this book, additional styles of neurofeedback have been developed and are undergoing clinical evaluation for efficacy with promising outcomes. These include: Z-Score training, full cap Z-Score training, Infra-slow, Infra-low, sLORETA, and specific to sLORETA, region of interest (ROI) training.

SUMMARY

Clinicians who rely entirely on QEEG claim they get excellent results training at the site that is deficient or excessive in some frequency range. That has not been entirely our experience. Instead, our experience indicates that the best pattern of training is often along the lines of what the Othmers, the Lubars, Valdeane Brown, and Margret Ayers originally found. All of these clinicians start their training at the sensorimotor strip and move outward, although of late the Othmers are frequently starting at the temporal lobes. Unless our brain maps clearly indicate one simple area of trouble, we often begin our training at the motor strip. We have found that we get the fastest results with this strategy. Why the motor strip may be the most robust starting point is not well explained, although many solid theories have emerged.

Note: Many neurologists see the frontal areas of the brain as an extension of the motor strip and the parietal areas as an extension of the sensory strip in terms of structure and function. This perspective makes the sensorimotor strip the structural-functional center of the cortex even though it is not the executive area. Consequently, its influence over thalamic function may be greater than that of other areas due to higher densities of primary systems innervation. Training at the sensorimotor strip also has the advantage of reduced artifact.

For those starting out in the present environment, Z-Score training or using an automated protocol output such as the NewMind Database system may be the best, easiest, and most reliable solution. The drawback with Z-Score is it tends to be a black box solution and does not foster a basic understanding of standard neurofeedback as it has evolved. The BCIA board focuses on an understanding of standard neurofeedback as an essential basis for certification. Never-the-less, these approaches provide specific guidance and built-in controls with respect to protocol selection. As you gain knowledge and skill, you can branch out into more innovative protocols.

Buying Equipment: Service Is #1

When equipment problems occur, the value of your equipment decisions is immediately evident. Having quick and reliable service departments with competent service technicians is crucial. It also helps to have an extra backup machine. Richard once had to get an appointment with one manufacturer's service department, which took several days. They were very nice people, but it took him over 6 months to solve the problem. This hassle included shipping equipment back and forth and what seemed like endless phone calls. If Richard had only had one neurofeedback unit, he would have had to stop doing neurofeedback for those 6 months. Luckily, Richard had a background in electronics. Otherwise, he is not sure he would have had the patience to go the distance with this manufacturer and fix the problem. This situation can become a nightmare for clinicians who are not technically oriented.

Before you buy:

- Ask other clinicians about the service department of the companies you may be dealing with.
- Check to see how long they have been in business and their track record.
- Go to a conference or visit their offices and try out their equipment in real time.

Many clinicians who did not test equipment or see it in action before they purchased it wish they had done so before purchasing.

Also, remember that machines are often built around the manufacturer's theoretical perspective with respect to EEG. Few, if any, pieces of equipment can do everything. Therefore, you should plan to buy at least two different pieces of equipment and make sure they do different, yet complementary tasks. This will expand your training capabilities and make room for changes in your technique as you grow.

When it comes time to set your equipment up for the first time, be prepared to have patience. We have never purchased a piece of equipment that did not require much time and attention before it was up and running in a clinically useful manner. Every machine has its quirks and it takes time to learn them. It is best to practice on yourself for a while until you get all the kinks worked out. We recommend a headset phone for this process, as it requires two hands to operate most equipment.

Note: Some programs are not happy unless they have exactly the right computer. We have built computers to specs just to avoid the "which computer is right" game.

REVIEW QUESTIONS

1. What differentiates a monopolar from a bipolar protocol?
2. Why is training by quadrants important?
3. Which conditioning type best describes neurofeedback?
4. What are common reference points in neurofeedback?
5. What are common grounds when using neurofeedback?
6. What is the importance of classical conditioning for generalized learning?

Chapter 7: Evaluation of Progress

THE CLINICAL PROGRESSION

Having your own protocols and established procedures makes a difference in how well your practice operates. We have developed a pattern of client management that has been very successful. Many clinicians come in the past to our practice to shadow our staff members and get a feel for how the office flows, what the paperwork looks like, and how the practice operates. Sometimes this process is crucial for clinicians to put together all they have learned at workshops, so that they can develop their own practices with confidence. Other practitioners intuitively grasp how they want to incorporate neurofeedback and integrate it easily.

In our book, *Becoming Certified in Neurofeedback* (Longo & Soutar 2019), we give examples of forms and office protocols that may be useful to those new to the field.

Our Procedures

When patients first contact us, we invite them in for an initial interview, so we can get acquainted and explain neurofeedback to them. It usually takes an hour to discuss their problem, explain neurofeedback, demonstrate a program, and discuss fees and schedules. Once they have decided to commit to doing sessions, they fill out the paperwork including history client rights and privileges, and financial responsibilities. As mentioned in Chapter 5, providing a brochure that describes QEEG, neurofeedback, homework, lifestyle changes, and expectations is a valuable way to assist patients and help them remember all that is discussed in the initial interview. Presently we provide them Rob Longo's book: *A Consumer's Guide to Understanding QEEG Brain Mapping and Neurofeedback Training* (Longo, 2018) This is an excellent introduction for new clients that provides detailed answers to all of their typical questions regarding brain mapping and QEEG. Clients tend to pass it along to acquaintances and other parents looking for help for their children and if you have a your clinical sticker and logo on it, it is very helpful at bringing in new interested customers.

During the next appointment, clients have a brain map or QEEG and a Test of Variables of Attention (TOVA) or the Integrated Visual and Auditory (IVA) continuous performance test, and fill out the Beck Depression Inventory or the NewMind Interactive Self Inventory which has anxiety and depression measures built into it. We may also do some memory testing and an HRV evaluation using Heart Math. Some clinicians prefer an HRV evaluation using more sophisticated equipment. We have observed effective evaluations with both approaches. In either case it is important to receive training in how to implement this technology effectively. These tests cover testing of the three primary frontal networks related to memory (dorsolateral), attention (anterior cingulate), and socio-emotional processing (orbital-frontal).

The NewMind Mapping system[1] provides the clinician an opportunity to have perspective clients/patients fill out online questionnaires that address physical health, cognitive and emotional functioning, personality traits, and a cognitive performance.

Often clients come in with complaints about their cognitive functioning. It is usually a good idea to use neurocognitive testing with these clients like CNS Vital Signs or NewMind Computerized Performance Tests in order to get a baseline evaluation of their actual performance. In many cases these can be done at home through the cloud for the convenience of the client and enhanced compliance for the clinician. Although certain memory and attentional regions may appear compromised due to excess slow-wave activity in delta and or theta or due to diminished activation such as low amplitude beta, clients may still perform surprisingly well due to the ability of the brain to compensate and reassign functional resources. Due to the brain's high level of complexity and the highly distributed nature of attention and memory networks, the brain has a very high level of resilience. In many cases these tests may reveal that the cognitive networks are not particularly compromised and that the majority of their deficit in function can be attributed to limbic based issues involving emotional processing and anxiety and depression. By retesting with the CPTs while training asymmetry for reductions in anxiety and depression you can confirm or disconfirm the degree of contribution of affect on the client's cognitive performance.

During the following appointment, we review the test results with the clients and correlate them with the client's symptoms. We review with them the list the symptoms we want to track, such as headaches, insomnia, low energy, etc., and then explain the protocol we will be using. In addition, we use the brain map to explain the process we will follow to obtain the desired results.

Keeping Records

Keeping good records is crucial to effective training, and may be a requirement of state regulations, licensure, accreditation requirements, etc. We take eyes-open or eyes-closed baselines at each session. These procedures often involve a 1- or 2-minute sample. Frequently, we chart client symptom changes and match them to changes in protocols to evaluate the effectiveness of our protocols (see Appendix D: Forms) We keep hard copies of these records in client files rather than rely upon computer-based client management programs, which may experience serious problems. This method also allows us to enter data into a

---

1   https://www.newmindmaps.com/

general database management program like Excel, which can be later transferred to statistical programs like SPSS or SAS. This way, our data analysis is not limited. If you are unfamiliar with these programs, most grad students are good with them and can be hired at very reasonable fees to do the work for you. More and more neurofeedback programs provide better statistical output that requires the use of other programs unless you are interested in doing research. Appendix D Forms, shows NewMind's Training Session Report form to use an example, but it is best to create your own form based on your office needs.

The NewMind Mapping System now generates an online summary of each neurofeedback session run when the clinician is using both NewMind Training Software and the NewMind Mapping system. Data in each report including date, time and length of session; Baseline data and post session averages, trend screen, training sites and parameters and offers the clinician the opportunity to note type and length of reinforcements, HRV data, photic data and a notes section (see Appendix D).

In addition, we record changes in client symptoms and have a checklist as part of the Training Session Report. A sample checklist is located in Appendix D. This checklist insures that the staff covers each important item. This information is placed in a folder with the bio-diagnostic, treatment plan, and protocol worksheet (Appendix D). Recently, we have begun to move this symptom evaluation to the internet, so clients can answer these questions from home. This process can be done by any clinician through the NewMind Maps site: www.newmindmaps.com.

The NewMind Mapping system also provides the clinician an opportunity to have clients/patients track progress in over 250 symptom choices and documents each neurofeedback session when used with NewMind Technologies software that includes protocol design, length of session, baseline and session averages data, types of reinforcement being used among other features.

IMPLEMENTING SINGLE CHANNEL PROTOCOLS

Once you have done an intake interview with your client and established his or her problems, you will use these symptoms as your subjective indicators of progress. If they have insomnia, headaches, and low motivation, then you will watch how these indicators vary during the training process. Specific symptoms can be added to the Symptom Checklist. A symptom checklist is crucial for monitoring progress and helps maintain your client's confidence in the neurofeedback training process. You will be trying to correlate these indicators or symptoms with the QEEG or initial multiple-site analysis. You have done your analysis and decided on a protocol. Now it is time to begin training.

We used to do three 10-minute trials with eyes open during training except when we did Alpha-Theta, which is a thirty-minute eyes closed session. This was prior to the advent of training with videos using video contrast changes as reinforcement. When that technology emerged we shifted from active conscious efforts to achieve feedback outcomes to passive involuntary reinforcement. If we revert to using ten-minute trials with conscious effort it is usually with individuals with cognitive deficits due to TBI or stroke and we do as many 10-minute trials as we can within an hour's time. We can usually get three 10-minute trials in within the hour. Most clients get tired by the third trial and show progressively worse results. With children, we will do either three 7-minute trials or four 5-minute trials, depending on their problems and their age. With experienced clients, we may do two 15-minute trials if it fits their protocol.

At the outset of each session, we go over the client's list of indicators to see if any changes have occurred. We may ask the client about other indicators as well. On the top left of our Training Session Report is a list of common indicators that are reviewed each visit. Clients often begin to sleep better and dream more. They may find themselves less likely to respond in their usual way when their "buttons are pushed." It is always a good idea to ask questions and probe for things that have changed. Often, important changes occur without clients' knowledge; they may fail to mention them or to note their importance.

Having hooked our client up, we take a 1- to 3-minute baseline at the beginning of each session (see Diagram 51). A new baseline is important because baselines vary somewhat from day to day due to ultradian rhythms, amount of sleep, diet, level of anxiety, mood, and so forth (an ultradian rhythm is a biological rhythm with an ultra-short period and very high frequency—e.g., heartbeat, breath). Kaiser (2008) has reported that due to circadian rhythms total EEG amplitude tends to be highest in the theta and alpha ranges during the noon time period for most people and drowsiness tends to occur with increased delta frequencies between 3 and 5 pm during the circadian dip. Consequently, it makes sense to try and train most people at the same time each day to avoid distortions due to these effects. Individuals usually stay within a certain range, however, and the ranges vary most for those who have significant problems with sleep. Most literature says that it takes several minutes to get a good theta baseline for research purposes; however, we have found that 2 minutes is adequate for clinical work.

Some investigators feel that fixed thresholds are more efficacious than auto-thresholding. After decades of clinical work our affiliates and clinics have not found that to be the case. However, if you choose to use fixed thresholds, we have developed some guidelines over the last two decades that can be valuable in achieving optimal results with this approach. We typically set dichotomous thresholds based on the baselines of that day. If alpha is 8 μV and we want to set

Diagram 49: Implementing Single Channel Protocols

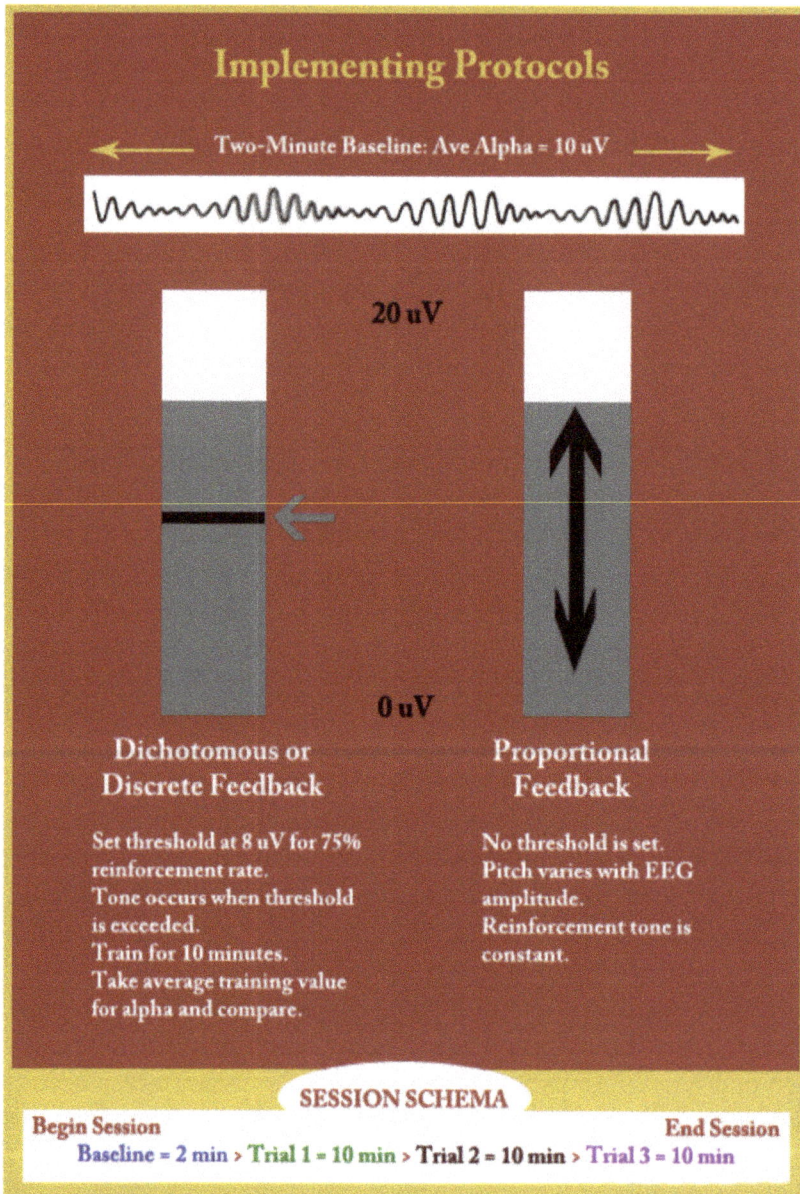

Implementing Protocols

Two-Minute Baseline: Ave Alpha = 10 uV

20 uV

0 uV

Dichotomous or Discrete Feedback

Set threshold at 8 uV for 75% reinforcement rate.
Tone occurs when threshold is exceeded.
Train for 10 minutes.
Take average training value for alpha and compare.

Proportional Feedback

No threshold is set.
Pitch varies with EEG amplitude.
Reinforcement tone is constant.

SESSION SCHEMA

Begin Session   End Session
Baseline = 2 min > Trial 1 = 10 min > Trial 2 = 10 min > Trial 3 = 10 min

a threshold for enhancement, then we set the threshold at 2 µV below that point, at 6 µV. If we wish to inhibit alpha, we set the threshold 2µV above that point, at 10 µV. This usually results in an 80% or better reinforcement rate. We call it "the 2 µV Rule." It works with most equipment, except BrainMaster®. When using BrainMaster®, you can watch the BrainMaster® rate of reinforcement on the fly and adjust it while training (see Diagram 50: Neurofeedback Trend Screen/Session Review Screen). This method is not always possible with other equipment that cannot be adjusted during training.

Diagram 50: Neurofeedback Trend Screen/Session Review Screen

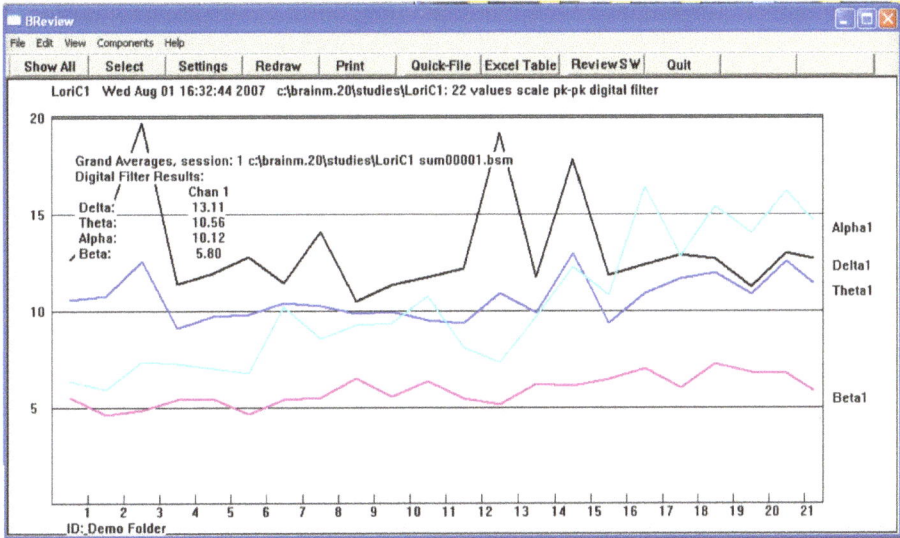

At the end of each trial we record their averages for each frequency that we are training. Often, we carefully watch other frequencies. For example, you may be training beta down, but also watch to see if alpha goes up and theta goes up or down. Compare the averages of each component band between each trial to see if the client is moving toward a normative distribution.

Note: You need to know if the average alpha on each trial is higher or lower than the baseline. Keep in mind:

- A .5 μV increase over baseline is significant.
- A 1 μV increase is very good.
- A 2 μV or more increase is excellent.

Digaram 51: Training Thresholds

Sometimes the client's alpha may not increase, but the beta will decrease. This change is significant as well. It is important to watch all the component bands to look for changes. Some programs provide training graphs with trend lines for each component band to show you all the subtle changes during training. It is our opinion that these programs provide a more effective evaluation of training efforts.

If the client can attain or exceed his or her baseline on the frequency in which the client is training during a trial in the first five sessions on a regular basis, then we feel confident the client will make good progress in the next 15 or so sessions.

Note: If clients fail to exceed baseline during these first trials, then we find it will often take them well over 30 sessions to achieve good results. We have come to this invaluable conclusion after years of clinical experience and analysis of client performance. This information is very helpful in offering clients an idea of their expected progress over the coming sessions.

Two Channel & Four Channel Training

Two channel training affords more information regarding the brain's status as well as more access to dynamics that influence the brain. Richard has published on this topic (Soutar, 2017) and presented extensively on it over the years at ISNR. We presently have hundreds of affiliated clinics using this approach because they find it very effective compared to other methods they have used and it is based on published standard neurofeedback research. Recently the University of St Louis completed a study showing very significant improvements in foster children utilizing this approach (Shauss et al., 2020). With two channel training we place sensors at homologous sites ie C3-C4, F3-F4 based on statistical analysis of QEEG maps. The 10-20 locations are rank ordered in deviance in all five neurometric dimensions and training begins with the most deviant or second most deviant set of homologous sites. The clinician determines which set of locations to train by training both sites and determining which set provided most change with the least amount of side effects.

In two channel training we monitor all of the main component bands rather than focusing on just the bands we are training. If training is effective the brain will tend to move in a normative direction. The caveat is that it does not do so in a linear fashion but through a series of cycles which progressively improve its efficiency and move toward the norm. The first dimension that most clearly reflects this movement is asymmetry. Individuals with disorders tend to have very divergent asymmetries. The left and right component bands are very far apart on the trend screen and converge into the same line progressively over the course of several sessions. We term this activity "convergence."

Diagram 52: Convergence

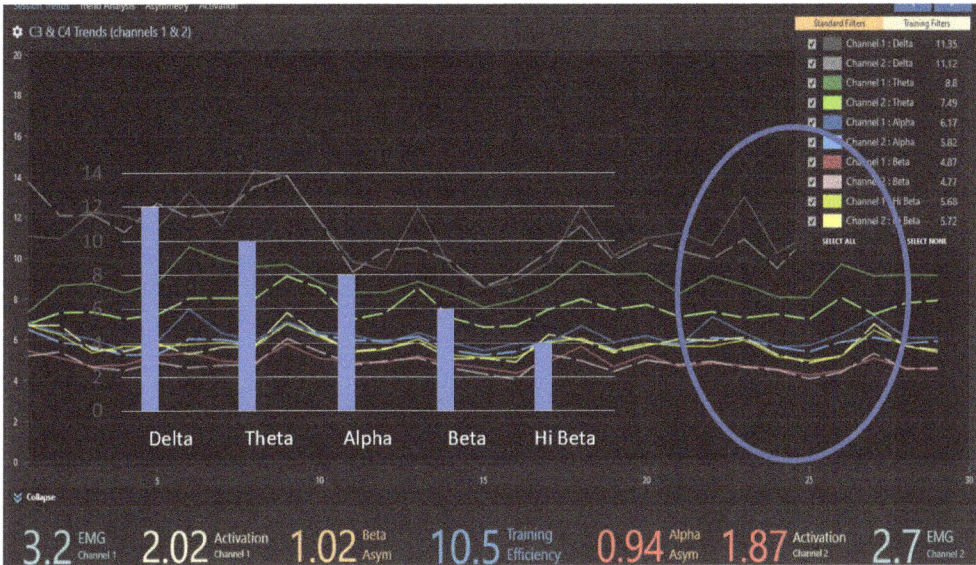

The second dimension that reflects effective training is "compression." This occurs when all of the components bands move together downward at the same time. After several initial sessions of this activity, they then begin to spread apart and move into more normative ranges.

Diagram 53: Compression

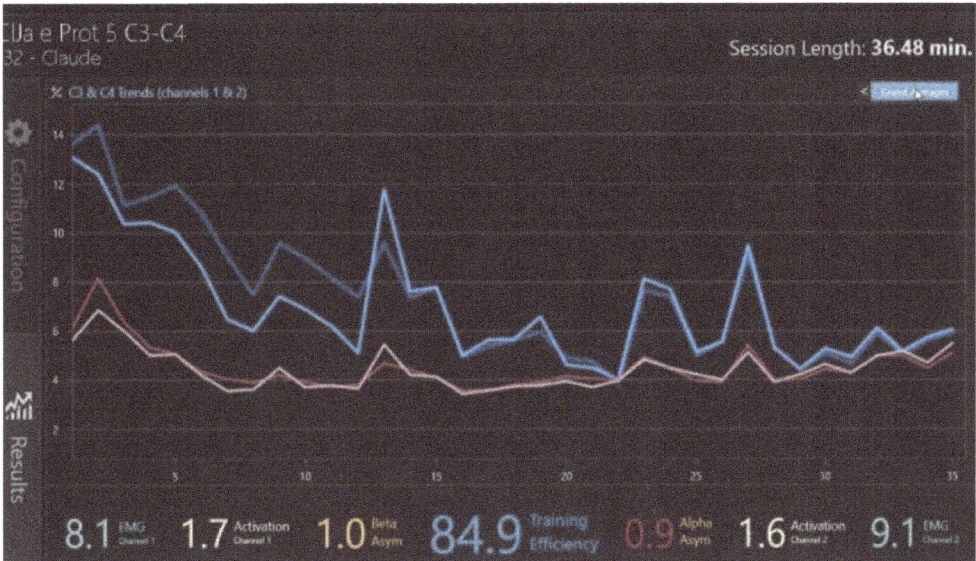

The approximate Eyes Open normative ranges are delta = 12, theta = 10, alpha = 9, beta = 6. The norms typically vary by about two microVolts. Note there is a normative layering pattern with delta the highest in amplitude, then theta, then alpha, then beta. Amplitudes tend to be about 30% lower at T3-T4 and F7-F8.

As of the writing of this book we are providing our affiliates with a single metric that combines these two metrics to provide on simple metric of training efficiency that we find very accurately reflects how well the client is training. There are older metrics such as percent of time a client meets criteria, often presented as points in many training softwares, and beta to theta ratios for those training to increase arousal and cognitive performance specifically. Another metric that is becoming popular and used by several vendors is Z-Score training, however research support for this approach has not been forthcoming (Coben et al., 2019). In spite of this many clinicians find it at least as effective as standard neurofeedback and some prefer the format.

The approach with four channel training is the same as for two channel training except that the clinician is monitoring all four locations at the same time. Those using the NewMind system can just select the two featured two channel protocols and run them simultaneously. For those interested in Z-Score training we recommend reading the chapter by Penny Jean Gracefire on the topic in the recent book edited by Collura and Frederick, *Handbook of Clinical QEEG and Neurotherapy* (2017).

In recent times there has been growing evidence of the efficacy of 4 channel training. We have been using 4 channel training for over a decade with excellent outcomes.

Plasticity

Plasticity is the lifelong ability of the brain to reorganize neural pathways based on new experiences. Plasticity may be the most valuable measure of progress in terms of EEG information available without a brain map. From our perspective plasticity is reflected in the brains ability to flexibly respond to training such that all component bands freely move in various directions in and out of normative ranges as the brain processes information. Pre-post QEEG comparisons are available in a printable format from the NewMind mapping system. What you will find instead is that most clients with disorders have a very rigid EEG, so that when they up-train one frequency, all the other frequencies go up as well in proportion to the one on which they are focused. As clients get better, they are able to up-train the frequency of interest with less of an effect on other frequencies. If they are up-training alpha, then the other frequencies should go down in relationship to alpha. Other frequencies may go up in amplitude somewhat, but their ratio to alpha should be less. So, whether we are training one or two frequencies at a time, we always carefully watch the other frequencies. The same goes for down training a frequency band. Asymmetry shifts freely as well but within a more narrow range than those with disorders. This is visually easy to identify when training with a trend screen.

Doing What Works

When choosing a protocol, you may try several variations at the outset to see which one is most effective. If a client has too much central beta, then you may try down-training beta, or uptraining alpha—whichever provides the best result. In this case, a brain map may reveal that the client's amplitude in beta is 3 to 4 standard deviations above the database mean. This indicates that the client's EEG may be putting out all that it can in every frequency and that up-training is almost impossible. Without the brain map, you would not know that this is the case, but by trying different variants of the same protocol you can see that down-training beta works best.

Once you decide on a protocol, you can probably try it for five sessions or so to see if the results are consistently good. You should watch for changes in client indicators. If results are not emerging, then you might consider another location and protocol.

Note: Remember that it takes more energy for the brain to produce high frequencies than low frequencies. Consequently, small changes in beta have more significance than changes in lower frequencies.

More recently we have provided statistically based protocols derived from maps but there are additional ways to consider protocols. One can look at the symptom and relate it to it the function of a Brodmann location. For instance, short term memory activity is correlated with activity in the Brodmann area that correlates with P3-P4. You may consider training an individual at those locations who complains of short-term memory issues if the component frequencies are significantly deviant or just because it is a hub for short term memory. On the other hand, memory is highly distributed in the brain and there may be other hubs that are actually causing the problem at P3-P4.

Training Off Site

When the initial multiple baseline analysis or brain map is done, you may find an area that is particularly abnormal. In attempting to run the appropriate protocol for several sessions, you may also find that the client is not making any progress moving above baseline. This situation is fairly common. To make more rapid progress, you may want to train at the next nearest site where the abnormality is a little lower. Often clients can initially do better at this site, and then when good progress is achieved, you can move back to the worse area and get better results. Again, this may be due to the highly distributive nature of many networks. For instance, the executive network is comprised largely of the frontoparietal networks involving the areas of P3-P4 and F3-F4 (Menon, 2015). You may be attempting to train F3-F4 because it is deviant in many neurometric parameters but find it is relatively unresponsive until you train the upstream (posterior) areas of P3-P4. If you find multiple regions that are unresponsive over many sessions or significant backsliding occurs you might consider investigating poor diet, sleep deficit issues or family system issues that may be confounding training.

It is not uncommon, for example, to train the brain working back to front since that is the direction in which the brain processes information. This is especially true if the QEEG shows evidence of deficiencies or abnormalities in the posterior regions of the brain.

The Brain's Wisdom

When training, much can be learned by watching the interaction between individuals and their brains. The more entrenched and intense the disorder, the less control they have over their brains. You can immediately see the disconnection in the way they train. The brain seems to have a will of its own, and it is a great struggle. Fighting this tendency directly is often a futile effort. It can actually interfere significantly with the process in the initial phases of training. This is why so many clinicians switched over to video contrast training and employing an involuntary method of operant conditioning.

When abnormal amplitude is present, it usually increases and decreases in a cycle very much like a swell in the ocean. In the past when we used more volitional training methods, we often watched frustrated clients fight against the peaks as they occur when they are trying to down-train a particular frequency band. We tried to get them to focus their energy on the dips when they are down-training and the peaks when they are uptraining. We compared it to surfing—when you catch the wave and ride it.

Clients train better on some days than on other days. Often, they become too concerned with the numbers and become frustrated or discouraged. When this discouragement happens, we tell our clients that it is the effort that counts and that being there training on a bad day is just as important as on a good day—perhaps even more so. We will often tell them that it is similar to going to practicing a sport or any other skill- you have good days and bad days but you slowly improve over time). We also remind them of the progress they have made so far.

Significant differences between sessions are often more apparent when the training times change. The circadian rhythm effects brain power and thus function; thus, a patient training on Monday and Thursday using the exact same protocol may have very different looking session trend screens if on session was run at 9 or 10 in the morning and the second was run 4 or 5 in the afternoon.

Frequency Of Training

The question clients ask is "How often should I come in?" because the answer directly affects their schedules and their pocketbooks. Many clients are disconcerted when they hear, "Twice a week at least." We have trained some people once a week; they do make progress, but it is much slower. This area is another area where we need more research. Training three times a week is even better. On the other hand, you should discourage clients from training every day. It is easy to lose sight of the fact that the reason many people have difficulty with memory and attention is because of emotional factors related to anxiety and depression which are far more common in the population than ADHD and usually comorbid with cognitive issues. Often changes may come too quickly for them, and they end up on an emotional roller coaster that is overwhelming.

It is helpful to view brainwave training as exercising the brain. When you overwork a muscle in the gym, it will cramp on you and be sore the next day. It is better to work it gently and give it frequent rests. The same applies to the brain. By giving it a day or two of rest in between workouts, you give the client's brain time for integration and growth. We know of no research to support this, but many of the clinicians with whom we have talked have adopted the same position. On the other hand, Bill Scott's (2005) research with the Cry Help addictions clinic in California suggests that this is not really necessary with regard to training attentional problems, so clinicians should not consider it an actual training limitation. In addition, most clients cannot afford to train every day and don't have the time. Making such a commitment can overwhelm them and cause them to give up early in the training.

The 30-Sessions Myth

We always hear stories of how people were "cured" in 15 sessions or 30 sessions. Some of the most competent neurofeedback specialists we speak with at conferences frequently do not find this miraculous recovery rate consistently accurate. There are two main reasons for this:

1. The concept of cure should not be considered applicable in biofeedback. We are not medical doctors and we don't cure diseases.

2. The amount a client "improves" depends on the measure of improvement used. Standard measurements vary in the field, and sometimes we are comparing apples to oranges.

Many long-term disorders take 60 or even 100 sessions to resolve, if you have high standards as a clinician and rigorous outcome measures. By promising a client significant results too quickly, you may be doing a disservice. Letting a client go prematurely may result in relapse. That is why we use objective measures to evaluate clients.

We have had an amazing recovery of function in many cases in as few as 15 sessions, but this is the exception. What we do experience is rapid improvement in symptoms in 10 or 15 sessions if the client is training well. However, we understand that this is often only the beginning of the client's full potential for recovery of mental order and function.

One of the ways to test the efficacy of Neurofeedback and when to discontinue sessions is to look at improvement and stability over time. This can be done by slowly reducing the number and frequency of sessions over time. For example, if the patient has been coming in twice per week and reaches 20 to 25 sessions, look at the reported progress. When the patient has reported symptom reduction to be consistent over 4-5 sessions, try reducing the frequency of sessions down to one session per week. If symptoms return and or worsen, go back to sessions twice per week for another 5-10 sessions. If the patient reports no increase in symptoms and progress stability after 4-5 weekly sessions have the patient come back in two weeks for a session. If symptoms return or worsen go back to 5-10 more once per week sessions. If the patient reports no return of symptoms and progress stability have them come back in for a session in two weeks. If there are no symptom increase and progress is stable, have the patient come back in for a session in three weeks. If symptoms do not increase and progress is stable, then consider discontinuation of neurofeedback.

Drop Outs

No matter how good you are or how effective your practice is, the time will come when a patient comes in for treatment, attends 10 sessions or so, and then drops out of treatment.

Examples

One patient we worked with was doing poorly in school. She was not promoted to the next grade. She began treatment in mid-summer and had trained for four sessions by the time she began school again in late summer. The teachers were amazed at how much better she was doing during the first few weeks of school. Her attention was better. Her grades improved. She was told that if she continued to do well, she would get promoted to the next grade by the Christmas holiday. She attended a total of eight sessions and then just stopped coming to treatment. When contacted, she said she was doing great, feeling better, and didn't feel the need to come back… objective achieved.

Another patient had nine sessions and wanted to be remapped because he was not feeling a sense of improvement. To honor his request, we conducted a second map, which in fact showed some improvement in several areas. Despite the findings, he did not return to treatment.

Possible Solutions

One of the best solutions is using a well-constructed symptom tracker. Most clients are slow to recognize their progress while others around them take notice far more quickly. Presenting them with graphs demonstrating changes in their own self-report of symptoms is a very powerful antidote to skepticism and impatience. NewMind assessments have specially developed symptom trackers that clients can fill out in the office using a tablet and rating themselves on their symptoms while being hooked up for training or even at home between sessions. We use a client portal in the cloud for this purpose. Most practitioners tell us that they cannot imagine doing neurofeedback without this resource once they become accustomed to using it and discovering its impact upon training. You can at least create your own paper versions if you do not have access to clinical software that allows you to do this type of tracking. Some practitioners suggest selling prepaid neurofeedback sessions in a package of 20 sessions. This encourages commitment at a fiscal level. The client is more likely to attend sessions as scheduled for 20 sessions. In many cases, this will result in both the practitioner and the client experiencing improvement.

There is no single best solution to the dilemma of patients who drop out of treatment or do not attend sessions on a regular basis. All of us need to be prepared for such and to come up with creative methods to encourage hesitant clients to continue in treatment.

Evaluating Progress

You should evaluate progress at every session by talking with clients about their subjective indicators and their present training levels. If progress is slow and you are around the twentieth session, you should take another brain map.

Using the NewMind protocol with two channels at the same time, some practitioners have had rapid changes occur (as fast as or faster than Z-Score training) that require a map every 15 sessions or even more often. Interesting information will often show up. We have not often found major changes in amplitude baselines during training, and it can be discouraging to have clients focus on them. The brain map usually shows changes that cannot be found during training baselines. Our position is that in the absence of a brain map, the ongoing evaluation in the form of NewMind's psychological assessments, symptom trackers and cognitive tests is the best measure of progress. After all, it is the symptoms that brought the client in, not his or her baselines.

Psychometric tests are especially valuable for evaluation. Initially, in the past, we used a Beck inventory for a client with issues regarding anxiety and depression. We found that this inventory correlates nicely with changes in the brain maps, as does the TOVA for clients with ADHD. These tests are fairly quick, inexpensive, and easy to administer, and they provide valuable information regarding changes. For individuals with short-term memory issues, we used the digit span section of the Wechsler Intelligence Scale for Children

(WISC), which is also quick and easy to use. Presently we have developed tests exclusively for the purpose of doing neurofeedback that are integrated into the mapping software and that are very user friendly and easy to access and use. Managing and integrating many testing formats can be time consuming and overwhelming to clinicians and we have found making the process as convenient as possible increases the clinical implementation of these very valuable assessment tools.

These types of tests can be used repeatedly with good results and help greatly in objectively documenting client progress. In the past we used components of the Memory Assessment Inventory (MAS) memory test to find out more details about memory problems if the client is suffering from TBI. Clients may quickly forget their progress and habituate to their new conditions. When the training is difficult, it is helpful to provide objective documentation of their progress. Presently we use the Computerized Performance Tests built into the NewMind software because it is automated, convenient and clients can repeat their cognitive tests at home as often as necessary in order to track their progress.

Quite often, we will use a personality inventory on clients who make slow progress. Frequently, this option can save valuable time and money. PTSD can often mimic other disorders and clients will forget or minimize the importance of traumas in their lives. For example, we were treating one client for depression. She recovered from the depression quite well, but her marriage became worse. She started to exhibit new maladaptive behaviors. We thought she had a personality disorder, but we gave her a Personality Assessment Inventory (PAI) and found she had PTSD. When we began treating her for PTSD, her progress rapidly improved.

Note: Research indicates that tests are generally more accurate in evaluating for particular conditions than even the most seasoned clinicians. If you can't do the testing yourself, then refer the client to someone who can.

Outsourcing

We have a psychologist for testing, a neurologist for trauma and organic disorders, an MD for medical problems, a psychiatrist for medications, and a counselor who specializes in violent children. They are not in our office, but we refer clients to them all the time. We have found professionals who believe that what we are doing is important and are willing to work with our clients in the capacity we wish. As we work with our clients' doctors, etc., we try to provide them with information on neurofeedback and meet them for lunch to get acquainted. As a result, we have built a reliable network for support that benefits all parties and makes it possible for us to provide the best service for our clients. We try to keep to our neurofeedback specialty as much as possible. We find this makes the training far more effective.

Ethics

Our field has an ethical standard that each of us must follow. The Biofeedback Certification Institute Alliance (BCIA, 2016) has a set of "Ethical Principles of Biofeedback." It is important to read and comply with these standards. As you continue your practice, you may have a client who comes to you for treatment after having left another professional's practice. The client may even complain about the professional's practice from an ethical concern. Should this occur, first contact that professional to understand both sides of the problem. For further information see Longo and Soutar (2019).

For example, assume a practitioner is treating an adolescent who sustained a TBI from playing hockey. In this scenario, the practitioner informs the client that during the course of neurofeedback treatment the client should refrain from playing hockey or any other sport that might result in another head injury, i.e., lacrosse, soccer, football, etc. However, the client, against the practitioner's advice, continues to play hockey and sustains another head injury. The practitioner then tells the client that neurofeedback treatment will not continue while the client engages in activity with a high risk for head injury. Then the client walks out of that practitioner's office and tries another practitioner.

In this case, the first practitioner followed a protocol that he or she believes in. The next practitioner might tell the client that s/he will continue treatment, but that continuing in a sport that puts the client at risk for a subsequent TBI is not in his or her best interest. This is just one example of the ethical concerns we all face. As Cory Hammond (personal communication, February 5, 2009) notes:

> *"Personally, I'd consider it unethical not to inform them strongly that continued head injuries could do further damage and undo progress. But I don't refuse to continue seeing them, but I keep telling them stories as we're working about cases where people have continued risky behavior and we've seen the results."*

Organizations such as AAPB and ISNR often provide workshops on ethics every year or so. There are two primary reasons for this. Frist, if a practitioner is licensed, they are often required by the state licensure board have 3 or more hours of ethics training for license renewal. When neurofeedback practitioners become BCIA certified in neurofeedback, they are required to have ethics training every renewal period which is currently every four years.

The second reason for attending ethics training is to keep up with the various challenges that may present themselves to neurofeedback clinicians. When we do ethics training we routinely review various and key elements of best ethical practice as well as new and challenging issues that can lead a practitioner in a wrong direction. Scope of practice, types of neurofeedback protocols, and use of new equipment and devices are just a few examples.

Some of the more general concerns among seasoned clinicians include:

Scope of Practice

Does the state licensing board under which you are licensed provide for doing neurofeedback under that license's scope of practice? Streifel and Whitehouse argue (2003):

> Practitioners should know the laws of their individual state in reference to who is and who is not legally allowed to provide biofeedback, psychotherapy, and other health care related services. Laws in some states restrict the provision of some health care services such as biofeedback and psychotherapy to members of specific disciplines, and some do not allow licensed practitioners to supervise unlicensed personnel in the provision of these restricted services. What do the relevant laws in your state say governing the provision of biofeedback, psychotherapy, and related services? It is critical that you know what the provisions of your state laws are. Colorado has licensing laws governing the practice of specific disciplines like psychology, social work, nursing, and physical therapy, but it allows unlicensed practitioners to register themselves as unlicensed psychotherapists and to provide such services as biofeedback (Streifel & Whitehouse, 2003, p. 8).

Scope of practice has become a growing issue in the neurofeedback field as practitioners often cite conditions that can be improved with neurofeedback. In a recent listserve post in 2019 one practitioner wrote:

> *"The new ...program ... with the cerebellum is going to open the doors to treating many disorders such as autism, Parkinson's disorder, dystonias and many other movement disorders as well as epileptic disorders that we could barely address using conventional Neurofeedback in the past. Very hopefully the presentations at this meeting in March and the publications that these new techniques will lead to should have a significant impact not only on the practice of medicine but hopefully on the training of new physicians by being exposed to these methodologies as part of their medical training in the future. "*

The author of this statement is not a physician and the majority of neurofeedback providers are not medical doctors. Claiming to treat medical disorders without a medical license can result in disciplinary actions and even legal action by state licensing boards.

Additionally, portions of the statement are not true. Disorders such as autism, epileptic disorders, and Parkinson's have been successfully treated for over a decade using traditional neurofeedback involving one and/or two channel training. At the time of this writing, there is no research involving clinical trials to treat such disorders nor research comparing the efficacy of "new techniques" to conventional /traditional neurofeedback methods. To date, the majority of clinical studies involve 1, 2, and 4 channel neurofeedback protocols.

Sherlin and Longo (2019) in their workshops on Ethics at ISNR accentuate the point that scope of practice concerns are one of the major and more problematic ethical concerns in neurofeedback.

Claims about Training Outcomes

As noted above, it is important to be honest and clear with potential clients about the benefits and potential outcomes of neurofeedback. All of us will eventually be faced with a difficult case where the patient's progress is slow, and the patient drops out or requires a higher number of neurofeedback treatment sessions to achieve some benefit.

To make claims that one can treat a specific disorder with X number of sessions is not ethical, especially if the clinician does not have a complete history including physical health history of a particular patient. In our clinical experience individual clients / patients who have a history of one or more of the following may be slow to respond to neurofeedback and/or not receive and lasting benefits; a history of taking multiple psychotropic medications, use of recreational drugs such as THC and/or alcohol, multiple physical health problems, and/or social relationship stressors.

Educational Requirements for Members

This field is growing at a rapid pace. It seems that new science in the field of neuroscience is appearing every week. It is important to keep up with the discoveries, research, and general practice concerns when performing neurotherapy. BCIA requires you to pursue educational training but these authors believe it should be part of your everyday work to read the research and share it with fellow clinicians. It should be part of your commitment and ethical standards. It is an unacceptable fact that the majority of medical physicians are seventeen years[2] behind the research and it undermines their effectiveness and the confidence of their patients. As a newly developing field we need to do better than our fellow healthcare professionals. Indeed, we typically find that neurofeedback practitioners are a cut above the rest when it comes to knowing and applying research and we are proud of that standard. There are many listserves available for this purpose. The NewMind group has met three times weekly over the internet for over a decade providing a platform for active information sharing, reviewing all aspects of mapping and training on a regular basis and promoting a sense of support and community identity

2   *https://www.ncbi.nlm.nih.gov/pmc/articles/PMC3241518/*

that is crucial for clinicians who are often isolated in a newly developing field that is often confronted with unreasonable and undeserved skepticism by other professionals who, as we have indicate, do not keep up on the research. We encourage everyone to form or join these types of group activities to enhance your effectiveness as a practitioner.

Professional Responsibility and Liability

Make sure you have insurance and that your insurance provider is aware of the elements of your practice. As noted above, make sure that doing neurofeedback is within your scope of practice, and if need be, that you are practicing under the direct supervision of a qualified professional.

Continuing Education Requirements

It is important to keep up with current trends and the science within our field. If you become BCIA certified, you will be required to attend a specified number of hours of CEU trainings. Joining organizations such APPB and ISNR helps you maintain current education on neurofeedback. Both organization host annual conferences and have publication arms including professional peer reviewed journals and book publication.

Standards of Practice

This is a part of our ethics, and all neurofeedback practitioners should be aware of and follow the ethics for our field as outlined by BCIA (2016); and ISNR[3].

Advertising

As we have noted above and throughout this book, it is important that you do not advertise your work with false claims and information. Many clinicians use information from general websites and those of colleagues. For example, ISNR's website notes; Research demonstrates that neurofeedback is an effective intervention for ADHD and epilepsy. Ongoing research is investigating the effectiveness of neurofeedback for other disorders such as Autism, headaches, insomnia, anxiety, substance abuse, TBI and other pain disorders, and is promising[4]. In fact, neurofeedback is used to address these disorders above others. However, if you are a licensed professional counselor and post on your business website and list these disorders in a brochure stating that you treat these disorders with neurofeedback, you would be liable for a scope of practice violation because LPCs cannot "treat" medical disorders.

---

3   *https://isnr.org/interested-professionals/isnr-code-of-ethics*
4   *https://isnr.org/what-is-neurofeedback*

Licensure

Most manufacturers require that you be licensed in order to buy their equipment. To protect yourself, you should be licensed, and if you are not, you should be operating under the supervision of a licensed professional. If you are interested in becoming BCIA certified, in or to be a certified clinician you must be licensed. If you are not licensed but wish to be certified as a neurofeedback technician, you must work under the direct supervision of a BCIA certified clinician.

Mentoring

Mentoring is the best way to learn the principles and practice of QEEG and neurofeedback. If you plan to be BCIA certified, you will be required to go through a formal mentoring process that is documented. The authors of this book have been working with BCIA to make this process as smooth as possible. We have even published a book of guidelines for those seeking mentoring and certification titled, *Becoming Certified in Neurofeedback* (Longo & Soutar, 2019).

As regards the use of technicians with inadequate training, and who are not fully supervised by licensed people:

If you work in a practice, clinic, or hospital setting where you have technicians working under you, it is important that they have adequate training, guidance, and ongoing supervision. In our practice, we require our technicians to engage in a specified number of hours of observation of our work, followed by a specified number of hours of practice under our direct supervision. They are required to complete readings and manuals and then pass a competency exam. Once they are practicing as technicians, as noted above, they still need to be under your direct supervision.

It is important not to conduct the sale, rental or lease of home training units without ongoing supervision of the use of those units; supervision includes structuring things so that there is assurance that the home training units are not being used by parents on people other than their own children (see ISNR.org/Home/Remote/Telehealth Training Best Practices). To that end NewMind has created software especially designed for training and monitoring individuals who are training at home because of travel restrictions or financial challenges. These units can be monitored and controlled at a distance from the clinician's office. Training data and trend screens are available online for evaluation. Clients cannot begin a session without filling out a progress tracker and notes from parents are encouraged to be entered into the training assessments as well. Practitioners should look for training systems that provide similar supportive technology to ensure high quality training at home.

Do not bill insurance, Medicare, or Medicaid for biofeedback/neurofeedback or QEEG services by representing them as psychotherapy or psychological testing. Be sure to use the appropriate codes that have been created already for these services. At the time of this writing, ISNR is working with the AMA to establish CPT codes that would be used for billing insurance companies directly for neurofeedback. It is anticipated this process could become effective as early as 2022.

Suggested Reading on Ethics

There are two excellent articles in the Journal of Neurotherapy authored by Cory Hammond that address ethics and standards of practice in our field. These are listed below:

Hammond, D., Walker, J., Hoffman, D., Lubar, J., Trudeau, D., Gurnee, R., & Horvat, J. (2004). Standards for the use of quantitative electroencephalography (QEEG) in neurofeedback: A position paper of the International Society for Neuronal Regulation. *Journal of Neurotherapy*, 8(1), 5–27.

Hammond, C., & Kirk, L (2008). First do no harm: Adverse effects and the need for practice standards in neurofeedback. *Journal of Neurotherapy*, 12(1), 79–88.

In addition, there are articles published by Seb Striefel (1989, 1995, 2004) on the topic of ethics and biofeedback that practitioners should review before sitting for the BCIA test or beginning their neurofeedback practices.

REVIEW QUESTIONS

1. How many sessions on average should be run before expecting to see progress with a client?

2. If a client comes to your practice and complains about the ethics of a previous professional, what should you do?

3. Why is tracking a client's symptoms on a weekly basis important?

4. After starting neurofeedback, when should you consider remapping a client using QEEG?

5. Should we advise patients that neurofeedback is mostly experimental?

CHAPTER 8: ALPHA-THETA TRAINING

Alpha-Theta training is very similar to plain alpha training, but with some important exceptions. Alpha-Theta training is a more passive process than other forms of feedback. Its goal is to achieve a temporary and profound liminal (in-between) state between sleeping and waking. In this state, the mind can be deeply probed, instructed, and directed or conditioned. It also appears to be a state highly conducive to the integration of trauma. This training is quite effective with a variety of disorders, especially anxiety, and has often been referred to as slow wave training to distinguish it from fast-wave training such as the SMR training or theta to beta ratio training etc.

BACKGROUND

Alpha-Theta first came to the public's attention through the publication of a series of journal articles authored by Eugene Peniston and Paul Kulkosky (1989). They took a course from Elmer Green on neurofeedback at the Menninger Clinic in Topeka, Kansas and applied the technology in their own clinic in Arizona. Since that time, quite a few well-designed and executed replications have been published (Martins-Moutao, Kerson & Kamiya, 2017). In spite of this, a great deal of myth and misunderstanding continues to surround the protocol and how it should be implemented. In a conversation with Paul Kulkosky (personal communication), Richard has found that their original goal, to a large extent, was to up-train alpha in alcoholics who had too little of it present.

Much of the following background has been lost in the evolution of this protocol, but it is worth understanding. Elmer Green, a biophysicist, became involved in pioneering EEG training. He originally performed extensive alpha training followed by several weeks of theta training. His theory was that the initial extensive alpha training would allow individuals to maintain awareness longer than usual when placed in theta states of consciousness. As a consequence of this process, many of the individuals he worked with were having profound altered-state experiences including many that mimicked near-death experiences.

Gene Peniston was very impressed with Green's workshops and decided to try alpha combined with theta training on resident alcoholics; some accounts indicate that he got the idea while training himself with the protocol. Peniston formulated a unique combination of therapies that included neurofeedback. He emphasized that neurofeedback was only one component of his experiment and should not be considered the only important component. This statement was in response to many professionals who had concluded that neurofeedback was the most important component, since it was the most innovative feature of the design, and the design was so successful in its outcome.

The original experiment involved placing an electrode at O1 on the occipital cortex and providing alpha feedback for a 30-minute session. Subjects were instructed to focus on the tones and encouraged to not engage in any directed thinking, allowing the mind to be still. Individuals were left alone to train in a dimly lit room. Beta was turned off after a five-minute baseline and subjects were left alone in the room to train. They engaged in an abstinence visualization, that had been developed previously in a separate session, prior to each session.

Peniston (1989) appears to have set the alpha threshold at baseline and the theta threshold at an arbitrary 10 µV below the alpha baseline. The procedure was done 5 days a week for a total of 28 days. After each session, the experimenters asked the subjects what they experienced. However, the experimenters reportedly did not do extensive processing with them. The subjects were residents in the institution and may have been engaged in other group or individual counseling activities that were not reported.

The methods section is quite unclear about many details (Lowe & McDowall, 1992). At least one other researcher who attempted to replicate the study reported at an ISNR meeting that he found the original article insufficient in detail for replication and felt that this insufficiency contributed significantly to his failure to find the same results. Going back to Elmer Green's (1977) original writings regarding the subject, we find that his goal was to induce theta in the left occipital cortex and that he felt electrode placement was crucial.

In addition to the EEG training itself, some pre-training exercises were involved including relaxation exercises and hand-warming exercises. The hand-warming exercises involved attaching a thermistor (thermometer) to one hand and practicing raising hand temperature. Some research indicates that there is a correlation between theta production and hand-warming exercises. Peniston (1989) trained prospective clients in visualization, temperature training, rhythmic breathing, and autogenic training before engaging in Alpha-Theta training.

RECENT RESEARCH

More recent literature on the topic and workshops that we have attended have described interesting variants of this original approach. Like so many other forms of feedback, the techniques have become rigid and ritualized as if they contain some kind of magic. However, little attention is given to the rationale underlying the process. Many practitioners presently do this type of training at Pz, P3, and even Cz. Literature from Nancy White's early workshops (personal communication) documents this shift in electrode placement. An interesting crossover phenomenon has also begun to dominate the procedure.

The crossover phenomenon involves a point in the training when subjects begin to experience higher levels of theta than alpha. As individuals train in alpha, they often become drowsy and their alpha frequency slows and drops in amplitude, while theta amplitude theoretically increases. At a certain point, theta becomes higher than alpha. This occurrence indicates the production of hypnagogic or hypnopompic images. A hypnagogic image is a dreamlike image, often vivid and resembling a hallucination, experienced by a person in the transition state from wakefulness to sleep. These images reportedly hold key information that needs to be integrated by the individuals. Post-session interviews with clients focus on bringing these issues to the foreground of their awareness, so they can process them. Consequently, trainers tend to count crossovers and hyper-focus on this occurrence as an indicator of successful training.

Recent research on this topic indicates that there is not a direct correlation between crossovers and these images. However, if you include spontaneous visualizations, then there is an increased correlation. Either way, it may be dangerous to conclude that individuals are repressing material merely because they are not demonstrating crossovers.

Other problems arise with this approach as well. Many individuals have baselines with theta already higher than alpha. This scenario makes it impossible to have a crossover unless you train them in alpha alone. You could attempt to up-train them until their baselines changed; however, baselines may not change that significantly after many sessions even though there is significant improvement in presenting problems. With these individuals, we find that up-training alpha alone results in hypnagogic images, spontaneous significant visualizations, and abreactions. Thus, you need to be prepared to address these experiences when they occur as a result of alphatheta training as described below.

Many variations regarding threshold settings exist as well. Settings for alpha thresholds vary to produce between 50% and 80% reinforcement rates. Settings for theta vary to produce between 20% and 60% reinforcement rates. This situation is interesting because Ratio Strain should occur below 70% reinforcement rates. Ratio Strain is a term used in behavior modification to indicate a point in a reinforcement schedule at which extinction begins to occur because the reinforcement is so difficult to obtain. This scenario means that reinforcement is so low that the operant behavior is poorly elicited. In other words, you are no longer using operant conditioning. A 40% reinforcement rate may be useful, however, in that theta typically increases as alpha decreases and the theta tone may occur during crossover and heighten the subject's awareness while in theta. Again, the underlying theory is that the client needs to produce more alpha initially to enter a state of drowsiness and reverie in order to get into the theta state.

What we observe occurring during a session is that alpha decreases in the first few minutes as the client becomes drowsy and theta begins to increase. The theta tone begins to sound more frequently and the client begins to shift focus to theta uptraining. After a brief period of a few minutes the client typically experiences a burst of what Elmer Green termed "Paradoxical Alpha" and the alpha tone begins to sound more frequently bringing the client back into a more alert state. Soon the client again becomes more drowsy and alpha diminishes again. The client continues to shift back and forth between theta stage 1 sleep and alert alpha awareness which allows them to spend more time in a twilight state between sleeping and waking which is similar to some meditation states.

The consequences of Alpha-Theta training can be very uncomfortable for clients. Abreaction is common, especially in clients with PTSD. Clients may cry, twitch, become restless, moan, and so forth. The common method of dealing with this situation is to leave them alone as much as possible and get them to continue to focus on training. Many practitioners believe these experiences generate a type of systematic desensitization. By this we mean that the client allows themselves to experience past memories of traumas and associated emotions and feelings with progressively less intensity while in the crossover state. When the session ends, it is important to discuss what the client experienced, but it is not necessary to do an in-depth analysis. It is a good idea to be sure that PTSD clients have access to a counselor, so they can process some of the material that surfaces. For those without PTSD, post-session periods of moodiness or anxiety that can be uncomfortable may occur.

Note: Clients need monitoring in this area and reassurance that the discomfort will pass in a few days.

Most practitioners have their clients do a 10-minute post session of SMR enhancement at Cz with theta down-training to get clients clear and to help them integrate material that emerges in the session. We have also used SMR after visualization sessions and find it very effective for the same reason. Some practitioners, like Bill Scott (2002), inhibit 3–5 Hz to reduce abreactions and report that this strategy is effective and does not seem to interfere with the training. When questioning Bill Scott about this innovation, he explained that he came up with this idea when he was training some Native Americans who kept falling asleep during the sessions. He originally thought he could train delta down to keep them awake. It not only helped keep them awake, but he felt that their abreactions began to reduce significantly in intensity and frequency.

Abreactions can occur outside the office; it is important to warn your clients of this possibility. Some people with histories of severe trauma are physically and emotionally incapacitated for days. Prepare them for this possibility and have them come in or contact their counselors if this occurs. In addition, make sure their counselors know what is going on, so they can assist you—especially if you are not their primary therapist. At NewMind, we have clients sign a form (see Appendix D) that explains the possible side effects of the therapy and basic client responsibilities.

Many practitioners such as Martin Wuttke (personal communication) insist that clients do preliminary SMR training or deal with abnormal brainwave activity before engaging in Alpha-Theta training. He also trains individuals in diaphragmatic rhythmic breathing as well. Alpha-Theta training is often contraindicated for individuals with ADHD, schizophrenia, epilepsy, stroke, and head trauma. Bill Scott (2005) reports that he trains individuals from all these categories but does fast-wave training with them first until their TOVAs show normal results. We have found that individuals with high theta have all they can handle in terms of abreactions with alpha training alone.

If you plan to work with individuals with addictions, it is important to get them to stop "using" for the process to be successful. They should also be attending a support group of some kind. The recommended training is daily for 30 days. If they "use" during the training period, they may experience flu-like symptoms or have severe hangovers. This is a commonly reported experience among most clinicians but may be due to other psychological factors not yet identified.

For example, one client who failed to go to meetings went ahead and drank his beer, but found that it tasted funny and did not have the expected effect. Consequently, he went out and bought a bottle of Jack Daniels to do the job. His wife reported that the training also made his hangover worse than usual. Needless to say, he dropped out of the training.

SESSION PROGRESSION

Bill Scott (2005) perfected several methods while performing his research. The following information is taken from that research.

Prior to doing Alpha-Theta training, it is helpful to get a complete history and a TOVA. If the TOVA indicates any attentional problems, these problems should be addressed first. The TOVA is used as a guide to design the protocol. Other measures of neuropsychological and psychological status may be of value as well.

Scott would usually train beta 16–20 Hz up on the left side with inhibits on 23–38 Hz and 2–7 Hz. SMR is uptrained on the right side with the same inhibits. Scott trains one side (hemisphere) at a time during the sessions. He trains more on the side of the brain that appears weakest on the TOVA based on his interpretation of the TOVA. If a client performs poorly on omissions, then Scott will train more on the left side. If the client scores poorly on commissions, then Scott will train more on the right side. The montage he uses is C3-Fpz for left side training and C4-Pz for right-side training. Amplitudes tend to be low because he uses bipolar montages. A great deal of artifact occurs due to eye blinks when training on the left side.

Today we usually do two or four channel training based upon a QEEG initially before engaging in Alpha-Theta training. This typically involves 15 to 20 sessions of neurofeedback or more. Another method in use is Z-Score training, which is similar except it utilizes norms from a database as a reference to set dual threshold ranges for each component band. Most clinicians find that this initial training helps stabilize clients and reduces abreactions as well as enhancing the efficiency of Alpha-Theta training and diminishing the intensity of side effects.

Note: Originally, we were skeptical of the value of training at all with the level of artifact we experienced, but Scott encouraged us to ignore it. To our surprise, clients improved greatly in spite of the artifact.

One of the most surprising things to come out of Bill Scott's (2005) research regards training session frequency. Scott found he could not only train people every day, but even twice a day. This frequency means he was able to normalize an individual's TOVA in 14 or 15 days!

Remediation of attentional problems can be very rapid, but for most people this training schedule can be a significant burden. At NewMind we still tend to train people two or three times a week but are willing to do more intensive training. We do have some people who are training every day.

Once a client's score on the TOVA falls into normal range, it is time to make preparations for the deep states training. Some form of relaxation training is very helpful. We have used finger temperature, skin conductivity response (SCR— also known as SCL, EDR, and GSR), HeartMath® or heart rate variability training, and breath work. At this point we have found that breath work is most effective for us. This training tends to accelerate clients' learning curves when it comes to moving into deep states during neurofeedback. For breath work, we use either HRV or RESPERATE®.

Another important area of preparation is visualization. We have professionally made relaxation and visualization CDs created by Barbara Soutar (available at www.newmindmaps.com), which were designed specifically for this purpose. These visualizations are integrated with audio visual entrainment (AVE) to assist individuals' movement from state to state. We find the entrainment accelerates the learning process for most individuals, but we also use the CDs effectively without entrainment. Many people are not used to actively visualizing scenes and need some initial practice. The CDs provide that practice. In addition, since more salient issues tend to surface during the relaxation and visualization practice, clients become more aware of the issues that they need to work on during Alpha-Theta training.

Beyond this unique potential utilization of visualization, it is a valuable addition for clients to use a short visualization prior to each session that is consistent with their goals. Goals can be solutions to problems, abstinence, performance, and insights into behavior. Usually, trainers instruct clients to focus on their visualizations at the beginning of the sessions and then to let go and focus on the neurofeedback.

This method of short pre-session visualization can be a good approach, but it is not the only way to use visualization. You should not be afraid to innovate with the process, if you feel intuitively that an adjustment could be effective in assisting change. Visualizing vivid dreams or using Jungian methods of symbolic visualization construction based on themes derived from the clients self-narrative can also be very effective. Once clients have practiced visualization and have decided on a specific visualization to use, they are ready to begin formal training.

After clients are hooked up and the filters are set with the correct frequencies and thresholds, they begin with their visualization for a minute or two, and then focus on the tones. Inevitably, most people start to experience an alpha drop out as they drift into deeper states. They also begin to lose self-awareness. At a certain point, the theta grows higher than the alpha. When this occurs, as we previously mentioned, they begin to experience more theta reinforcement than alpha. This point is a good time to tweak the threshold by increasing or decreasing it, so that they are actively getting theta reinforcement.

Clients will experience periodic resurgences of alpha that bring them back into greater self-awareness and then slide back into theta. The beta inhibit will assist those clients with anxiety from getting overly aroused when this shift occurs. Clients tend to swing back and forth like this until they begin to drift into stage 1 sleep. At this point, delta will begin to rise in amplitude. As your client nods off, you can note the delta level and readjust it, so a sound of some kind will rouse the client. We use an alarm clock sound in one of our programs that goes off when delta goes above its baseline value. Elmer Green (personal communication) used to tie one of the client's fingers to a mercury switch and have the client hold his or her arm up by resting the elbow on the chair. When the client drifted off, the arm would drop, and the mercury switch would set off a doorbell. When clients experience a complete cycle like this, you will know how to set their thresholds exactly. Bill Scott tends to sit through the session and "ride" the thresholds the whole time. If clients tend not to fall asleep, then we dispense with the delta tone altogether. You can also rattle your paperwork or make other sounds to rouse them. It is also important to keep in mind that as long as they are hooked up, they are not in a normal sleep mode because their brain is still processing auditory feedback even though their frontal lobes are exhibiting diminished conscious activity.

At NewMind, we tend to just let clients train alone, although we constantly check on them to make sure they are doing well and that the electrodes have not fallen off. Many clients will train better with no one present in the room as was the case in the original research methods reported. Clients will swing back and forth between full awareness and sleep. Over a series of several sessions, they will get better and better at balancing in a deep state between sleep and waking. This deep state is really the goal of the training.

Diagram 54: Threshold, shows the different frequencies and how to set the thresholds as discussed. Client EEG averages tend to look like the pattern shown. After training with their eyes closed for a few minutes, the pattern tends to shift to the pattern shown in at the bottom (see Diagram 55: Thresholds After Eyes Closed). Delta tends to be highest only when they move into very deep states approaching sleep, with theta next highest and alpha the lowest. Clients will shift back and forth from the top pattern to the bottom pattern as they train. It is during these shifts that they will have crossovers.

Crossovers vary in length and importance, as previously mentioned. They tend to begin somewhere between the fifth and the tenth sessions. The longer the crossover, the less likely clients are to recall any associated images and the more likely they are to drift into sleep. The images may or may not have pertinence to them at the time. Our most seasoned clients can drop into long crossovers without going into sleep like states and remain there for 5–10 minutes at a time. This may or may not be valuable, depending on the goal of the training.

When clients finish the session, it is a good idea to review their experiences, both physical sensations and psychological events. Specific probes such as "did you feel any unusual physical sensations" or "Did you have any brief intense dream like images" etc. Frequently, clients will have unusual experiences while they are outside of the office. Some clients have no hypnagogic experiences at all, but instead have intense and sometimes lucid dreams while sleeping at home at night. These dreams may sometimes hold the key to fundamental issues and may be of value to review and discuss. If relevant, they may be used as visualization material.

Although this initial didactic discussion of Alpha-Theta training is very helpful in explaining the basic theory behind Alpha-Theta training, it is no substitute for a good workshop, mentoring and hands on training. We recommend that every clinician who plans to utilize this form of Alpha-Theta training also train themselves extensively using this protocol. This will enhance your understanding of how it works and how it is experienced by your clients in a manner that will greatly assist you in employing it clinically.

Diagram 54: Thresholds After Eyes Open

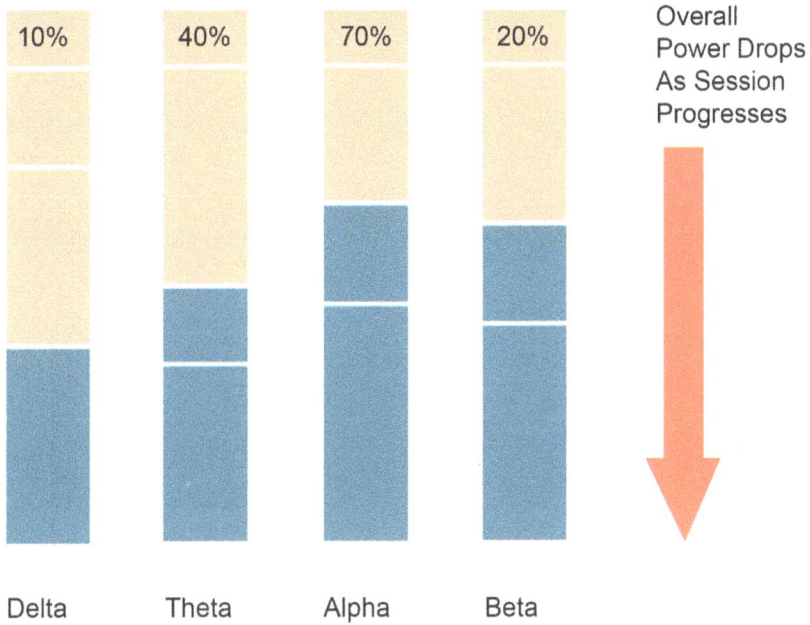

| 10% | 40% | 70% | 20% |

Overall
Power Drops
As Session
Progresses

Delta   Theta   Alpha   Beta

Set Initial Thresholds A Above And Adjust During Session
Adjust Theta To Be Highest After Alpha Drops
Adjust Delta To Sound When Client Drifts Into Sleep

Diagram 55: Thresholds After Eyes Closed

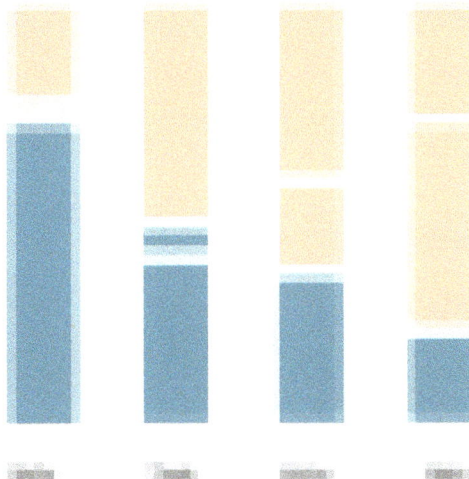

REVIEW QUESTIONS

1. What is the value of Alpha-Theta training?

2. What creates crossover?

3. What is a hypnagogic image?

Chapter 9: Audio Visual Entrainment & Photic Stimulation

DEFINITION OF AVE

Photic stimulation is a procedure whereby flashing light pulses are used to stimulate the optic nerve in an effort to influence brainwave activity. Traditionally this has been done as a standard procedure in evaluating individuals with seizure activity utilizing powerful freestanding light devices in an effort to induce interictal epileptiform discharges. The lamps required for this type of testing need to be very bright in order to induce epileptiform activity and are usually a high intensity type of xenon gas lamp manufactured specifically for this purpose. Because of the ability of bright light pulses to induce abnormal EEG patterns, many researchers over the years have become very interested in how pulsing light might influence brainwave activity in other ways. Other innovators, like Dave Siever (Siever, 2000) have drawn on the decades of research in this area to develop lower intensity devices that appear to provide a variety of benefits for end users. When combining intermittent photic stimulation along with intermittent audio stimulation a synergistic effect occurs which appears to further enhance these benefits. Siever calls this type of device an Audio-Visual Entrainment device (AVE).

In the past two decades progressively more vendors have emerged offering variations on this type of low intensity intermittent stimulation in the form of popular devices for consumers to use. They vary in form and function as well as claims regarding the benefits they offer. In particular they offer a variety of preset frequency patterns that purportedly have effects unique to their proprietary formulations.

Richard began working closely with Dave Siever in 1999 at the clinical level combining his technology with neurofeedback after hearing about the work of Len Ochs (Kravitz, 2006) with this combination of technologies. Richard began using the new QEEG technology of the time to investigate the effects of AVE upon the brain of healthy individuals as well as individuals with a wide variety of disorders. The results were encouraging and agreed with the research Siever was conducting and publishing at the time, so we continued to use this technology as well as share our findings at the ISNR and AAPB meetings with other practitioners over the years.

One of our key findings that rather quickly came to light was that the photic component of AVE accounted for about 90% of its effect upon the EEG. In light of this finding, we primarily implemented the use of this technology moving forward using only the Photic stimulation component. At the same time we continued to send clients home with devices to further condition their brainwave patterns that employed the full AVE components of both light and sound stimulation. This strategy appeared to enhance their neurofeedback training in the clinic as well as assist them in managing their symptoms as the neurofeedback training gradually took hold. We found they enjoyed the combination of music and photic stimulation and were more likely to regularly use the devices when both types of stimulation were available.

RESEARCHING AVE

The typical AVE device involves a standalone box connected to a pair of glasses with LEDs embedded in the lenses and a set of earphones. The end user can control the frequency and intensity of both the light and sound pulses produced. It is often possible to control the pulsing wave shape utilized so that sinusoidal, square or sawtooth waveforms are available. Usually there are preselected programs providing the proprietary combinations that are purported to benefit the user. Most manufacturers have no research to back these claims up and most of it is based on subjective report. In addition, users can usually plug in their cell phone to the device and use a music app to play music through the headset along with the pulse tones which provides a more pleasant experience. This also provides the opportunity to offer prerecorded audio programs with affirmations and visualizations. As far back as 1999 we were using guided visualizations to control the frequencies of the MindAlive® DAVID devices and providing progressive relaxation sequences as well. These audio visualizations are still available from the NewMind website.

AVE and photic devices can be used to stimulate higher frequency brainwave activity and increase arousal or they can be used to generate lower frequency brainwave activity to reduce arousal. This can easily be confirmed by any practitioner by merely observing the raw EEG trace and inspecting the session review screen of any individual they are training. Some individuals are more responsive than others depending on a variety of factors discussed below. Based on decades of clinical observation and recorded notes, we have concluded that those with the greatest amount of disorder appear to be the least responsive. Drugs in particular appear to reduce efficacy as is the case with neurofeedback. It should be kept in mind that AVE and photic technologies are coercive technologies and can force a change in EEG pattern when neurofeedback cannot. The change in pattern, however, disappears the moment the device is turned off.

Some of the AVE devices, such as the MindAlive® series by Dave Siever, also come with additional technologies that appear to enhance the effect of this technology. One such technology is Cranio-Electrical Stimulation (CES) that involves applying a small electrical stimulus across the scalp. This technology purportedly stimulates endorphins and some neurotransmitter activity. Further research is required to validate this technology but it presently looks promising as an adjunctive technology, however it cannot be used at the same time as neurofeedback training as the electrical pulses are picked up by the neurofeedback sensors and this generates significant artifact that makes neurofeedback impossible.

USING AVE

Photic stimulation produces a pulsed electromagnetic field (PEMF) effect, usually between .5 and 6 milligauss depending on the unit being used, as well as a photobiological stimulation effect upon the prefrontal region of the brain as the light that flashes also penetrates the skull. The impact of this "photobio" effect varies with light color, with the near infrared light having the most penetrating effect (Hamblen, 2016). The additional impact of these effects have yet to be studied but are clearly present based on measures that any clinician can take and observe using a field meter.

The primary mechanism of action, based on extensive research is well established. Stimulation of the optic nerve generates frequency pulses that travel to the lateral geniculate nucleus of the thalamus, through the radiata and into Brodmann areas 18 and 19 of the occipital cortex. This activity tends to stimulate the neurons in this region and drive these networks to oscillate at a frequency similar to the photic driving frequency. A controversy still exists as to whether the photic stimulation drives these neurons or whether it merely stimulates a mimetic activity (Collura, 2002). This is the exogenous vs endogenous debate. The question arises as to whether the exogenous activity converts to an endogenous activity. It is clear that the majority of the driving effect dissipates as soon as the photic activity is turned off but a residual effect appears to remain for approximately 15 minutes (Frederick et al., 1999). When monitoring changes with pre-post QEEG it is common to find that 10Hz stimulation tends to normalize the distribution of all five neurometric dimensions within 30 seconds of photic onset or less. Again, this normalization of distribution dissipates within seconds of discontinuing the photic stimulation. All of this is readily observable with standard equipment by any practitioner wishing to spend the time to investigate. What varies is the degree to which each neurometric dimension responds between individuals and between disorders. Further investigations in this arena would be highly useful.

It is possible to train hemispheres somewhat independently. Each eye has a left and right eyefield that crosses over to the contralateral hemisphere. So the left eyefield trains the right hemisphere and vice versa. There is some overlap in the nerve pathways so it is not exclusive but it does have some independent impact. The photic glasses can be programmed in some photic units to take advantage of this physiological feature. For instance you can entrain the left eyefield in SMR frequencies that will drive primarily the right hemisphere while at the same time train entrain the right eyefield in the betas frequencies to drive the left hemisphere. This type of protocol can be especially effect with depression as it trains brain asymmetry.

Disorders That Respond

A wide variety of disorders reportedly respond with varying degree to AVE and Photic Stimulation. It has been found to reduce anxiety and depression, insomnia, high blood pressure, trigeminal neuralgia, attention deficits, memory, PMS, migraines, chronic fatigue and many forms of pain. We have experienced considerable clinical success with all of these disorders and if this technology was a drug it would be widely used. It is inexpensive and fairly effective at managing these disorders. It is not a cure however and should be used purely for management purposes or to generate more plasticity in the brain in order to enhance the efficacy of clinical neurofeedback. Generally, the more severe the symptomology the less impact it will have on the client. We have witnessed clients with severe migraine abort their migraine within 20 minutes after employing this technology and do so episode after episode. We have also seen some migraines fail to respond completely. Not all migraines have the same etiology.

Training Methods

Using AVE and Photic devices as home units for training support is quite straight forward. The NewMind QEEG brainmaps tell you exactly what frequencies to use in the protocol output section. You can also use these devices for relaxation and calming as well as aiding in sleep onset. We have developed the ZION units with Dave Sievers help to simplify the process as much as possible. Clients can usually put on the glasses and head set and click the "on" button and then their protocol button and begin training without further ado. Many of the other units available involve a lot of manual reading, experimentation with many button sequences required to generate the correct protocol. Many units also will list one frequency and use many other frequencies besides.

The ZION unit only generates the frequency that it indicates and does not vary from that frequency. This is an important feature for clinical applications. If units are generating a lot of frequency variations in their protocols, the clinician will not be able to reliable determine which protocol to use and what occurred if the protocol did not generate the intended results. We would be happy to recommend other devices, but we cannot find any others that we find clinically reliable, hence our own development program.

We have utilized white light for training for decades because the light color has a minimal effect with the exception of red square wave light which has been known to be more likely to generate epileptiform activity in some individuals prone to neuronal instability. In addition we tend to use sinusoidal pulse waveforms to target specific frequencies because they tend to reproduce less unwanted harmonics. There are times however when we will employ square wave pulses when we are looking for a multiple harmonic effect as when we want to downtrain a frequency during neurofeedback sessions. More on that below.

An additional procedure we recommend for implementing protocols is to place a sensor at Cz and monitor the component bands while having the client run the recommended protocol. Confirm that it is having the anticipated intended effect. For instance, if you are looking for the theta to decrease, then it should trend down during some portion of the session. If the beta increases, that may be an equivalent outcome.

Using Photic stimulation during training is a different procedure. Both NewMind and Brainmaster® offer a variety of possibilities in this area as does Clearmind equipment. The software allows you to train each hemisphere independently at the same time you train each hemisphere separately with neurofeedback. You can therefore match the neurofeedback protocol to the entrainment Protocol. NewMind and Brainmaster® also allow you to trigger the photic glasses so they entrain only when you are above or below a component band threshold. In addition, NewMind software allows you to increase the intensity of the frequency as it approaches and exceeds the threshold to produce a proportional training effect. NewMind also provides a left to right light feature for those wishing to use the glasses for EMDR while monitoring brainwave activity. Unfortunately none of the other vendors have developed this technology and integrated it with neurofeedback software, although I have urged them to do so, but that should not prevent you from using a stand-alone device in conjunction with your neurofeedback equipment to take advantage of the synergy these two technologies can produce in the clinical environment when training.

As you can see there are many possibilities for combining these two technologies to provide more enhanced outcomes. We are constantly researching and developing new methods and software for photic technology and expect it to continue being a key component of neurofeedback training in the future.

EARLY RESEARCH: THE FOUNDATIONS

In this section we will review the research behind AVE and Photic technologies for those interested in the detail of the supporting investigations. Much of the early research regarding entrainment focused on establishing the existence of entrainment and exploring the essential features of the basic phenomena. Kawaguchi et al. (1993) noted that these early studies focused on the existence of the driving response, responsivity, latency of response (cortical resistance to entrainment), and variability of response.

Loomis, Harvey, and Hobart (1936) found that individuals with strong alpha rhythms had a narrow frequency range in which entrainment took place, whereas those individuals with low alpha had a much wider frequency range of entrainment. This discovery was repeatedly explored over the next several decades. James Toman (1941) followed up this research with findings that replicated the earlier work.

Walter and Walter (1949) determined that photic stimulation can cause EEG patterns to match the frequency of the driving stimulus. Gastaut and Hunter (1950), on the other hand, concluded that a difference probably exists between spontaneous brain rhythms and photic driven rhythms and consequently developed a new line of investigation on this interesting distinction to be pursued in future research which Tom Collura later picked up (Collura, 2002). Garoutte and Aird (1958) also found considerable variation in subjects regarding how well EEG binds to photic stimulation rhythms.

Barlow (1959) continued to investigate whether entrainment resulted in a change in natural EEG, or if the response occurred in special networks related to intrinsic EEG phenomena. After concluding that entrainment was actually taking place, he noted that the frequencies of entrainment did not generate mirror images in the EEG, and there could be a highly variable relationship between input and response. He theorized that both EEG and "sensory after discharge" occur in nonspecific systems to generate alpha, but that the two systems might still be separate. Tweel and Lunel (1965) also found that although the amplitude of the EEG response could often be independent of the intensity of photic stimulus, typically it reflected input character in terms of amplitude and frequency. They also found that out-of-phase stimulation in both eyes produced cancellation effects.

Ulett (1957) studied susceptibility to entrainment in low and fast frequency ranges of anxiety-prone individuals. He found that the driving response fluctuated from day to day based on mood. There was a relationship examined between colors seen during photic driving, amount of movement perceived in eyes-closed patterns, and Rorschach responses, with rigid personalities exhibiting less of both colors and movement.

Ultett (1957) also reported:

- Shifts in blood oxygen saturation occurred at specific frequencies.
- Photic stimulation could cause visual hallucinations related to past experiences along with irregular bursts of slow-wave activity.
- Specific frequencies could cause subjective dysphoria in some individuals.
- Specific frequencies could cause myoclonus or paroxysmal activity and could lower seizure thresholds.

- Photic shock or intense bursting pulses was thought to be more effective and less destructive than regular shock therapy.
- Sleep deprivation increased myoclonic and paroxysmal responses to photic driving.
- Metabolic changes could alter responses to photic driving.

He even reported on research in which it was found that photic stimulation paired with sound can generate the same rhythm when the sound is played back. These findings suggest a multitude of confounds that can be present when experimenting with photic stimulation and that are not usually considered in more modern research. This evidence seriously calls into question the internal validity of many of these studies.

Dieter and Weinstein (1995) agreed that photic driving in the alpha range increased EEG alpha beyond natural levels and acknowledged that photic theta pulses produced altered states with hypnagogic phenomena. Iwahara et al., (1974) found that the entrainment effect was the result of a combination of EEG, photic driving effect, and a blocking effect. The blocking effect resulted in a reduction in EEG amplitude due to the stimulus that was present but was not usually considered. They felt this research supported the idea that the photic driving effect was a different phenomenon than just the increase in basic EEG activity and that the research supported earlier researchers who had concluded that it occurred in different circuits than networks that typically produced the endogenous EEG.

Townsend et al., (1975) began exploring Sinusoidal Modulated Light (SML) and determined that it is different than photic driving. SML at the alpha frequency is more specific in its action upon the EEG with less activity occurring outside the alpha range. The degree of entrainment at the cortex depends on the proximity of the driving stimulus frequency to the dominant alpha frequency. Entrainment also reduces frequency variability without appreciably altering morphology. The average evoked EEG response amplitude is highest at the dominant resident alpha frequency. He also concluded that the driving response occurs in other networks and alters natural EEG through this mechanism. Unfortunately, he and previous researchers fail to discuss what these networks might be, how they relate to natural EEG networks, and how they specifically alter EEG. The theory behind all this research was apparently not well developed.

Takahashi and Tsukahara (1976) experimented with colors and frequencies to determine what would be most likely to induce a seizure or photo-convulsive response. They determined that the color red in conjunction with 15 Hz was most likely to induce this phenomenon.

RECENT RESEARCH

Moving into later research, we find that brain imaging becomes more important and that there is a continued focus on physiology. Fox and Raichle (1985) reported that regional cerebral blood flow increased in the striate cortex by 28% due to photic stimulation. Mentis et al., (1997) reported that photic stimulation activates the frontal area of the brain. Diehl et al., (1998) found that significant cerebral blood flow increases due to photic stimulation.

Pigeau and Frame (1991) found that subjects with high amplitude alpha baselines showed best entrainment at frequencies closest to their spontaneous peak alpha frequencies. Low alpha baseline subjects, however, didn't appear dependent on this same phenomenon. Subjects with low amplitude alpha baselines, on the other hand, were more responsive across the alpha range and more responsive across all frequencies. The authors concluded their research with the theory that high and low alpha baselines may represent the degree of coupling between two different alpha sources in the cortex and subcortex. Strongly coupled thalamo-cortical connections could be reducing cortical activity, which shows up as high alpha with a strong spontaneous peak alpha frequency (lack of plasticity). Low-amplitude alpha may represent weaker thalamo-cortical connections and less stable spontaneous peak alpha frequency. Of special interest is the neurophysiological theory proposed with regard to the phenomena studied, and the suggestion that the path of entrainment is through the lateral geniculate nucleus into the visual cortex via geniculo-calcarine radiation.

Kawaguchi et al., (1993) investigated inter- and intra- hemispheric synchrony and found that repetitive flashes enhance these phenomena, but they are not consistent during photic driving. They concluded that the lateral geniculate nucleus is the main player in setting up resonance between EEG and photic driving.

Patrick (1996) used AVE in place of neurofeedback on ADD using EEG monitoring to confirm a client's ability to duplicate AVE experience (small group). Morse (1993) reported that AVE with recorded music works better than AVE alone.

Rosenfeld et al., (1997), building especially on Pigeau and Frame (1992), found that high baseline alpha showed no entrainment at 10 Hz, and low baseline alpha showed transient entrainment (stopped when stimulus stopped). However, only 25% of the variance was explained by the variance in the baseline. They further found that training just off the spontaneous peak alpha frequency tended to inhibit rather than enhance alpha production. They indicated that high alpha baseline subjects showed no entrainment at 22 Hz stimulation and that low alpha baseline subjects did show transient entrainment. Furthermore, beta entrainment also produced increased alpha in some individuals. They concluded that effects of entrainment cease once stimulus is terminated. They argued that there was insufficient evidence to show what had been called "sensory after discharge" or entrained EEG and that spontaneous EEG arises from the same pathways. Lubar's lab (Lubar, 1997, 1998; Timmerman, Lubar, Rasey, & Frederick, 1999) found that dominant alpha frequency training with AVE increased eyes-open beta and reduced delta. Budzynski (1999) performed a pilot study that indicated that AVE can shift dominant alpha frequency upward. Shealy (1990) reported that 10 Hz AVE increases serotonin levels by 20% and beta-endorphins by 14%. He found that the optimal session length is 20–30 minutes and that most people prefer violet light. He also reported that variable frequency is best for dealing with pain.

RESEARCH ON THE USE OF AVE WITH SPECIFIC DISORDERS

In addition to the impact photic stimulation has on physiological and psychological features associated with anxiety, other exploratory research efforts indicate it has considerable potential with a variety of other disorders.

Solomon (1985) found AVE to be effective with muscle-contraction headaches but not with migraines (small group study).

Anderson (1988) found AVE effective with migraines (small group study).

Norton (1997) found AVE useful for treating PMS (small group study).

Carter and Russell (1993) used AVE successfully with Learning Disorders.

Montgomery et al., (1994) used AVE successfully with closed head injury, aneurysms, and stroke.

Kumano et al., (1996) found AVE effective with depression in a highly criticized study (single case design). Cantor and Stevens (2009) on the other hand did a well-designed small groups study that also should significant reductions in the symptoms associated with depression.

David Noton (1995, 1996) found that PMS symptoms were reduced by 50%.

Rozelle and Budzynski (1996) found that EEG-driven photic stimulation gives good results with stroke victims.

Michael Joyce (1998) was successful using it with ADD, and D. J. Anderson (1989) regularly stopped migraines with AVE.

David Trudeau (1999) reported a successful case using 18 Hz AVE for 60 sessions with chronic fatigue syndrome.

Dave Siever (1999) reported on using AVE alpha and/or delta (n = 51) in a study of people with fibromyalgia in which he found good results and also another study with TMJ.

Tom Budzynski (2002) reported use of AVE in the case of an Alzheimer's patient that appeared to show promise in slowing the progress of decline. Gaspar et al. (2013) did a meta analysis of the literature of photic as it relates to Alzheimers Disease and concluded it may have significant potential to reduce symptomology. During photic stimulation the authors found interhemispheric coherence higher in older individuals in the harmonic response in the 30 Hz and 40 Hz range when stimulated at 5 Hz. AD patients had lower coherence in the harmonic response in the 10 Hz and 20 Hz range in response to 5 Hz stimulation. AD patients had lower coherence in the harmonic response in the 10 Hz and 20 Hz range in response to 10 Hz stimulation. Alpha response to alpha photic stimulation.

Pastor et al. (2003) find that the photic stimulation on the 40 Hz range produces a lesser response than 10 Hz, 15 Hz, or 35 Hz. On the other hand, Ross et al. (2014) found that any binaural tone stimulation, even low frequencies, evoke a 40 Hz response (Fujioka, Jamalie, Miyazaki, Ross, Thompson, 2014).

In children, using 15 and 40 Hz alternating frequencies, there is a study in ADHD with 35 sessions, with outcomes in WISC improvement and concentration capacity (Olmstead, 2005)

Kohdabashi et al. (2005) stimulated alpha in .5 Hz increments in a range from 8 to 10.5 Hz with each photic burst lasting 10 seconds in length and repeated 10 times before moving to the next increment. Photic stimulation resulted in minimal change compared to controls suggesting a widespread loss of functional interactions in the alpha band. Temporoparietal regions exhibit low glucose consumption and low oxygen consumption as well as lower cerebral blood flow. EEG in these areas show high delta and theta and low beta and alpha.

Williams, Ramaswamy, & Oulhaj (2006) found best frequencies for improving memory in indiviuals over 67 was to train using frequencies between 10 Hz and 10.5 Hz.

Gaspar et al. (2013) did a meta analysis of the literature of photic as it relates to Alzheimers Disease and concluded it may have significant potential to reduce symptomology.

Tang et al. (2014) demonstrated that AVE reduced pain and improved sleep. They used a 30 minute program that slowly descends from alpha into delta.

Roberts et al. (2018) 5.5 Hz Enhanced episodic memory performance.

PAST RESEARCH FINDINGS AND RULES OF ENTRAINMENT

It is clear from this research that AVE has considerable potential for a wide variety of disorders when used on its own; however, our main interest is whether it can be used to accelerate the neurofeedback process. It seems to be effective in most of the same disorders as neurofeedback and is likely to be of value in the same domains. This similarity causes us to consider the rules of entrainment when using it in conjunction with neurofeedback. Where and when will it assist and where could it create problems? We constructed the following axioms of entrainment from the above research and our own clinical experience.

General Findings of AVE

- The effects of entrainment are highly variable between clients
- The effects of entrainment vary between sessions
- Individuals with low alpha baselines are most affected by entrainment
- With respect to EEG. For these individuals:
  - Training is fairly effective across the spectrum
  - There are more effects outside the target frequency
- Individuals with high alpha baselines are least affected by entrainment
- With respect to EEG. For these individuals:
  - Training is most effective within the alpha range
  - Training is most effective at the dominant alpha frequency
- Most of the entrainment effects with respect to EEG dissipate quickly after the entrainment device is shut off
- There does appear to be some residual effect on beta amplitudes, which may last over 24 hours
- Training next to a dominant frequency may cause cancellation effects
- Training next to a dominant frequency may reduce EEG amplitude
- AVE is more effective with music
- Clients prefer violet light
- It may be possible to classically condition a client's entrainment pattern to music

Seizure Concerns

- AVE can temporarily enhance paroxysmal patterns in the EEG

- Red frequencies are most likely to contribute to paroxysmal patterns
- Frequencies over 15 Hz are likely to contribute to paroxysmal patterns
- Square waves are more likely to contribute to paroxysmal patterns than sine waves

Morphology

- Square waves are more likely to generate harmonics
- Sine waves are more specific in entrainment effects

Physiology

- AVE reduces autonomic arousal
- AVE increases frontal activity
- AVE increases cerebral blood flow
- High baseline alpha may indicate strongly coupled thalamo-cortical connections
- Low baseline alpha may indicate weakly coupled thalamo-cortical connections

Personality Theory

- High responsivity to AVE in terms of color and movement may be correlated with flexible personality
- Low responsivity to AVE in terms of color and movement may be correlated with rigid personality
- The above axioms suggest a wide range of variables not reported or taken into account in most of the experimental designs executed so far
- Case studies should carefully screen for all these factors

  - Baseline Alpha Levels
  - mood
  - sleep patterns
  - metabolic changes
  - drugs taken
  - color of light used
  - type of wave pattern employed
  - personality profile
  - use of music

These factors constitute possible confounds with regard to both training and research and must be taken into consideration. The findings to date would seem to clearly emphasize the importance of regarding the brain not as a linear, passive system, but as a non-linear, reactive system with regard to outside stimuli. In the prevailing zeal to deal with objective phenomena, many seem to lose sight of the fact that EEG is coupled to very subjective phenomena. As stable as EEG phenomena may be with respect to averaged readings of power and frequency, it is still profoundly variable on an instantaneous basis and reflects subjective changes of state. These changes of state are linked to very subjective factors.

Client Reactivity To Photic Stimulation and Client History: Further Confounds

The research on AVE dealing with variables such as high and low alpha baselines does not as a rule extend its discussion into areas regarding what generates these differences in alpha baselines and appears to assume that they are normal variants. This is a dangerous assumption to maintain, as recent research suggests that high amplitude slow alpha and low amplitude fast alpha are often correlated with depression and anxiety disorders, respectively. This scenario is often the case even at a subclinical level.

The prevailing theory, of course, is that altering these baselines can reduce disorder and symptoms. However true this may be, the reverse should also be considered. Factors outside the clinic can cause symptoms to increase and generate reduced client responsivity with respect to training. Internal environments are also likely to generate similar reactivity. In this sense, history often works through the reactive process to generate forces that compromise training efforts. There are clients who do not respond to AVE or neurofeedback.

De Goode et al. (1972) indicated that expectation and cognitive set considerably influence alpha training. Lynch and Paskewitz (1971) noted that alpha only occurs in situations where subjects cease to attend to stimuli that normally block this activity, such as cognitive, somatic, emotional, and environmental events. Anxiety and depression both have ruminative features involving repetitive negative self-talk and related emotions. It may very well be these features that influence alpha baselines by engaging and occupying attentional networks.

We have had anxiety clients increase their alpha instantaneously by suspending their ruminative activities for a few moments. In similar situations, others have decreased their abnormally high amplitude alpha. In cases where individuals are so emotionally involved with internal ruminations that they cannot disengage, it is likely they will not do well with neurofeedback. It is also likely that this applies to AVE. We have, however, observed variations in responsivity to neurofeedback and AVE. Initially, many clients will generate higher amplitudes of alpha during AVE than during neurofeedback. This suggests that attentional networks are influencing outcomes. Clients may be overusing active attentional networks during neurofeedback, and consequently blocking alpha in their efforts to focus and concentrate on the stimulus tone.

The Role of Active and Passive Attentional Networks

Othmer et al. (1999) and Sterman (1996) observed that it may not be necessary that a conscious awareness of training take place for neurofeedback effects to emerge. More recently, Birbaumer (2006) demonstrated with MRI imaging that neurofeedback could be an entirely involuntary process. In some instances, it may be that conscious efforts at training may not always be as successful as those efforts that bypass it, as in cases when clients try too hard. Kamiya (1979) discovered through experimental procedure that initial training using conscious intent results frequently in an achieved average alpha that is less than baseline. Successive trials usually, but not always, result in training averages higher than baseline. This evidence suggests that conscious efforts alter the training pattern of neurofeedback and vary its impact on subconscious operant processes. The variety of factors influencing this conscious effort may be quite large and could include a considerable number of interaction effects as well. In addition, the human unconscious response may also have considerable impact on training efficacy. The consequences for AVE may be similar as well.

An under-acknowledged assumption in previous decades is that EEG and neurofeedback are being investigated in a passive brain system, that is, the brain passively responds to a stimulus. Investigators have not clearly acknowledged that they are dealing with an active system that may respond in accordance with a number of variables so complex as to qualify as a nonlinear chaotic system. Nunez and associates (1996; 2006) have recognized the non-linear characteristics present, but also have failed to recognize intentional and preconscious components driving that system. Whether the observer-subject is a consequence of the system or not has yet to be determined, but in either case the observer-subject surely constitutes a metasystem with its own unique characteristics.

This observer-subject system is often more reactive in a manner based on its history rather than immediate stimuli. As interaction with a stimulus accumulates, memories may alter the meaning and value of any given stimulus and thus the appropriate response. This consideration calls for a different perspective than that which presently operates frequently in the EEG experimental environment. Although it is traditionally acknowledged in psychology that a subject's awareness of the purpose of an experiment can confound the internal validity of that experiment, those who have been conducting experiments with EEG, as well as clinical protocols, often assume that EEG operates independently from subject awareness. They appear to assume that EEG could be consistently responsive to training independent of subjective factors known to influence it. The most curious part of this fact is that it even needs to be mentioned to psychologists engaged in research.

The implications of this consideration are that the presence of the subject's observer system can alter the nature of the object of experimentation or treatment, which in this case is the brain. The responses of the brain from this perspective arises from a proactive system with regard to the independent variable and can alter the definition, and consequently the effectiveness, of the independent variable, that is beyond or outside of the experimenter's definition. The subject's observer system can instantly alter the response pattern of the brain. It can anticipate, be proactive, and marshal resources to resist training or entrainment at a conscious or pre-conscious level of operation. This resistance process may be due to activities and responses of the observer that occur outside the clinical setting.

Our clinical experiments indicate that subjects can frequently produce high levels of alpha EEG during entrainment while failing to produce similar results using neurofeedback. Successive trials usually continue to produce this result until the average neurofeedback amplitude equals the average photic driven amplitude. Paradoxically, photic or AVE at this point often proves to be less effective than neurofeedback, with clients producing higher amplitudes without AVE. This also supports the notion that subjects are learning to use their attentional networks in such a way as to sustain attention, but not generate an alpha blocking effect. Active attentional shifts cause a reduction in grand average alpha over the course of a session as well as instantaneous alpha amplitude, but sustained attention without active processing increases it. It is not uncommon to find that some individuals with very busy minds, or heavy automatic thinking, produce very high alpha while meditators with very little automatic thinking also produce high alpha. The brain is idling for two different reasons. Automatic thinking requires very little effort, so that much of the cortex is disengaged while a small area is very busy. In meditation, the brain in general is significantly less engaged in active or automatic thinking and thus producing high levels of alpha idling. This outcome suggests the possibility that AVE engages a passive attentional network that the client eventually learns to employ with neurofeedback as well over successive trials. At this point, clients not using AVE are able to more effectively use this network than with the AVE. Consequently, their neurofeedback average amplitude is higher. What remains to be explained is why AVE amplitudes tend to decrease after this point.

Research literature from the late twentieth century provides evidence of an active and passive attentional system (Posner & Raichle, 1994). Active networks are employed to learn new skills and passive networks are engaged to execute those learned skills. Once alpha production has become an acquired skill, it can be done with the passive network, which interferes less with alpha production because it does not involve as much active processing. The exact roles of the cingulate, globus pallidus, and other neural structures have yet to be worked out. It is these networks, however, that would be the primary vehicles through which an observer-subject system would confound entrainment or neurofeedback. More investigation regarding the relationship between EEG, attentional networks, and mood would further clarify existing relationships.

As previously mentioned, variance due to observer effect may be a consequence of immediate factors such as mood or automatic thinking and rumination level as they affect EEG through attentional networks as well as through the autonomic system as it relates to arousal, or it may be due to social contextual factors extending beyond the immediate force of their influence. It may be impossible to clearly separate all of these variables. Lubar and Lubar's (1999) original observations regarding the influence of familial factors on the efficacy of training in the clinic further support this perspective. Trauma within the family system carries over into the clinical setting and emerges as resistance in the neural system to outside influences, including neurofeedback and AVE. Similar effects are apparent in pharmacological interventions when dosage is increased to deal with increase in symptoms due to external stressors. The biological system has a preference for a particular neurochemical balance and resists efforts to shift that balance. The consequence of those efforts is often increased side effects.

Researchers such as E. Roy John and associates (1988) have in the past noticed immediate and dramatic shifts in QEEG configurations when cognitions commanding powerful emotional correlates temporarily generate QEEGs that mimic disorder. As we have said, our clients have demonstrated an ability to exert direct and immediate control over their EEG in such a manner as to apparently normalize their readings. The problem is that they cannot sustain that control over extended periods of time. They become distracted and fall back into automatic patterns of function. They have habituated to pathological network patterns.

CONCLUSION

Photic stimulation and AVE appear to offer a significant contribution with respect to enhancing neurofeedback training and more recently are being recognized as potentially powerful standalone interventions as well. In the last decade, and especially in the last few years, there is a heightened interest in these technologies emerging in fields outside of neurofeedback using fMRI to cofirm efficacy. Anyone with QEEG equipment can observe the powerful effect photic alone has upon the brains electrical fields, but many questions remain regarding the permanence of that effect. That permanence is guaranteed when used in conjunction with neurofeedback as changes due neurofeedback are based in learning and if photic accelerates or enhances this learning process, then there are great advantages to be had by integrating it with neurofeedback. The research already appears to support the value of its use in the home to help enhance the effect of neurofeedback in the office, especially for anxiety, depression and attention issues.

It is important for practitioners to keep in mind that responses to neurofeedback and AVE vary from day to day and trial to trial and from client to client much in the same way as neurofeedback or drugs. This variance is due to a wide variety of extraneous variables frequently not accounted for in the literature. These variables may be a consequence of physiological factors or diurnal effects, or they may be a consequence of psychological factors such as cognitions and mood. The neuronal resistance to photic intervention is often active and seeking to maintain allostasis, with the brain responding robustly in the opposite direction of the training intentions. It is hypothesized that a preconscious system is proactively resisting intervention, preferring instead a state that has its origination in other social-psychological factors relating to the individual's history of observations and responses to the environment. These factors must be measured and accounted for if research efforts are to reflect accurately the effects of neurofeedback and AVE interventions and if widely effective protocols are to be developed.

APPENDICES

APPENDIX A ～ SELECTED DISTRIBUTORS OF NEUROFEEDBACK & ACCESSORIES (IN ALPHABETICAL ORDER)

Alpha Stim

Electromedical Products International, Inc.
2201 Garrett Morris Parkway
Mineral Wells, TX 76067
Phone: 800.367.7246
Email: info@epii.com
Website: https://www.alpha-stim.com

Applied Neuroscience, Inc.

228 176th Terrace Drive
St. Petersburg, FL 330708
Phone: 727.244.0240
Fax: 727.392.1436
Website:http://www.appliedneuroscience.com
Email: QEEG@appliedneuroscience.com

Association of Applied Psychophysiology and Biofeedback

4400 College Blvd. Suite 220
Overland Park, KS 66211
Phone: 800.477.8892
Email: infor@aapb.org
Website: https://www.aapb.org

Biofeedback Certification International Alliance (BCIA)

5310 Ward Road Suite 201
Arvada, CO 80002
Phone: 720. 502.5829

Biofeedback Resources International, Corp.

109 Croton Ave Suite 240
Ossining, NY 10562
Phone: 914.762.4646
Website: www.biofeedbackinternational.com
Email: harry@biofeedbackinternational.com

Bio-Medical Instruments, Inc.

38875 Harper Ave
Clinton Township, MI 48036
Phone: 586.756.5070
Fax: 586.756.9891
Website:http://www.bio-medical.com
Email: sales@bio-medical.com

Brainmaster® Technologies, Inc.

195 Willis Street
Bedford, OH 44146
Phone: 440.232.6000
Fax: 440.232.7171
Sales & Support: 440.232.7300
Website: www.brainmaster.com
Email: sales@brainm.com

Cambridge Brain Science

15 Toronto Street Unit 600
Toronto, Ontario
Canada M5C 2E3
Phone: 888.774.8084
Website: www.cambridgebrainsciences.com
Email: pr@cambridgebrainscience.com

CNS Vital Signs

598 Airport Boulevard Suite #1400
Morrisville, NC 27560
Phone: 888.750.6941
Fax: 888.650.6795
Website:http://www.cnsvs.com
Email: support@cnsvs.com

Deymed Diagnostic

1720 N. 7th Avenue
Payette, ID 83661
Phone:208.642.9300
Website: www.deymed.com

EEGer

18017 Chatsworth #254
Granada, CA 91344
Phone: 818.886.2585
Fax: 888.650.6795
Website:http://www.eeger.com

EEG Info

22020 Clarendon St. Suite 305
Woodland Hills, CA 91367
Phone: 818.456.5965
Toll Free: 866.334.7878
Fax: 818.373.1331

Website: http://www.eeginfo.com

EEG Spectrum International, Inc.

21601 Vanowen Street, Suite 100
Canoga Park, CA 91303
Phone: 818.789.3456
Fax: 818.728.0944
Website: http://www.eegspectrum.com
Email: info@eegspectrum.com

Electro-Cap, International

1011 W. Lexington Road
P.O. Box 87
Eaton, OH 45320
Phone: 800.527.2193
Fax: 937.456.7323
Website: http://www.electro-cap.com
Email: eci@electro-cap.com

Foundation for Neurofeedback & Neuromodulation (FNNR)

2131 Woodruff Rd, Suite 2100-121
Greenville, SC 29607
Phone: 864.501.4146
Email: admin@thefnnr.org
Website:http://www.thefnnr.org

Integrated Neuroscience Services

86 West Sunbridge Drive
Fayetteville, AR 72703
Phone: 479.225.3223
Email: admin@integratedneuroscienceservices.com
Website:http://www.integratedneuroscienceservices.com

International QEEG Certification Board

148 Sheffield G.
West Palm Beach, FL 33417
Phone:561.247.1347
928 Broadway, Suite 305
New York, NY 10010
Phone: 917.405.8168
Email: IQEEGCB@gmail.com

International Society for Neurofeedback & Research (ISNR)

13876 SW 56th Street, PMB #311
Miami, FL 33175
Phone: 703.848.1994
Email: office@isnr.org
Website:http://www.isnr.org

Lenyosys

2881 E. Oakland Park Blvd
FOrt Lauderdale, FL 33306
Phone: 888.619.2929
Email: info@lynyosys.com
Website:http://www.lenyosys.com

Mind Alive, Inc.

9008-51 Avenue
Edmonton, Alberta, Canada
T6E 5X4
Toll Free (within US & Canada): 800.661.6463

US: 780.465.6463
Fax: 780.461.9551
Website: http://www.mindalive.com
Email: info@mindalive.com

NewMind Technologies

701 Macy Drive
Roswell, GA 30076, USA

Sales & Support: +1 (844) 405-3553
Website: http://www.newmindtraining.com
Email: Sales@newmindtech.com

Neurofield, Inc.

P.O. Box 506
Bishop, CA 93515
Phone: 760.872.4200
Website: http://www.neurofield.com
Email: contact@neurofield.com

Nova Tech EEG, Inc.

8503 E. Keats Ave
Mesa, AZ 85209
Phone: 480.219.3048
Website: http://www.novatecheeg.com
Email: rebecca@novatecheeg.com

Ochs Lab

7300 Healdsburg Avenue, Suite C
Sebastopol, CA 95472
Phone: 707.823.6225
Fax: 707.823.6266
Website: http://www.ochslabs.com
Email: cathywills@ochslabs.com

Stens Biofeedback- Stens Corporation

3020 Kerner Blvd., Suite D.
San Rafael, CA 94901
Toll Free: 800.257.8367
Website: http://www.stens-biofeedback.com
Email: http://ww.stens-biofeedback/contactus

Thought Technology, LTD.

USA
20 Gateway Drive
Plattsburgh, New York 12901
Toll Free: 800.361.3651
Fax: 514.489.8255

Canada
2180 Belgrave Avenue
Montral, Quebec, Canada
H4A2L8
Phone: 514.489.8251
Website: http://www.thoughttechnology.com

Email: mail@thoughttechnology.com

Vielight, Inc.

346 A. Jarvis Street
Toronto, Ontario
Canada M4Y 2G6
Phone: 855.875.6841
Website: http://www.vielight.com
Email: info@vielight.com

APPENDIX B ~ SELECTED TRAINERS IN NEUROFEEDBACK

Richard Soutar

NewMind Center
702 Macy Drive
Roswell, GA 30076
Phone: 678.516.5942
Website: www.newmindcenter.com
Email: drs@newmindcenter.com

John Demos

Neurofeedback of South
Vermont, LLC
P.O. Box 325
Westminster, VT 05158
Phone: 802.732.8060
Website: www.eegvermont.com
Email: workshop@eegvermont.com

Stegfried & Sue Othmer - EEG Info

6400 Canoga Ave., Suite 210
Woodland Hills, CA 91367
Phone: 818.456.5965
Toll Free: 866.334.7878
Fax: 818.373.1331
Website: www.eeginfo.com

EEG Spectrum International, Inc.

15400 SE 30th Place, Suite 205
Bellevue, WA 98007
Phone: 425.643.2495
Toll Free: 800.400.0334
Fax: 425.644.7452
Website: http://www.
eegspectrum.com
Email: evash@eegspectrum.com

Lynda Thompson

The ADD Centre
50 Village Centre Place
Mississauga, ON
Canada, L4Z 1V9
Phone: 905.803.8066
        416.488.2233
Fax: 905.803.9061
Website: www.addcentre.com
Email: addcentre@gmail.com

Stress Therapy Solutions

3401 Enterprise Parkway, Suite 340
Beachwood, OH 44122
Phone: 216.766.5707
Toll Free: 800.447.8052
Fax: 440.439.3015
Website: www.
stresstherapysolutions.com
Email: stsinc@pantek.com

Jon Anderson

Stens Biofeedback-Stens Corporation
3020 Kerner Blvd., Suite D.
San Rafael, CA 94901
Toll Free: 800.257.8367
Website: http://www.stens-
biofeedback.com
Email: stephen@stens-
biofeedback.ccsend.com

APPENDIX C ~ SELECTED QEEG DATABASES

NxLink

NYU Medical Center School of Medicine

Brain Research Laboratory
Website: www.nyu.edu/brl/research.QEEG_database.html

NeuroGuide

Applied Neuroscience, Inc.

Website: www.appliedneuroscience.com

SKIL

Sterman Kaiser Imaging Labs

Website: www.skiltopo.com

The Brain Resource International Database

Brain Resource Company

Website: www.brainresource.com

Institute of the Human Brain

HBIMed Brain Diagnostics

Website: www.hbimed.com

APPENDIX D ~ Forms

NewMind Neurofeedback Center

SYMPTOM CHECKLIST   SESSION #_____

At the beginning of each session use this checklist to help evaluate and track your progress. Rate yourself. On a scale of 1 to 10 regarding each of the items below, use 1 as low, little or poor and use 10 as high, a lot, or excellent. Use a marker to trace over each dotted line to create a bar graph.

	1 LO	5 AVERAGE	10 HI

Concentration   ---

Short Term Memory--

Quality of Sleep---

Appetite---

Motivation/Energy--

Positive Moods--

Patience--

Assertiveness   ---

Restlessness---

Worry/Negative Thinking ---

Negative Mood*---

Negative Emotions---

Pain/Physical Discomfort --

Fatigue--

Irritability---

Impulsivity**--

*An emotion lasts for 20min to an hour, a mood lasts for several hours, days, or weeks.

** Impulsivity includes disorganization, foot in mouth, impulse buying, blowing up at people. This test is also available on our website and clients can fill it out from home.

https://www.newmind-maps.com/

NewMind Neurofeedback Center
Physiological History Questionnaire

Have you experienced any of the following symptoms?

Place a number (for frequency) at the beginning of the item, then place a letter (for severity) at the end of each item.

1=rarely	A=unbearable
2=sometimes	B=very unpleasant
3=often	C=unpleasant
4=very often	D=mild
5=all of the time	E=very mild

Example: _____ Back pain _____

_____Abdominal bloating_____

_____Abdominal pain   _____

_____Always sickly_____

_____Amnesia_____

_____Anxiety attacks_____

_____Aphonia (loss of voice above a whisper)___

_____Back pain_____

_____Bulimia_____

_____Burning pains in rectum/ vagina/mouth _____

_____Chest pains_____

_____Constipation_____

_____Diarrhea_____

_____Dizziness_____

_____Dysmenorrhea (painful menstruation)_____

premarital_____

_____Dysmenorrhea-other_____

_____Headaches_____

_____Heart palpitations_____

_____Insomnia_____

_____Joint pain_____

_____Labored breathing_____

____Lump in throat_____

____Menstrual irregularity___

____Nausea_____

_____Other bodily pains____

____Paralysis_____

____Phobias_____

_____Ringing in ears_____

___Sexual indifference___

___Shaking or tremor___

_____Spasms_____

____Suddenweight fluctuation_____

_____Dyspareunia (painful sexual intercourse)_____Tics-verbal or motor_____

_____Dysuria (painful urination)___   _____Excessive menstrual bleeding___

_____Unconsciousness_____   _____Extremity pain_____

_____Urinary retention_____   _____Weight loss_____

_____Fainting spells_____   _____Visual blurring_____

_____Fatigue_____   _____Vomiting_____

_____Fits or convulsions___   _____Food intolerances_____

_____Frigidity (absence of orgasm)_____   _____Weakness_____

_____Had to quit working because felt bad_____

_____Vomiting all nine months of pregnancy_____

___ Trouble doing anything b/c felt bad_____

Other Medical Problems

_____Alcoholism_____

_____Chronic illness_____

_____Diagnosed illness_____

_____Diagnosed mental disorder_____

_____Drug addiction_____

_____Emotional abuse_____

_____Physical abuse_____

_____Sexual abuse_____

NewMind
Training Session Report

CLIENT _____   DATE _____

TIME _____AM _____ PM

CLINICIAN _____   INTER-PROTOCOL # _____

TOTAL SESSIONS # _____

PRESENTING PROBLEM STATUS   STATUS NOTES
Sleep   Headaches _____
Awareness of dreams   Focus   _____
Nightmares   Concentration_____
Boundary clarification   Attention _____
Reduced emotional reactivity   Memory_____
Enhanced calmness   Moodiness_____
Energy level   Irritability _____

(PROTOCOL) **SCREEN NAME** _____

BASELINE 1   **BASELINE 2**
SITE _____   NOTES _____   SITE _____   NOTES _____

(FREQ)   EO   EC   (FREQ)   EO   EC

_____ F1 _____   F1 _____   _____ F1 _____   F1 _____
_____ F2 _____   F2 _____   _____ F2 _____   F2 _____
_____ F3 _____   F3 _____   _____ F3 _____   F3 _____
_____ F4 _____   F4 _____   _____ F4 _____   F4 _____

TRIAL 1   **TRIAL 2**   **TRIAL 3**   **TRIAL 4**
NOTES _____   NOTES _____   NOTES _____   NOTES _____
PROTOCOL _____   PROTOCOL _____   PROTOCOL _____   PROTOCOL _____
SITE _____   SITE _____   SITE _____   SITE _____
TIME ____   TIME ____   TIME ____   TIME ____
EO   EC   EO EC   EO EC   EO   EC
VE: L ___   R ___   VE: L ___   R ___   VE: L___ R ___   VE: L ___   R ___

___ GOALS ___   ___ GOALS ___   ___ GOALS ___   ___ GOALS ___
F1 F2 F3 F4   F1 F2 F3 F4   F1 F2 F3 F4   F1 F2 F3 F4

UV

___ ___ ___ ___   ___ ___ ___ ___   ___ ___ ___ ___   ___ ___ ___ ___

%

___ ___ ___ ___   ___ ___ ___ ___   ___ ___ ___ ___   ___ ___ ___ ___

        L   R   L   R   L   R   L   R
(FREQ) TRIAL 1 **RESULTS**   TRIAL 2 **RESULTS**   TRIAL 3 **RESULTS**   TRIAL 4 **RESULTS**
_____ F1 _____ _____   F1 _____ _____   F1 _____ _____   F1 _____ _____
_____ F2 _____ _____   F2 _____ _____   F2 _____ _____   F2 _____ _____
_____ F3 _____ _____   F3 _____ _____   F3 _____ _____   F3 _____ _____
_____ F4 _____ _____   F4 _____ _____   F4 _____ _____   F4 _____ _____

SESSION NOTES

_____

_____

NewMind Center
Protocol Worksheet

Date _____ Patient verbalizes awareness of protocol change _____
Client _____ *Clinician's initial* _____ *Patient initial* ____
Protocol _____ EO   EC
Rational _____
Sx changes _____

Client-specific indicators

_____   _____
_____   _____
_____   _____
_____

Date _____ Patient verbalizes awareness of protocol change _____
Client _____ *Clinician's initial* _____ *Patient initial* ____
Protocol _____ EO   EC
Rational _____
Sx changes _____

Client-specific indicators

_____   _____
_____   _____
_____   _____
_____

Date _____ Patient verbalizes awareness of protocol change _____
Client _____ *Clinician's initial* _____ *Patient initial* ____
Protocol _____ EO   EC
Rational _____
Sx changes _____

Client-specific indicators

_____   _____
_____   _____
_____   _____
_____

Date _____ Patient verbalizes awareness of protocol change _____
Client _____ *Clinician's initial* _____ *Patient initial* ____
Protocol _____ EO   EC
Rational _____
Sx changes _____

Client-specific indicators

_____   _____
_____   _____
_____   _____

Soutar & Longo - Informed Consent

The purpose of this form is to obtain your voluntary consent to participate in one or more methods of quantitative electroencephalography (QEEG) brain mapping, peripheral biofeedback, neurofeedback, other forms of relaxation and stress reduction interventions, and to disclose potential benefits and risks associated with these interventions. (Business Name) provides various educational interventions, assessment protocols, and health care services, a few of which are still considered by some to be experimental.

QEEG Brain Mapping

To determine an appropriate neurofeedback training plan, a QEEG performed by (Business Name) using the (Company) expert referential database system will be conducted.

(Business Name) will assess your need for having a QEEG. To engage in neurofeedback, you will be required to have a QEEG assessment. In other instances, to help verify a disorder, your doctor, or another health care professional, may recommend you have a QEEG. A QEEG consists of placing a cap on your head with 20 electrodes/sensors. Each site will be cleansed, and a special gel will be placed under each sensor to insure proper conductivity to read your brainwaves. Preparation and the assessment procedure take approximately 1 hour.

Benefits: QEEG may help me further understand and/or confirm the problems/symptoms, disorders, and/or diagnosis for which I am seeking assessment and health care services.

Side Effects/Risks: QEEG may result in my feeling anxious/apprehensive, and/or uncomfortable during the procedure, and sad/disappointed regarding findings from the procedure. The cap may cause you to have a mild headache.

Forensic Services: QEEG brain mapping for purposes of neurofeedback is not a medical procedure and is not done at (Business Name) for purposes of medical diagnosis. Data collected is not done in a manner that meets the Daubert[1] criteria for admissibility of evidence in court. (Business Name) does not provide forensic services or diagnosis for TBI. We do not accept invitations for depositions. Those seeking a diagnosis for TBI or any other diagnosable medical or mental disorder should seek services of an appropriate health care professional such as a physician or a forensic neuropsychologist. Your signature below indicates you agree not to request or seek such services from us presently or in the future, or through third parties such as legal counsel or insurance companies.

---

1   https://www.theexpertinstitute.com/working-experts-understanding-five-daubert-factors/

Client/Patient Rights. You have the right to:

- Decide not to receive QEEG brain mapping services from us. If you wish, we can provide you with the names of other qualified QEEG providers.

- End the QEEG at any time.

- Ask questions about protocol and procedures used during the QEEG procedure, and to ask questions about QEEG techniques if you feel unsure of them.

- Have all that you say treated confidentially and be informed of state law placing limitations on confidentiality in the QEEG relationship. Under certain circumstances, we are required by law to reveal information obtained during a QEEG assessment to other persons or agencies without your permission. Also, we are not required to inform you of our actions in this regard. These situations are as follows: (a) if you threaten bodily harm or death to yourself or another person, we are required by law to notify the victim and appropriate law enforcement agencies; (b) if a court of law issues a subpoena; (c) if you are having a QEEG or being tested by a court of law, the results of the QEEG assessment must be revealed to the court; (d) if you have given us information concerning non-accidental injury and neglect to minors or incompetent adults; or (e) if you are in the process of filing a workman's compensation claim or file such in the future.

Equipment/Software: QEEG measures will involve the use of the. (Business Name) software and hardware (equipment type). (Business Name) products are FDA registered. QEEG maps are produced using (report system).

Neurofeedback Training

Neurofeedback involves several electrodes/sensors being placed on the scalp and earlobes. The sensors detect brain wave activity including alpha, beta, delta, and theta brainwaves. Individual brainwaves are measured and displayed on a computer screen revealing your brainwave activity. Through instruction you can learn to train down or train up certain brainwaves associated with stress management, attention, cognitive and/or emotional deficits, and related disorders. In some cases, neurofeedback must be considered as experimental. Treatments last from 10–30 minutes and may occur two or more times per week for an average of 30–40 sessions, and in some cases, more than 40 sessions.

Benefits: Neurofeedback (NFB) is known to assist individuals by decreasing symptoms associated with brain and central nervous system dysfunction. Other benefits include the possibility of reducing problem behaviors and increasing peak performance. In many cases, neurofeedback is experimental when used to a treat certain disorders. Please feel free to ask for a more detailed explanation regarding your problem area or treatment interest.

Side Effects/Risks: Neurofeedback will not interfere with most other treatments. Neurofeedback has few side effects when administered properly. The most common side effects of neurofeedback include improved sleep, more awareness of dreams, feeling calmer, more energetic, and more focused. Temporary side effects such as headaches, insomnia, anxiety, feeling giddy, agitated, or irritated may occur during or right after a neurofeedback session. However, these side effects can be adjusted and eliminated immediately in most cases. It is also possible that you might fall asleep during or after neurofeedback sessions.

Client Rights. You have the right to:

- Decide not to receive neurofeedback services from us. If you wish, we can provide you with the names of other Board Certified neurofeedback providers in your area.

- End neurofeedback sessions at any time.

- Ask questions about protocols and procedures used during neurofeedback training, and to ask questions about techniques if you feel unsure of them.

- Have all that you say treated confidentially and be informed of state law placing limitations on confidentiality in the neurofeedback relationship. Under certain circumstances, we are required by law to reveal information obtained during training to other persons or agencies without your permission. Also, we are not required to inform you of our actions in this regard. These situations are as follows: (a) if you threaten bodily harm or death to yourself or another person, we are required by law to notify the indicated victim and appropriate law enforcement agencies; (b) if a court of law issues a subpoena; (c) if you are being treated with neurofeedback, at the direction of an attorney or medical doctor for legal purposes, the results of the training or tests must be revealed to the court; (d) if you have given us information concerning non-accidental injury and neglect to minors or incompetent adults; or (e) if you are in the process of filing a workman's compensation claim or have plans to file such in the future.

Equipment/Software: Neurofeedback treatment will involve the use of the (Business Name) software and hardware (equipment type). (Business Name) products are FDA registered.

Other Methods: Other treatment methods may not work as rapidly as the methods and modalities described above. Alternative methods of treatment and/or therapy include traditional medical treatments, medications, the use of supplements, the use of relaxation techniques, and/or group and individual therapy.

Choosing the Right Intervention: The interventions described above are voluntary, not mandatory. You will not be pressured to participate. You may withdraw from or stop receiving neurofeedback training sessions at any time without consequence.

Consent

I voluntarily consent to participate in and undergo the assessment and/or intervention methods and modalities described above. I understand that I am free to withdraw my consent and to discontinue participation in the interventions/modalities/methods described above at any time. The natural consequences and potential risks and benefits have been fully explained to me by (Business Name).

Permission

My signature below indicates that I have read, reviewed and understand this informed consent (and/or I have had the form and its contents read to me and explained to me), and I consent to participate in the procedures described above. I understand I may ask questions at any time, and may request to stop interventions at any time.

I have read and understand my rights.

_____   _____

Signature   **Date**

Longo & Soutar - Client Bill of Rights and Responsibilities Regarding Biofeedback and Neurofeedback

We want to encourage you, as a client of (Business Name), to speak openly with your clinical provider, take part in your assessment and treatment choices, and promote your own safety and well-being by being well informed and involved in your biofeedback (BFB) and neurofeedback (NFB) treatment services. You are encouraged to think of yourself as a partner in your care, and therefore to know your rights as well as your responsibilities during your course of treatment. (Business Name) provides various educational interventions, assessment protocols, and treatment services, a few of which are still considered, by some, to be experimental.

Client Rights:

- You have the right to receive considerate, respectful, and compassionate treatment in a safe setting, free from all forms of abuse, neglect, or mistreatment, regardless of your age, gender, race, national origin, religion, sexual orientation, gender identity, or disabilities. You have the right to inquire about and discuss ethical issues related to your care at all times, and to voice your concerns about the care you receive.

- You have the right to be told by your treatment provider about your diagnosis and possible prognosis, the benefits and risks of treatment, and the expected outcome of treatment. You have the right to give written informed consent before any non-emergency procedure begins, and to understand the costs of assessment and treatment before you begin.

- You, your family, and friends with your permission, have the right to participate in decisions about your treatment, including the right to refuse/withdraw from treatment.

- You have the right to decide not to receive BFB/NFB treatment from us. If you wish, we can provide you with the names of other BFB/NFB providers in your area.

- You have the right to ask questions about protocol and procedures used during all BFB/NFB sessions, and to ask questions about NFB/BFB techniques. You have the right to prevent the use of certain training techniques if you feel unsure of them, and to participate in setting goals and evaluating progress towards meeting them.

- You have the right to have all that you say treated confidentially and be informed of state law placing limitations on confidentiality in the NFB/BFB relationship. Under certain circumstances, we are required by law to reveal information obtained during NFB/

BFB to other persons or agencies without your permission. Also, we are not required to inform you of our actions in this regard. These situations are as follows: (a) if you threaten bodily harm or death to yourself or another person, we are required by law to notify the intended victim and appropriate law enforcement agencies; (b) if a court of law issues a subpoena; (c) if you are in NFB/BFB training or being tested by a court of law, the results of the treatment or tests must be revealed to the court; (d) if you have given us information concerning non-accidental injury and neglect to minors or incompetent adults; or (e) if you are in the process of filing a workman's compensation claim or file such in the future.

Client Responsibilities—You Are Expected to:

1. Provide complete and accurate information, including your full name, address, home telephone number, date of birth, and employer when it is required.
2. Provide complete and accurate information about your health and medical history, including present condition, past illnesses, hospital stays, medicines, vitamins, herbal products, and any other matters that pertain to your health, including perceived safety risks.
3. Ask questions when you do not understand information or instructions. If you believe you cannot follow through with your treatment plan, you are responsible for telling your treatment provider. You are responsible for outcomes if you do not follow the treatment plan.
4. Provide complete and accurate information about your finances and your ability to pay your fees in accordance with the arrangement you established previously with (Business Name).
5. Set and keep appointments with your provider and be on time for your appointments. Appointments cancelled without at least 24-hour notice are subject to a $50 charge.
6. Help plan your therapy goals and keep your NFB/BFB provider informed of your progress toward meeting your goals.
7. Inform your NFB/BFB provider of any problems you have which may influence your progress or which may be potentially harmful to yourself or others.
8. Notify (Business Name) if you intend to discontinue training.

I have read and understand my rights.

_____   _____

Signature   **Date**

Soutar & Longo - Client Acknowledgements

Benefits of Neurofeedback

The FDA recognizes that all interventions pose risks and benefits. Typically, the benefits of neurofeedback far outweigh the risks and although on occasion, it can result in non-serious adverse events. As a form of biofeedback, it falls under the category of other low risk activities such as progressive relaxation, hypnosis, breathing exercises, meditation, yoga, and massage. The benefits are usually experienced as improved focus, enhanced concentration, increased energy, higher quality sleep, decreased moodiness, diminished agitation, and reduction in anxiety, as well as reductions in other physical symptoms typically related to stress such as headaches.

Risks of Neurofeedback

Training with neurofeedback can occasionally result in adverse response(s) that temporarily increase symptoms that are typically associated with relaxation and calming of the central nervous system such as fatigue, headaches, lightheadedness, dizziness, irritability, moodiness, weeping, insomnia, agitation, and difficulties with focus and anxiety. These reactions, if they occur, are temporary and typically only last 24–48 hours. Once clients/patients become more relaxed and aware, they tend to integrate past emotional issues and these symptoms subside.

I have participated in a QEEG brain map, have read the notations above, and I would like to pursue neurofeedback training. I understand that:

1. NFB is not a quick fix or cure all, but reduces symptom severity over time through training to improve central nervous system (CNS) regulation.
2. The average number of NFB sessions to achieve enduring change is 40 sessions. This will vary depending on the client/patient's diagnosis, general health, and other factors.
3. On average, most people require 10 - 15 sessions to experience symptom changes. If symptom changes do not occur within 15–20 sessions it is may be due to any one of several factors including but not limited to metabolic conditions, medications, life stress issues, toxins, or a severe medical disorder.
4. Side effects may result from prescribed drugs when dosage is not reduced over sessions which must be guided by the prescribing professional.
5. Some agitation or irritability may occur for a couple of weeks following the 15th session. In some cases, this may not occur while in others onset could occur after only a few sessions. If this occurs, please report this to your neurofeedback practitioner immediately.
6. The chronic use of psychotropic drugs impedes progress.
7. For clients/patients taking psychotropic medications and wanting to reduce or eliminate such; reducing dependence on pharmaceuticals is a key objective of the training program.
8. That client must make efforts to manage diet, exercise, sleep and stressful activities to achieve the best results.
9. Failure to work with practitioners to make lifestyle changes can reduce or mitigate effects of NFB training.
10. Hair analysis or organic acid tests will be required if progress is slow.
11. Clients are expected to complete weekly progress reports the day before their NFB Training sessions. Completion of weekly progress reports helps guide us in providing the best quality of care.

I have read and understand the items outlined above:

_____   _____

Signature   Date

Longo & Soutar - Authorization for
Release of Information (HIPAA)

Name: **Date of Birth:**   **Client # :**

(Business Name) is authorized to release protected health information about the above-named individual to the entities named below. The purpose is to inform the professionals or persons listed below in keeping with the patient's instructions.

Entity to Receive Information Check each person/entity that you approve to receive information	Description of information to be released. Check each that can be given to the person/entity on the left in the same section.
Voice Mail	Results of QEEG **/**Assessments NFB Treatment Sessions Other
Spouse (provide name & phone number)	Results of QEEG **/**Assessments NFB Treatment Sessions Other
Parent (provide name & phone number)	Results of QEEG **/**Assessments NFB Treatment Sessions Other
Other (provide name & phone number)	Results of QEEG **/**Assessments NFB Treatment Sessions Other
Your E-mail:	Results of QEEG **/**Assessments NFB Treatment Sessions Other
Other E-mail: Name of Person E-mail will go to:	Results of QEEG **/**Assessments NFB Treatment Sessions Other

Personal Information: I understand that I have the right to revoke this authorization at any time and that I have the right to inspect or copy the protected health information to be disclosed as described in this document. I understand that a revocation is not effective in cases where the information has already been disclosed but will be effective going forward.

I understand that information used or disclosed because of this authorization may be subject to redisclosure by the recipient and may no longer be protected by federal or state law.

I understand that I have the right to refuse to sign this authorization and that my treatment will not be conditioned on signing. This authorization shall be in effect until revoked by the individual named above.

_____   _____

Signature of Person or Personal Representative   **Date**Description of
Personal Representative's Authority (attach necessary documentation)

Longo - Financial Policy

The following information offers some guidelines regarding our financial policy.

- We do not take health insurance and are not a Medicaid/Medicare provider.

- **Please be prepared to pay for services at the time they are rendered.**

- Please be aware that **you are ultimately responsible for the timely payment of your account**.

- A $35.00 bank fee will be charged for any returned checks.

- Past due accounts of 90 days or more may be subject to collections.

- Except in cases of emergencies, **we require a minimum 24-hour notice if you cannot keep your scheduled appointment**. We reserve the right to charge for appointments canceled or broken without a 24-hour notice. Our fee for missed appointments (those without a 24-hour cancellation) is $50.00 per session hour.

- For your convenience, we accept cash, personal check, MasterCard, Visa, Discover Card, and American Express.

If you have any questions regarding our policy, please feel free to ask us. We are here to help you!

I have read and agree to the conditions as outlined:

_____   _____

Signature   **Date**

QEEG Brain Mapping Preparation Checklist

Below is a sample of a QEEG Preparation Checklist you might be given.

The following instructions are for the patient to review and follow before they come in for a QEEG, and will help assure that the best results possible are acquired. **PLEASE PAY ATTENTION to bolded print.**

1. Illness. If you are sick, please call to reschedule even if you only have a cold.

2. Sleep. You should get a good night's sleep before the QEEG. (Let us know if you have any sleep problems or disturbances.)

3. Hair and Scalp. Your hair needs to be clean and dry. Use a pH neutral detergent shampoo such as Neutrogena Anti-Residue or Suave Clarifying shampoo the night before or the on the day of your scheduled appointment. Wash your hair three times. If you have a hair weaves, toupee, or corn-rows, please remove them (if they are removable), before your appointment. **No chemical treatments may be administered (coloring, perms, relaxers, etc.) within 48 hours before the QEEG. DO NOT use oils, lotions, mousse, gels, or hairsprays. Hair must be free of beads, weaves, etc. Make sure your hair is completely dry before coming for the QEEG.**

Please bring a comb or brush.

4. Medications. The QEEG assessment is often cleaner and easier to read if there are no medications in the brain. If the client is taking stimulant medication (i.e., ADHD medication), it is preferable to do the QEEG recording after the patient has stopped taking the medication for *up to 48* hours prior. **The client MUST check with his/her prescribing physician or health care provider to determine if it is possible to stop taking the stimulants 48 hours prior to the QEEG. If 48 hours is not advisable, 12–24 is the next preferred length of time. Do not make changes in any other medication(s) unless authorized by your physician. If you are taking medications for anxiety, depression, or sleep, please do NOT stop taking these medications without first consulting with your prescriber. If you prescriber approves, please bring these medications with you the day of your QEEG and take them after the QEEG assessment has been conducted.**

5. Over the Counter Medications and Supplements. *Unless prescribed by a physician or licensed health care provider,* client should avoid taking any over the counter medication or supplements for 2 or 3 days prior to the QEEG. This includes medications and supplements such as such as: acetaminophen (Tylenol), Advil (Motrin/ibuprofen), aspirin, analgesics, antihistamines/allergy medications (Benadryl, Claritin, Allegra, Zyrtec), cough and cold medicines, herbs, nasal sprays, nutraceuticals (sports drinks, Gator Aid, etc.), food **supplements (including amino acids), vitamins, or other similar products).** If you have any questions about these items, please contact your QEEG practitioner.

6. Caffeinated Beverages. The client should ***NOT*** drink excessive amounts of coffee, tea, or caffeinated beverages in the morning of the testing (i.e., one cup is fine) and the patient should ***NOT*** drink soft drinks with excessive amounts of caffeine in them, i.e., Red Bull, highly caffeinated soft drinks, for at least 15 hours prior to the QEEG.

7. Alcohol and Drugs. Alcohol should be avoided 24 hours prior to your session. Marijuana should be avoided 24–72 hours prior to your session.

8. Contact Lenses. Portions of the QEEG require that your eyes be closed for up to 15 minutes. If you wear contact lenses, please be prepared to remove them if they create discomfort with your eyes closed.

9. Please bring a complete list of medications you take on a daily or regular basis with you when you come for your QEEG.

The day of the QEEG, the client should:

1. Eat a high protein breakfast.

2. **Women should not wear any makeup on the forehead or ear lobes**.

3. Drink plenty of water the day before the QEEG recording.

4. Use the restroom to prior to the start of the QEEG.

5. **No jewelry on neck or ears.**

6. **Nicotine should be avoided 3 hours prior to your session.**

7. **Bring any medications or supplements you would like to take after your QEEG is complete.**

On the day of your QEEG brain map appointment, plan to spend a minimum of 90 minutes in the office. In addition, you will likely need several minutes to fix your hair following your appointment. Facilities are provided.

PLEASE NOTE: Lack of sleep, medications, low blood sugar, and movement of the eyes, tongue, head or body, may affect the results.

Neurofeedback Session Notation Form

Example of neurofeedback session note using SOAP format.

Patient's Name: **ID#:**   **Date of service:**

Subjective (client/family report and/or clinical interview data):

Objective: Psychophysiological monitoring using EEG.

Observations:

Impressions/assessment/comments:

Plan:

Protocol name/ID:
Sites **A1**   **R1**   A1   **G**   Cz   **R2**   A2   **A2**   Threshold
Training Protocol: CH#1   CH#2
Run Length: Seconds _____   Number of Runs: _____

Rewards: Multimedia: Station: Vol: Practitioner:

	Delta	Theta	Alpha	LoBeta	Beta	HiBeta	Hz	Hz
Channel 1 Pre								
Channel 1 Post								

Comments:

	Delta	Theta	Alpha	LoBeta	Beta	HiBeta	Hz	Hz
Channel 2 Pre								
Channel 2 Post								

Comments:

Session #   *Total Sessions:*

_____

Therapist's Signature

Appendix E ~ Suggested Reading List

Neurofeedback – Historical, Technical, General, and Related Topics

The flowing books on Neurofeedback, and related topics, are relatively easy to read but informative with regard to history and technique.

Amen, D. G. (2001). Healing ADD: *The breakthrough program that allows you to see and heal the 6 types of ADD*. NY: Berkley Books.

Arntz, W., Chasse, B., & Vicente, M. (2005). *What the bleep do we know: Discovering the endless possibilities for altering your everyday reality*. Deerfield Beach, FL: Health Communications, Inc.

Austin, J. H. (1998). *Zen and the brain: Toward an understanding of meditation and consciousness*. Cambridge, MA: The MIT Press.

Begley, S. (2007). *Train your mind change your brain: How a new science reveals our extraordinary potential to transform ourselves*. NY: Ballentine Books.

Brizendine, L. (2006). *The female brain*. New York, NY: Broadway Books.

Buzsaki, G. (2006). *Rhythms of the brain*. New York: Oxford University Press.

Cade, M. C., & Coxhead, N. (1989). *The awakened mind: Biofeedback and the development of higher states of awareness*. Dorset, England: Element Books.

[Cade was one the first to use EEG to guide changes in behavior and consciousness. He was among the first to identify key features of the EEG relating to meditative states. A classic in the field.]

Campbell, D. (1997). *The Mozart effect: Tapping the power of music to heal the body, strengthen the mind and unlock the creative spirit*. New York, NY: Avon Books.

Campbell, T. C., & Campbell, T. M. (2004). *The China study: Starting implications for diet, weight loss, and long-term health*. Dallas, TX: BenBella Books.

Dispenza, J. (2007). *Evolve your brain: The science of changing your mind*. Deerfield Beach, FL: Health Communications, Inc.

Doidge, N. (2007). *The brain that changes itself: Stories of personal triumph from the frontiers of science*. New York, NY: Penguin Books

Doidge, N. (2015). *The brain's way of healing*. New York, NY: Viking.

Femi, L., & Robbins, J. (2008). *The open-focus brain: Harnessing the power of attention to heal mind and body.* Trumpeter, 2008.

[Les Femi understands attention and how it relates to consciousness better than almost anyone out there. His workshops on open focus attention are a revelation about how we use attention without knowing it. His specialty area is 4 channel coherence training and he has been doing it for decades. Jim Robbins, a science writer for the New York Times who personally explored many of the paradigms of neurofeedback, was especially attracted to this approach.]

Gladwell, M. (2005). *Blink: The power of thinking without thinking*. NY: Little,

Brown and Co.

Green, E. E., & Green, A. M. (1977). *Beyond biofeedback*. San Francisco: Delacarte.

[Elmer pioneered this whole field and created his own equipment and methods. We still have not followed through in replicating the research and equipment he devised decades ago. This book is a fascinating story of his journey and a must read for anyone in the field.]

Katz, L. C., & Rubin, M. (1999). *Keep your brain alive*. NY: Workman Publishing Co.

Kotulak, R. (1996). *Inside the brain: Revolutionary discoveries of how the mind works*. Kansas City, Missouri: Andrews McMeel Publishing.

LeDoux, J. (1996). *The emotional brain: The mysterious underpinnings of emotional life*. New York: Simon & Schuster.

Lipton, B. (2005). *The biology of belief: Unleashing the power of consciousness, matter, and miracles*. Santa Rosa, CA: Mountain of Love/Elite Books.

Moyers, B. (1993). *Healing and the mind*. NY: Doubleday.

Promislow, S. (2005). *Making the brain body connection: A playful guide to releasing mental, physical, & emotional blocks to success*. Vancouver, BC, Canada: Enhanced Learning & Integration, Inc.

Robbins, J. (2000). *A symphony in the brain*. New York, NY: Grove Hills.

[This is the book you give to all your clients who want to know more about neurofeedback.]

Schiffer, F. (1998). *Of two minds: The revolutionary science of dual brain psychology*. NY: Free Press.

Schore, A. N. (1994). *Affect regulation and the origin of the self: The neurobiology of emotional development*. Hillsdale, NJ: Erlbaum.

Schwartz, J. M., & Begley, S. (2002). *The mind & the brain: Neuroplasticity and the power of mental force*. NY: Regan Books.

Siegel, D. J. (1999). *The developing mind: Toward a neurobiology of interpersonal experience*. NY: Guilford Press.

Siegel, D. J. (2007). *The mindful brain: Reflection and attunement in the cultivation of well-being*. New York, NY: W.W. Norton & Company.

Stein, P., & Kendall, J. (2004). *Psychological trauma and the developing brain: Neurologically based interventions for troubled children*. NY: The Hawthorne Maltreatment and Trauma Press.

Steinberg, M. S., & Othmer, S. (2004). *ADD the 20-Hour solution: Training minds to concentrate and self-regulate naturally without medication*. Bandon, OR: Robert D. Reed Publishers.

Soutar, R., & Crane, A. (2000). *Mindfitness training: Neurofeedback and the process*. New York: iUniverse:

[Discusses a lot of the theoretical underpinnings of peak performance training. Not a how to manual.]

Soutar, R. (2006). *The automatic self: Transformation & transcendence through brainwave training*. New York: iUniverse.

[Written for the general public, this book explicates its theme on many levels and is a favorite of clinicians while at the same time a mysterious waste of time to the technical people in the field. It reviews the profound implications of the manner in which the nervous system

manages information and behavior. It then discusses how neurofeedback can fundamentally alter the consequences of this human dilemma. Although the premise is not new and may seem simple and obvious, clearly most people have not understood it well or the world would be a different place.]

Swingle, M. K. (2015). *I-minds: How cell phones, computers, gaming, and social media are changing our brains, our behavior, and the evolution of our species.* Portland, OR: Inkwater Press.

Teicher, M. H. (2002). Scars that won't heal: The neurobiology of child abuse. *Scientific American, 286*(3), 68-75.

Whitaker, R. (2010). *Anatomy of and epidemic: Magic bullets, psychiatric drugs, and the astonishing rise of mental illness in America.* New York, NY: Broadway Paperbacks.

Wise, A. (1997). *The high performance minds.* New York: G. P. Putnam's Sons.

[Anna's work has been a great unacknowledged contribution to the field and is essential for anyone planning to do Deep states training with neurofeedback.]

Ziegler, D. (2002). *Traumatic experience and the brain: A handbook for understanding and treating those traumatized as children.* Phoenix, AZ: Acacia Publishing.

Neurofeedback – Overview

Budzynski, T. H., Budzynski, H. K., Evans, J. R., & Abarbanel, A. (2008). *Introduction to quantitative EEG and neurofeedback advanced theory and applications* (2nd ed.). Amsterdam, Elsevier: Academic Press.

Evans, J. R. (Ed.) (2007). *Handbook of neurofeedback: Dynamics and clinical applications.* NY: The Hawthorne Medical Press.

Evans, J. R., Dellinger, M. B., & Russell, H. L. (2020). *Neurofeedback: The first fifty years.* Cambridge, MA: Academic Press.

Longo, R. E. (2018). *A consumer's guide to understanding QEEG brain mapping and neurofeedback training.* Bloomington, IN: iUniverse.

Longo, R. E., & Soutar, R. (2019). *Mentoring for neurofeedback certification: A guide for mentors and mentees.* Greenville, SC: FNNR.

Othmer, S. (2008). *Protocol guide for neurofeedback clinicians.* Woodland Hills, CA: EEGInfo.

Neuroscience & the Brain

Amen, D. G. (2005). *Making a good brain great.* NY: Three Rivers Press.

Amen, D. G. (1998). *Change your brain change your life: The breakthrough program for conquering anxiety, depression, obsessiveness, anger and impulsiveness.* NY: Three Rivers Press.

Braverman, E. R. (2004). *The edge effect: Achieve total health and longevity with the balanced brain advantage.* NY: Sterling Publishing Co. De

De Haan, M., & Gunnar, M. R. (2009). *Handbook of developmental social neuroscience.* NY: Guilford Press.

Hill, R. W., & Castro, E. (2002). *Getting rid of ritalin: How neurofeedback can successfully treat attention deficit disorder without drugs.* Charlottesville, VA: Hampton Roads Publishing Co., Inc.

Larson, S. (2006). *The healing power of neurofeedback: The revolutionary LENS technique for restoring optimal brain function.* Rochester, VT: Healing Arts Press.

Swingle, P. G. (2008). *Biofeedback for the brain: How neurotherapy effectively treats depression, ADHD, autism, and more.* NJ: Rutgers University Press.

Heavier and More Clinically Oriented

Chapin, T. J., & Russell-Chapin, L. A. (2013). *Brain-based treatment for psychological and behavioral problems.* New York, NY: Routledge.

Collurra, T. F. (2014). *Technical foundations of neurofeedback.* New York, NY: Routledge.

Collurra, T. F., & Frederick, J. A. (Eds.) (2017). *Handbook of clinical QEEG and neurotherapy.* New York, NY: Routledge.

Cantor, D. S., & Evans, J. R. (2014). *Clinical neurotherapy: Applications of techniques for treatment.* New York, NY: Academic Press.

Demos, J. N. (2019). *Getting started with EEG neurofeedback* (2nd ed.). New York, NY: W. W. Norton & Company, Inc.

[When John called me up and said he was planning to write an easy to read introduction to neurofeedback for clinicians entering the field, I sent him Doing Neurofeedback and pointed him in the direction of some good research. He went to scads of workshops by everyone on the field and took copious notes. The result is this highly proclaimed and excellent book which every practitioner should read before they lift an electrode.]

Fisher, S. F. (2014). *Neurofeedback in the treatment of developmental trauma: Calming the fear driven brain.* New York, NY: W. W. Norton & Company, Inc.

Hill, R. W., & Castro, E. (2009). *Healing young brains: The neurofeedback solution.* Charlottesville, VA: Hampton Roads Publishing Company.

LeDoux, J. (2015). *Anxious: Using the brain to understand and treat fear and anxiety.* New York, NY: Viking.

Martins-Mourao, A., & Kerson, C. (Eds.). (2017). *Alpha-Theta neurofeedback in the 20th century: A handbook for clinicians and researchers.* Greenville, SC: Foundation for Neurofeedback and Neuromodulation Research.

Nunez, P. L. (Ed.). (1995). *Neocortical dynamics and human EEG rhythms.* New York, NY: Oxford University Press.

Nunez, P. I., & Srinivasan, R. (2006). *Electric fields of the brain: The neurophysics of EEG* (2nd ed). New York, NY: Oxford University Press.

Stoler, D. R., & Hill, B. A. (1998). *Coping with mild traumatic brain injury: A guide to living with the challenges associated with concussion/brain injury.* New York, NY: Avery.

Thatcher, R. W. (2012). Handbook of quantitative EEG and EEG biofeedback:

Scientific foundations of quantitative EEG and biofeedback with tutorials. St. Petersburg, FL: Anipublishing.

Thompson, M., & Thompson, L. (2003). *The neurofeedback book: An introduction to basic concepts in applied psychophysiology.* Wheat Ridge, CO: AAPB.

Neuroscience

Some good basic reading on neurocognitive science that applies to clinical neurofeedback:

Cozolino, L. (2002). *The neuroscience of psychotherapy: Building and rebuilding the human brain.* New York: Norton.
[One of the best books written on the relationship between talk therapy and resulting changes in neurophysiology.]

Damasio, A. (1994). *Descartes' error: Emotion, reason, and the human brain.* New York: Avon Books. [Demasio was among the first to define how the emotional brain impacts the frontal lobes in terms of executive function and social behavior. A very readable text.]

Damasio, A. (1999). *The feeling of what happens.* New York: Harcourt Brace.
[A very good sequel on consciousness and self-construction.]

Goleman, D. (1995). *Emotional intelligence.* New York: Bantam Books.
[This book was the first definitive book explaining the important role of emotion and limbic structures in social behavior. This is a must read for all clinicians.]

LeDoux, J. (1996). *The emotional brain: The mysterious underpinnings of emotional life.* New York: Simon & Schuster.
[Le Doux is an excellent writer and able to make complex topics simple to understand. He is a leading researcher in fear conditioning and how it relates to anxiety and PTSD. The material here will provide you with an excellent basis for better understanding the anatomy and physiology of anxiety.]

LeDoux, J. (2002). *The synaptic self: How our brains became who we are.* Viking: New York.
[A good sequel to The emotional brain.]

Posner, M. I., & Raichle, M. E. (1997). *Images of mind.* New York: Scientific American Library.
[This was very popular reading at ISNR years ago and still stands up well today. It provides excellent pictures and diagrams and covers the topic of attention in a detailed and informative manner that is very useful to neurofeedback clinicians and individuals involved in QEEG and MiniQ.]

Schore, A. N. (1994). *Affect regulation and the origin of the self: The neurobiology of emotional development.* Hillsdale, NJ: Lawrence Erlbaum Associates.
[Schores's book is acknowledged universally as the definitive treatise on the topic of trauma and how it impacts development, socialization and emotion functioning.]

Schwartz, J. M., & Begley, S. (2002). *The mind and the brain.* Harper Collins: New York.

[This is one of the best books on OCD I have read. It explains the disorder right down to the "worry circuit" they have identified as the source of obsessive thinking. It is also an excellent book on the brain in general as well as providing interesting theoretical ideas toward resolving the mind-brain problem.]

Heavier Reading

Crosson, B. (1992). *Subcortical functions in language and memory*. The Guilford Press, NY.

[Those interested in memory and language function will find all the details regarding structures and networks that are associated. Be prepared for a complex and dry rendition that raises more questions than it answers.]

Chow, T. W., & Cummings, J. L. (1998). Frontal-subcortical circuits. In B. L. Miller & J. L. Cummings (Eds.), *The human frontal lobes* (pp. 3-44). New York: The Guilford Press.

[For those interested in finding out every little detail about how executive function operates and drive the rest of the brain, this is the book. This text reviews all of the structures and networks as well as most of the MRI research regarding brain function.]

Kaplan, G. B., & Hammer, R. P. (2002). *Brain circuitry and signaling in psychiatry: Basic science and implications*. Washington, DC: American Psychiatric Publishing.

[You definitely want this one for your bookshelf. It covers many of the major disorders and the networks identified as being involved as well as a good review of the research regarding the impact of drugs on these disorders. Well written and easy to understand with lots of diagrams and pictures to help.]

Electrophysiology

Books that are pertinent to QEEG and fairly heavy reading-nuff said:

Nunez, P. L. (Ed.) (1995). *Neocortical dynamics and human EEG rhythms*. New York: Oxford University Press.

Lubar, J. (2004). *Quantitative electroencephalographic analysis (QEEG) databases for neurotherapy: Description, validation, and application*. Binghamton, NY: The Haworth Medical Press.

Entrainment

Siever, D. (1999). *The rediscovery of audio-visual entrainment technology*. Alberta, Canada: Comptronic Devices Ltd. [If you are interested in entrainment, this is the book to get. Period.]

REFERENCES

Alper, K. R., Prichep, L. S., Kowalik, S., Rosenthal, M. S., & John, E. R. (1998). Persistent QEEG abnormality in crack cocaine users at 6 months of drug abstinence. *Neuropsychopharmacology, 19*, 1-9. https://doi.org/10.1016/S0893-133X(97)00211-X

Alstott, J., Breakspear, M., Hagmann, P., Cammoun, L., & Sporns, O. (2009). Modeling the impact of lesions in the human brain. *PLoS computational biology, 5*(6), e1000408. https://doi.org/10.1371/journal.pcbi.1000408

Peniston, E. O. (1998). *The Peniston-Kulkosky brainwave neurofeedback therapeutic protocol: The future psychotherapy for alcoholism/PTSD/behavioral medicine*. The American Academy of Experts in Traumatic Stress. Retrieved May 1, 2010, from https://www.aaets.org/traumatic-stress-library/the-peniston-kulkosky-brainwave-neurofeedback-therapeutic-protocol-the-future-psychotherapy-for-alcoholism-ptsd-behavioral-medicine

Anda, R. F., & Felitti, V. J. (2012, August 27). *Adverse childhood experiences and their relationship to adult well-being and disease : Turning gold into lead*. https://www.thenationalcouncil.org/wp-content/uploads/2012/11/Natl-Council-Webinar-8-2012.pdf

Andersen, S. L., Tomada, A., Vincow, E. S., Valente, E., Polcari, A., & Teicher, M. H. (2008). Preliminary evidence for sensitive periods in the effect of childhood sexual abuse on regional brain development. *The Journal of Neuropsychiatry and Clinical Neurosciences, 20*(3), 292–301. https://doi.org/10.1176/jnp.2008.20.3.292

Anderson, P., & Andersson, S. A. (1968). *Physiological basis of the alpha rhythm*. New York, NY: Appleton Century Crofts.

Amen, D. G. (1998). *Change your brain, change your life*. New York, NY: Random House. Applied Neuroscience (n.d.). Medical legal services. https://appliedneuroscience.com/medical-legal-services/

Applied Neuroscience (n.d). *Medical legal services.* https://appliedneuroscience.com/medical-legal-services/

Applied Psychophysiology Education. (n.d.). *Courses.* http://www.aped.training/

Association for Applied Psychophysiology and Biofeedback, Inc. (2008). Retrieved May 1, 2010, from: News & Media Coverage http://www.aapb.org/news.html

Baehr, E., Rosenfeld, J. P., & Baehr, R. (1997). The clinical use of an alpha asymmetry protocol in the neurofeedback treatment of depression:

Two case studies. *Journal of Neurotherapy, 3*, 10-23. https://doi.org/10.1300/J184v02n03_02

Bassett, D. S., Meyer-Lindenberg, A., Achard, S., Duke, T., & Bullmore, E. (2006). Adaptive reconfiguration of fractal small-world human brain functional networks. *Proceedings of the National Academy of Sciences of the United States of America , 103*(51), 19518-19523. https://doi.org/10.1073/pnas.0606005103

Beck, A. T. (1979). *Cognitive therapy and the emotional disorders*. Cleveland, OH: Meridian.

Begley, S. (2007). *Train your mind, change your brain: How a new science reveals our extraordinary potential to transform ourselves*. New York, NY: Ballentine Books.

Brain Paint. (2007*). Bill Scott's biography sketch*. Retrieved May 1, 2010, from Brain Paint: http://www.brainpaint.com/index_files/about-billscott.htm

Brown, V. W. (1995). Neurofeedback and Lyme's disease: A clinical application of the five-phase model of CNS functional transformation and integration. *Journal of Neurotherapy, 1*(2), 60- 73. https://doi.org/10.1080/J184v01n02_05

Brown, V. (2010). *Author page*. Retrieved May 1, 2010, from Future Health: http://www.futurehealth.org/populum/authors productpage.php?sid=418

Buckner, R. L., Andrews-Hanna, J. R., & Schacter, D. L. (2008). The brain's default network: Anatomy, function, and relevance to disease. *Annals of the New York Academy of Sciences, 1124*, 1-38. https://doi.org/10.1196/annals.1440.011

Buzsaki, G. (2006). Rhythms ofthe brain. New York, NY: Oxford University Press.

California Institute of Technology. (2009, March 12). Neuroscientists map intelligence in the brain. *ScienceDaily*. www.sciencedaily.com/releases/2009/03/090311124020.htm

Chabot, R. J., Di Michele, F., & Prichep, L. , (2005). The role of quantitative electroencephalography in child and adolescent psychiatric disorders. *Child and Adolescent Psychiatric Clinics of North America, 14*, 21-53. https://doi.org/10.1016/j.chc.2004.07.005

Chabot, R. (1998). Quantitative EEG profiles and LORETA imaging of children with attention deficit and learning disorders. Presentation at 1998 SNR Conference.

Changeux, J. P. (1985). *Neuronal man: The biology of mind*. Princeton, NJ: Princeton University Press.

Chow, T. W., & Cummings, J. L. (1998). Frontal-subcortical circuits. In B. L. Miller & J. L. Cummings (Eds.), *The human frontal lobes: Functions and disorders* (pp. 3-26). New York, NY: The Guilford Press.

Cohen, G., Johnston, R. A., & Plunkett, K. (2000). *Exploring cognition: damaged brains and neural networks: Readings in cognitive neuropsychology and connectionist modeling.* East Sussex, UK: Psychology Press.

Crane, A., & Soutar, R. (2000). *Mind fitness training: Neurofeedback and the process.* Lincoln, NE: Writer's Club Press.

Criswell, E. (1995). *Biofeedback & somatics: Toward personal evolution.* Novato, CA: Freeperson Press.

Crossen, B. (1992). Subcortical junctions in language and memory. New York, NY: The Guilford Press.

Evans, J. R. (2007). *Handbook of neurofeedback: Dynamics and clinical applications.* New York, NY: The Hawthorne Medical Press.

Evans, J. R., & Abarbanel, A. (Eds.). (1999). *Introduction to quantitative EEG and neurofeedback.* San Diego, CA: Academic Press.

Duffy, F. H., Iyer, V. G., & Surwillo, W. W. (1989). *Clinical electroencephalography and topographic brain mapping: Technology and practice.* New York, NY: Springer-Verlag Publishing.

Dyro, F. M. (1989). *The EEG handbook.* Boston, MA: Little Brown Company.

Davidson, R. J. (1995). Cerebral asymmetry, emotion, and affective style. In R. J. Davidson, & K. Hugdahl (Eds.), *Brain asymmetry* (pp. 361-387). Cambridge, MA: MIT Press.

Davidson, R. J., Jackson, D. C., & Kalin, N. H. (2000). Emotion, plasticity, context, and regulation:Perspectives from affective neuroscience. *Psychological Bulletin, 126*(6), 890-909. https://doi.org/10.1037/0033-2909.126.6.890

DeBeus, R., Ball, J. D., DeBeus, M. E., & Herrington, R. (2003). Attention training with ADHD children: Preliminary findings in a double blind placebo controlled study. Presented at the International Society for Neuronal Regulation Annual Conference, Houston, Texas.

Damasio, A. (1994). *Descartes' error: Emotion, reason, and the human brain.* New York, NY: Avon Books.

Damasio, A. (1999). *The feeling of what happens: Body and emotion in the making of consciousness.* New York, NY: Harcourt Brace.

Demos, J. N. (2005). Getting started with neurofeedback. New York, NY: W. W. Norton & Company.

Diamond, M. C., Scheibel, A. B. , & Elson, L. M. (1985). *The human brain coloring book (Coloring concepts)*. New York,NY: Harper Collins.

Drevets, W. C., Price, J. L., Simpson, J. R., Jr, Todd, R. D., Reich, T., Vannier, M., & Raichle, M. E. (1997). Subgenual prefrontal cortex abnormalities in mood disorders. *Nature, 386*(6627), 824–827. https://doi.org/10.1038/386824a0

EEGInfo. (n.d.). *Infra-low frequency neurofeedback.* Research papers. Retrieved March 15, 2020, from https://eeginfo.com/research/infra-low_neurofeedback.jsp

Engels, A. S., Heller, W., Mohanty, A., Herrington J. D., Banich, M. T., Webb, A. G. & Miller,

G. A. (2007). Specificity of regional brain activity in anxiety types during emotional

processing. *Psychophysiology*, 44, 352-363. https://doi.org/10.1111/j.1469-8986.2007.00518.x

Femi, L. G. (1978). EEG biofeedback, multichannel synchrony training, and attention. In A. A. Sugarman & R. E. Tarter (Eds.), *Expanding dimensions of consciousness* (pp. 152- 182). New York, NY: Springer Verlag.

FitzGerald, M. J., & Folan-Curran, J. (2002). *Clinical neuroanatomy and related neuroscience*. New York, NY: W. B. Saunders.

Pulvermueller, F. , Preissl, H., Eulitz, C., Pantev, C., Lutzenberger, W., Elbert, T., & Birbaumer, N. (1994). Brain rhythms, cell assemblies and cognition: Evidence from the processing of words and pseudowords. *Psycoloquy, 5*(48). From: http://www.cogsci.ecs.soton.ac.uk/cgi/psyc/newpsy?5.48

Gunkelman, J. (1998). Drug exposure and EEG/QEEG findings. Future Health Presentation Handout. Future Health. Palm Springs, California.

Gunkleman, J. (1999). QEEG patterns, sources and NF interventions. SNR Workshop. Myrtle Beach, Florida.

Gläscher, J., Tranel, D., Paul, L. K., Rudrauf, D., Rorden, C., Hornaday, A., Grabowski, T., Damasio, H., & Adolphs, R. (2009). Lesion mapping of cognitive abilities linked to intelligence. *Neuron, 61*(5), 681–691. https://doi.org/10.1016/j.neuron.2009.01.026

Green, E. (1992). Alpha-theta brainwave training: Instrumental vipassana? Montreal Symposium. Montreal, Canada.

Green, E. E., Green, A. M., & Walters, D. E. (1970). Voluntary control of internal states: Psychological and physiological. *Journal of Transpersonal Psychology, 2*(1), 1-26.

Green, E., & Green, A. M. (1977). *Beyond biofeedback*. San Francisco, CA:

Delacorte.

Hughes, J. R., & John, E. R. (1999). Conventional and quantitative electroencephalography in psychiatry. *Journal of Neuropsychiatry and Clinical Neuroscience, 11*(2), 190-208. https://doi.org/10.1176/jnp.11.2.190

Hughes, S. W., & Crunelli, V. (2005). Thalamic mechanisms of EEG alpha rhythms and their pathological implications. *The Neuroscientist, 11*(4), 357-372. https://doi.org/10.1177/1073858405277450

Hagmann, P., Cammoun, L., Gigandet, X., Meuli, R., Honey, C. J., Wedeen, V. J., & Sporns, O. (2008). Mapping the structural core of human cerebral cortex. *PLoS biology, 6*(7), e159. https://doi.org/10.1371/journal.pbio.0060159

Hammond, D. C., & Kirk, L. (2008). First, do no harm: Adverse effects and the need for practice standards in neurofeedback. *Journal of Neurotherapy, 12*(1), 79-88. https://doi.org/10.1080/10874200802219947

Hammond, D. C., Walker, J., Hoffman, D., Lubar, J. F., Trudeau, D., Gurnee, R.,& Horvat, J. . (2004). Standardsfor the use of quantitative electroencephalography (QEEG) in neurofeedback: A position paper of the International Society for Neuronal Regulation. *Journal of Neurotherapy, 8*(1), 5-27. https://doi.org/10.1300/J184v08n01_02

Hartmann, T. (1993). *Attention deficit disorder: A different perception*. Grass Valley, CA: Underwood Books.

Homan, R. W., Herman, J., & Purdy, P. (1987). Cerebral location of international 10-20 system electrode placement. *Electroencephalography and Clinical Neurophysiology, 66*(4), 376-382. https://doi.org/10.1016/0013-4694(87)90206-9

International EEG Certification Board. (n.d.). *Certification process.* https://qeegcertificationboard.org/certification-process/

John, E. R., Karmel, B. Z., Corning, W. C., Easton, P., Brown, D., Ahn, H., John, M., … Schwartz, E. (1977). Neurometrics. *Science, 196*(4297), 1393–1410. https://doi.org/10.1126/science.

John, E. R., Prichep, L. S., Fridman, J., & Easton, P. (1988). Neurometrics: computer-assisted differential diagnosis of brain dysfunctions. *Science, 239*(4836), 162–169. https://doi.org/10.1126/science.

Johnstone, J. (2001). Effect of antidepressant medications on the EEG. *Journal of Neurotherapy, 5*(4), 93-97.

Kaplan, G. B., & Hammer, R. P. (2002). *Brain circuitry and signaling in psychiatry: Basic science and implications*. Washington, DC: American Psychiatric Publishing.

Knyazev G. G. (2012). EEG delta oscillations as a correlate of basic homeostatic and motivational processes. *Neuroscience and Biobehavioral Reviews, 36*(1), 677–695. https://doi.org/10.1016/j.neubiorev.2011.10.002

Kolb, B., & Whishaw, I. Q. (1996). Fundamentals of human neuropsychology (4th ed.). Alberta, Canada: University of Lethbridge/Worth Publishers.

Kurzweil. (2016, July 20*). New brain map provides unprecedented detail in 180 areas of the cerebral cortex*. Retrieved November 19, 2018, from http://www.kurzweilai.net/new-brain-map-provides-unprecedented-detail-in-180-areas-of-the-cerebral-cortex

Longo, R. E., & Soutar, R. (2019). *Mentoring for neurofeedback certification: A guide for mentors and mentees.* Greenville, SC: FNNR.

Lubar, J. F. (1991). Discourse on the development of EEG diagnostics and biofeedback for attention-deficit/hyperactivity disorders. *Biofeedback & Self-Regulation, 16*(3), 201-225. https://doi.org/10.1007/BF01000016

Lubar, J. F. (1995). Neurofeedback for the management of attention deficit/ hyperactivity

disorders. In M. S. Schwartz (Ed.), *Biofeedback: A practitioner 's guide* (2nd ed.) (pp. 493-522). New York, NY: Guilford.

Lubar, J. F. (1997). Neocortical dynamics: Implications for understanding the role of neurofeedback and related techniques for the enhancement of attention. *Applied Psychophysiology and Biofeedback, 22*, 11-126. https://doi.org/10.1023/a:1026276228832

Lubar, J. F., & Lubar, J. (1999). Neurofeedback assessment and treatment for attentiondeficit/hyperactivity disorders. In J. R. Evans & A. Abarbanel (Eds.)*, Introduction to quantitative EEG and neurofeedback* (pp. 243-310). New York, NY: Academic Press.

Larson, S. (2006). *The healing power of neurofeedback: The revolutionary lens technique for restoring optimal brain function.* Rochester, NY: Healing Arts Press.

LeDoux, J. (1996). *The emotional brain: The mysterious underpinnings of emotional life.* New York, NY: Simon & Schuster.

McCormick, D. A. (1999). Are thalamocortical rhythms the Rosetta Stone of a subset of neurological disorders? *Nature Medicine, 5*(12), 1349-1351. https://doi.org/10.1038/70911

McEwen, B. (1987). Influence of hormones and neuroactive substances on immune function. In C.W. Cotman, R. E. Brinton, A. Galaburda, B.Mcewen & D. M. Schneider (Eds.), *The neuro-immune endocrine connection* (pp. 33- 47). New York, NY: Raven Press.

McIntosh, A. R., & Korostil, M. (2008). Interpretation of neuroimaging data based on network concepts. *Brain Imaging and Behavior, 2*(4), 264–269. https://doi.org/10.1007/s11682-008-9031-6

Melgari, J. M., Curcio, G., Mastrolilli, F., Salomone, G., Trotta, L., Tombini, M., … Vernieri, F. (2014). Alpha and beta EEG power reflects L-dopa acute administration in parkinsonian patients. *Frontiers in Aging Neuroscience, 6*, 302. https://doi.org/10.3389/fnagi.2014.00302

Monastra, V. J., Lynn, S., Linden, M., Lubar, J. F., Gruzelier, J., & LaVaque, T. J. (2005). Electroencephalographic biofeedback in the treatment of attention-deficit/hyperactivity disorder. *Applied psychophysiology and biofeedback, 30*(2), 95–114. https://doi.org/10.1007/s10484-005-4305-x

Montgomery, D. D., Robb, J., Dwyer, K. V., & Gontkovsky, S. T. (1998). Single channel QEEG amplitudes in a bright, normal young adult sample. *Journal of Neurotherapy, 2*(4), 1-7. https://doi.org/10.1300/J184v02n04_01

Moss, D. (Ed.) (1998*). Humanistic and transpersonal psychology: A historical and biographical sourcebook.* Westport, Connecticut: Greenwood Press.

Nunez, P. (1995). *Neocortical dynamics and human EEG rhythms*. New York, NY: Oxford University Press.

Niedermeyer, E., & Silva, F. H. (1999). Electroencephalography: Basic principles, clinical applications and related fields (4th ed.). New York, NY: Lippincott Williams & Eilkins.

Ochs, L. (2010). Author's page. Retrieved May 1, 2010, from Future Health: http://www.futurehealth.org/populum/authorsproductpage.php?sid=424

Othmer, S. (2008). *Protocol guide for neurofeedback clinicians.* Woodland Hills, CA: EEG Info.

Othmer, S. (1994). *Training syllabus*. http://www.eegspectrum.com/

Othmer, S., Othmer, S. F., & Kaiser, D. A. (1999). EEG biofeedback: An emerging model for its global efficacy. In J. R. Evans, & A. Abarbanel (Eds.), *Introduction to quantitative EEG and neurofeedback* (pp. 243-310). New York, NY: Academic Press.

Pascual-Marqui, R. D. (2007, November 9). *Instantaneous and lagged measurements of linear and nonlinear dependence between groups of multivariate time series: Frequency decomposition*. Retrieved August 16, 2010, from Arsiv.org: http://arsiv.org/abs/0711.1455

Patent Storm. (2010). *Electrode locator - US Patent 5518007 description*. Retrieved May 1, 2010, from Patent Storm: http://www.patentstorm.us/patents/5518007/description.html

Peniston, E. G., & Kulkosky, P. J. (1989). Alpha-theta brainwave training and beta-endorphin levels in alcoholics. *Alcoholism, clinical and experimental research, 13*(2), 271–279. https://doi.org/10.1111/j.1530-0277.1989.tb00325.x

Plutchik, R. (1980). Emotion: A psychoevolutionary synthesis. New York, NY: Harper & Row..

Posner, M. I., & Raichle, M. E. (1997). Images of mind (Scientific American Library). New York, NY: W. H. Freeman & Co.

Pulvermueller, F. , Preissl, H., Eulitz, C., Pantev, C., Lutzenberger, W., Elbert, T., & Birbaumer, N. (1994). Brain rhythms, cell assemblies and cognition: Evidence from the processing of words and pseudowords. *Psycoloquy, 5*(48). http://www.cogsci.ecs.soton.ac.uk/cgi/psyc/newpsy?5.50

Suffin, S. C., & Emory, W. H. (1995). Neurometric subgroups in attentional and affective disorders and their association with pharmacotherapeutic outcome. *Clinical Electroencephalography, 26*(2), 76-83. https://doi.org/10.1177/155005949502600204

Swingle, P. G. (2008). *Biofeedback for the brain: How neurotherapy effectively treats depression, ADHD, autism, and more.* New Jersey: Rutgers University Press.

Schwartz, J. M., & Begley, S. (2002). *The mind and the brain: Neuroplasticity and the power of mental force*. New York, NY: Harper Perennial.

Schachter, S., & Singer, J. E. (1962). Cognitive, social, and physiological determinants of emotional state. *Psychological review, 69*, 379–399. https://doi.org/10.1037/h0046234

Schiffer, F. (1998). *Of two minds: The revolutionary science of dual-brain psychology*. New York, NY:Free Press.

Schmahmann, J. D., & Pandya, D. N. (2006). *Fiber pathways of the brain*. New York, NY: Oxford University Press.

Schore, A. N. (1994). *Affect regulation and the origin of the self: The neurobiology of emotional development*. Hillsdale, NJ: Lawrence Erlbaum Associates.

Scott, W. C., Brod, T. M., Sideroff, S., Kaiser, D., & Sagan, M. (2002). Type-specific EEG biofeedback improves residential substance abuse treatment. Paper presented at American Psychiatric Association Annual Meeting 2002.

Scott, W. C., Kaiser, D., Othmer, S., & Sideroff, S. I. (2005). Effects of an EEG biofeedback protocol on a mixed substance abusing population. *The American Journal of Drug and Alcohol Abuse, 31*(3), 455–469. https://doi.org/10.1081/ada-

Siever, D. (1999). *The rediscovery of audio-visual entrainment technology.* Alberta, Canada: Comptronic Devices Limited.

Sheer, D. E. (1976). Focused arousal and 40 Hz EEG. In R. M. Knights & D. J. Bakker (Eds.), *The neuropsychology of learning disorders: Theoretical approaches* (pp. 71-87). Baltimore, MA: University Park Press.

Sherlin, L., & Congedo, M. (2005). Obsessive-compulsive dimension localized using low-resolution brain electromagnetic tomography (LORETA). *Neuroscience Letters, 387*(2), 72–74. https://doi.org/10.1016/j.neulet.2005.06.069

Soutar, R. G. (2006). *The automatic self: Transformation and transcendence through brainwave training.*Lincoln, NE: iUniverse.

Soutar, R. (2017). Perspective and method for a qEEG based two-channel bi-hemispheric compensatory model of neurofeedback training. In T. F. Collura & J. A. Frederick (Eds.), *Handbook of clinical QEEG and neurotherapy* (pp. 387-403). New York, NY: Routledge

Soutar, R., & Crane, A. (2000). *Mindfitness training: The process of enhancing profound attention using neurofeedback.* New York, NY: iUniverse.

Srinivasan, R., & Nunez, P. L. (2006). *Electric fields of the brain: The neurophysics of EEG* (2nd   ed.). New York, NY: Oxford University Press.

Sterman, M. B., & Bowersox, S. S. (1981). Sensorimotor electroencephalogram rhythmic activity: A functional gate mechanism. *Sleep, 4*(4), 408-422. https://doi.org/10.1093/sleep/4.4.408

Sterman, M. B., & Mann, C. A. (1995). Concepts and applications of EEG analysis in aviation

performance evaluation. *Biological Psychology, 40*(1), 115-130. https://doi.org/10.1016/0301-0511(95)05101-5

Sterman, M. B., Kaiser, D. A., & Veigel, B. (1966). Spectral analysis of event related EEG responses during short-term memory performance. *Brain Topography, 9*(1), 21-30. https://doi.org/10.1007/BF01191639

Stien, P. T., & Kendall, J. (2004). *Psychological trauma and the developing brain: Neurologically based interventions for troubled children.* New York, NY: Routledge.

Streifel, S. (1995). Professional ethical behavior for providers of biofeedback. In M. S. Schwartz (Ed.),*Biofeedback: A practitioner's guide* (pp. 685-705). New York, NY: The Guilford Press.

Streifel, S. (1989). A perspective on ethics. *Biofeedback, 17*(1), 21-22.

Svitil, K. (2009, March 11). *Mapping intelligence in the brain.* Caltech.https://www.caltech.edu/about/news/mapping-intelligence-brain-1516

Ruden, R. A. (1997). *The craving brain: The biobalance approach to controlling addictions.* New York, NY: Harper Collins Books.

Ruden, R. A., & Byalick, M. (1997). *The craving brain: A bold new approach to breaking free from drug addiction, overeating, alcoholism, and gambling.* New York, NY: Harper Collins Books.

Robbins, J. (2000). *A symphony in the brain: The evolution of the new brain wave biofeedback.* New York, NY: Grove Press.

Rotter, J. B. (1990). Internal versus external control of reinforcement: A case history of a variable. *American Psychologist, 45*(4), 489–493. https://doi.org/10.1037/0003-066X.45.4.489

Teicher, M. H. (2007, April 7). Childhood abuse, brain development and impulsivity. Keynote speech. Massachusetts Adolescent Sex Offender Coalition/Massachusetts Assocation for the Treatment of Sexual Abusers Joint Conference. Marlborough, MA.

Thatcher, R. W. (1998). Normative EEG databases and EEG biofeedback. *Journal of Neurotherapy, 2*(4), 8-39. https://doi.org/10.1300/J184v02n04_02

Thatcher, R. W., Walker, R. A., Biver, C. J., North, D. N., & Curtin, R. (2003). Quantitative EEG normative databases: Validation and clinical correlation. *Journal of Neurotherapy, 7*(3-4), 87-121. https://doi.org/10.1300/J184v07n03_05

Thatcher, R. W., Camacho, M., Salazar, A., Linden, C., Biver, C., & Clarke, L. (1997). Quantitative MRI of the gray-white matter distribution in traumatic brain injury. *Journal of Neurotrauma, 14*(1), 1–14. https://doi.org/10.1089/neu.1997.14.1

The Menninger Clinic. (2010). History. Retrieved May 1, 2010, from The Menninger Clinic: http://www.menningerclinic.com/about/Menninger-history.htm

Thompson, M., & Thompson, L. (2003). The neurofeedback book: An introduction to basic concepts in applied psychophysiology. Wheat Ridge, CO: AAPB.

Thornton, K. (2000). Rehabilitation of memory functioning in brain injured subject with EEG biofeedback. *Journal of Head Trauma Rehabilitation, 15*(6), 1285-1296.

Thornton, K. E., & Carmody, D. P. (2008). Efficacy of traumatic brain injury rehabilitation: interventions of QEEG-guided biofeedback, computers, strategies, and medications. *Applied Psychophysiology and Biofeedback, 33*(2), 101–124. https://doi.org/10.1007/s10484-008-9056-z

Travis, T. A., Kondo, C. Y., & Knott, J. R. (1974). Parameters of eyes-closed alpha enhancement. *Psychophysiology, 11*(6), 674–681. https://doi.org/10.1111/j.1469-8986.1974.tb01136.x

Training & Research Institute, Inc. (2004). The neurobiology of child abuse [PosterJ. Albuquerque, NM: Author. Retrieved from: http://trainingandresearch.com/58275.html

Walker, J. E., Norman, C. A., & Weber, R. K. (2002). Impact of qEEG-guided coherence training for patients with a mild closed head injury. *Journal of Neurotherapy, 6*(2), 31-43. https://doi.org/10.1300/J184v06n02_05

Watts, D. J. (2004). Small worlds: The dynamics of networks between order and randomness. Princeton, NJ: Princeton University Press.

Wise, A. (1997). *The high- performance mind.* New York, NY: G. P. Putham's Sons.

Ziegler, D. (2002). *Traumatic experience and the brain: A handbook for understanding and treating those traumatized as children.* Phoenix, AZ: Acacia Publishing.

LIST OF DIAGRAMS

All images are public domain or designed by the author(s) except for those noted within the text

LIST OF TABLES

INDEX

Symbols

A

B

www.ingramcontent.com/pod-product-compliance
Lightning Source LLC
Chambersburg PA
CBHW050105220326
41598CB00043B/7385